PATIENT-CENTRED IVF

Fertility, Reproduction and Sexuality

GENERAL EDITORS:

Soraya Tremayne, Founding Director, Fertility and Reproduction Studies Group and Research Associate, Institute of Social and Cultural Anthropology, University of Oxford.

Marcia C. Inhorn, William K. Lanman, Jr. Professor of Anthropology and International Affairs, Yale University.

Philip Kreager, Director, Fertility and Reproduction Studies Group, and Research Associate, Institute of Social and Cultural Anthropology and Institute of Human Sciences, University of Oxford.

PATIENT-CENTRED IVF
Bioethics and Care in a Dutch Clinic

Trudie Gerrits

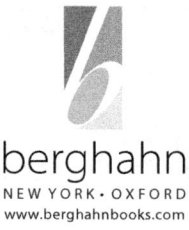

berghahn
NEW YORK · OXFORD
www.berghahnbooks.com

First published in 2016 by
Berghahn Books
www.BerghahnBooks.com

Library of Congress Cataloging-in-Publication Data
Names: Gerrits, Trudie, author.
Title: Patient-centred IVF : bioethics and care in a Dutch clinic /
  Trudie Gerrits.
Other titles: Patient-centred in vitro fertilization | Fertility,
reproduction and sexuality ; v. 33.
Description: New York : Berghahn Books, 2016. | Series: Fertility,
reproduction and sexuality ; volume 33 | Includes bibliographical
references and index.
Identifiers: LCCN 2016024965| ISBN 9781785332265 (hardback :
  alk. paper) |
ISBN 9781785332272 (ebook)
Subjects: | MESH: Fertilization in Vitro | Patient-Centered Care |
Reproductive Techniques, Assisted--ethics | Netherlands
Classification: LCC RG133.5 | NLM WQ 208 | DDC 176/.2--dc23 LC
  record available at https://lccn.loc.gov/2016024965

British Library Cataloguing in Publication Data
A catalogue record for this book is available
from the British Library.

Cover image: *Tulips*, geraldford (CC BY-SA 2.0 creativecommons.org)
https://www.flickr.com/photos/geraldford/8707684221/in/
album-72157630245291392/

ISBN 978-1-78533-226-5 (hardback)
ISBN 978-1-78533-227-2 (ebook)

Contents

Acknowledgements

This book could not have been written without the involvement, the advice, and the support of many other people. To start with, I want to express my gratitude to the women and men with fertility problems for allowing me to follow their quests for a solution closely and intensively. Thanks for the many experiences, viewpoints, and emotions you shared with me. Without your collaboration and trust I would never have been able to write this book.

The same goes for the staff of the fertility clinic of the Radboud University Medical Center (RUMC), in Nijmegen, the Netherlands, including the doctors, nurses, laboratory staff, the clinical psychologist and the social worker. Though you were not at all used to the presence of a medical anthropologist in your clinic, you allowed me to be present on many different occasions, including consultations, treatment sessions and staff meetings. Your explanations of medical subjects and the many other insights and opinions you shared with me enriched my understanding of the topic and as such has contributed to the contents of this book.

I am also grateful for the support I received from the RUMC support staff. Not only did you help me in contacting the couples in the initial phase of the fieldwork, but you were also accommodating throughout the whole research period in promptly providing me with any and all kinds of information or help I asked for.

This study was made possible by funding from the Amsterdam Institute of Social Science Research (AISSR) of the University of Amsterdam, which has supported my work, first through a PhD-fellowship, and later with sabbatical funding to support the writing of this book. Many thanks also go to the AISSR support staff who have given me practical and administrative support wherever needed throughout the years.

A special words of thanks to Anita Hardon, Didi Braat, Jan Kremer, and Ria Reis – a fantastic combination of medical anthropologists and gynaecologists specialized in medical assisted reproduction – who offered invaluable support in the early stages of this project. The way we worked together has increased my faith in interdisciplinary collaboration. Anita and Ria, I want to thank you in particular for the intellectual input throughout the years and your strong encouragement to 'stick to my own way' of presenting and analysing my data. Didi and Jan, thinking of you, notions of transparency and trust come to the fore. It is true that initially I had to convince you about the relevance and validity of the ethnographic study approach, but once you had accepted me at your clinic, you gave me all the space I needed to carry out the study. Discussing the study approach, the findings and analysis with you has made – at least this is what I hope – this book more readable for audiences beyond the social sciences.

Throughout the years, I have discussed the contents of the book with many other scholars, including Josien de Klerk, Christine Dedding, John Kinsman, Marie Lindegaard, Miranda van Reeuwijk, Erica van der Sijpt and Marian Tankink at the AISSR, and other colleagues at the Anthropology Department, Sjaak van der Geest, Stuart Blume, Anja Hiddinga and Winny Koster, in particular. I also want to thank Annemarie Jurg and Myra van Zwieten for their valuable comments at different stages of my study. Further, I want to mention the members of the international network of scholars involved in the study of infertility, childlessness, and reproductive technologies, whose meetings are enormously inspiring. In particular I want to express my gratitude to Marcia Inhorn and Soraya Tremayne – editors of the Fertility, Reproduction and Sexuality series of Berghahn Publishers – who have enormously encouraged and supported me to transform my thesis in the current book. Very special thanks to Marcia Inhorn and two anonymous reviewers who read the entire manuscript and who made excellent suggestions for its improvement.

Further, I want to thank Marian Verheul and Klazien de Klerk for the transcription of the lengthy interviews; I am grateful to Zoe Goldstein and Malissa Shaw who have both been involved in editing this book and Luca Koppen for composing the index. In addition, I want to thank all people from Berghahn Books, Dhara Patel, Charlotte Mosedale, Caroline Kuhtz and Ben Parker, for smoothly guiding me through all steps of the production of this book.

Finally, I want to thank my colleagues at the University of Amsterdam, including the members of my intervision group and others – of which I mention Rachel Spronk and Rene Gerrets in particular – for their encouragement to finish the book, their good collegial company and their 'listening ear' over the years.

On a personal note, I want to say words of thanks to my late mother, who passed away in the period when I was writing up the study. I am grateful to her, as she always encouraged me – and my brothers and sisters – to take the chances life offers you and to make the best of it. And at the end, there is my family – my husband Hans van den Hoogen and our children, Carmen and Jaap. For a large part of the children's life I have been working on this study, culminating in the current book. I want to thank them for their flexibility and understanding at times – when they were still young – when I was not fully available for them. Most of all, though, I want to express my happiness and delight at the two of them being in my life, and being the people they are. Hans has supported me, both practically and emotionally, wherever and whenever I needed it, for which I want to thank him. The good and easy life we share at home, together and with the children, at the one hand fuels the passion that I have for the topic of this book, but it also provides me with the energy to commit myself to life and work beyond the borders of family life.

TABLES AND BOXES

ABBREVIATIONS

AI	Artificial Insemination
AID	Artificial Insemination by Donor
CAM	Complementary and Alternative Medicine
CBS	Centraal Bureau voor Statistiek (Central Office for Statistics)
CMO	Commissie Mensgebonden Onderzoek (Medical-ethical Committee for Research Involving Human Beings)
CCMO	Centrale Commissie Medisch-Ethisch Onderzoek (Central Medical-Ethical Committee)
CRM	Clinic for Reproductive Medicine
CvZ	College van Zorgverzekeringen (Board of Health Insurers)
DET	Dual Embryo Transfer
Fiom	Dutch organization providing psychosocial care, information and advice (among others) in case of involuntary childlessness
Freya	Dutch patient organization for people with fertility problems
FSH	Follicle Stimulating Hormone
GnRH	Gonadotropin-Releasing Hormone
HSG	Hysterosalpingogram
HCG	Human Chorionic Gonadtrofin
ICSI	Intra Cytoplasmic Sperm Injection
IUI	Intra Uterine Insemination
IVF	In Vitro Fertilization
LH	Luteinizing Hormone
KLEM	Vereniging voor Klinisch Embryologen (Association for Clinical Embryologists)
NIAZ	Nederlands Instituut voor de Accreditatie van Ziekenhuizen (Netherlands Institute for the Accreditation of Hospitals)

NOGO	Nederlands Onderzoek naar Gedrag bij Onvruchtbaarheid (Dutch Study of Behaviour during Infertility)
NVOG	Nederlandse Vereniging voor Obstetrie en Gynaecologie (Dutch Association for Obstetrics and Gynaecology)
NVRB	Nederlandse Vereniging voor Reageerbuis Bevruchting (Dutch Association for Test-tube Fertilization) (now: Freya)
OFO	Oriënterend Fertiliteits Onderzoek (Initial Fertility Examinations)
OHSS	Ovarian Hyperstimulation Syndrome
PESA	Percutaneous Epididymal Sperm Aspiration
PCOS	Polycystic Ovarian Syndrome
PGD	Pre-implantation Genetic Diagnosis
PGS	Pre-implantation Genetic Screening
PND	Pre-Natal Diagnosis
RIVM	Rijksinstituut voor Volksgezondheid en Milieu (National Institute for Public Health and the Environment)
RUMC	Radboud Universitair Medisch Centrum (Radboud University Medical Centre)
SET	Single Embryo Transfer
TESE	Testicular Sperm Extraction
WHO	World Health Organization
ZON-Mw	Zorg Onderzoek Nederland-Medische Wetenschappen (Dutch intermediary organization for the promotion and financing of research in health and care innovations)

INTRODUCTION

Sylvia: 'We always said, all that hassle, we *thought* – we always emphasized that – we would not do it [in vitro fertilization, IVF]. We *thought*
so, that is what we always stressed. Because we had understood from
our environment, from people around us who were confronted with
the same problem, that it is not so easy to say "It does not matter; we
will see what will come". We thought, let us first go to the Canisius
[regional clinic, not offering IVF], maybe it is just simple. . . But it
was not so obvious for us to go there. And then later we went to the
Radboud Clinic [the academic clinic where the study presented in this
book was carried out, offering IVF]. In fact, it always goes like that,
you simply go . . .'

Bob, Sylvia's husband, nods his head and says: 'You shift your
boundaries. Yes, that is it, you shift your boundaries. And that is what
we always heard. Now you look at it like this, but you do not know
how you look at it when you are in the midst of it yourself. I can easily
say "I do this and this and this". But that is not reality. Because once
you've taken the first step, then maybe you make different decisions'.
(A couple with fertility problems about to start their first IVF
treatment)[1]

Medicalization and Persistence

Having once entered the field of reproductive medicine, many
people with fertility problems find it hard to stop treatments
such as IVF before all medical options have been exploited. The

dominant picture in empirical studies is that people are drawn into a kind of 'medical treadmill', and many shift their initial borders regarding how far they would be prepared to go in their pursuit of a child (Franklin 1997; Verdurmen 1997; Pasveer and Heesterbeek 2001). Expressions such as sitting 'in a never halting express train' (Pasveer and Heesterbeek 2001: 114) or 'roller coaster' (Becker 2000: 165), being 'taken over' (Franklin 1997: 131) or feeling 'compelled to try' (Sandelowski 1991: 29), are frequently heard when people talk about their experiences with fertility treatments, indicating – as Bob and Sylvia express in the above interview excerpt – that once the first step into treatment has been taken, initial boundaries shift, and many feel overwhelmed by dynamics that they feel they cannot fully control.

People with fertility problems are often characterized as very persistent in their 'quest for conception' (Inhorn 1994), sometimes even being depicted as 'addicted' to treatment (Sandelowski 1991: 30–31). Only a small number discontinue treatment or do not start any treatment at all, even when these treatments would be paid for by health insurance.[2] The situation of those undergoing fertility treatment has also been depicted as ambiguous: they simultaneously want to continue and yet also to discontinue treatment (Pasveer and Heesterbeek 2001). Clearly, a tension exists between the eagerness of many infertile people to make use of assisted reproductive technologies (ARTs) – as they seem the only way to achieve their desired goal, a child of their own – and the demanding and controversial characteristics and dynamics of ARTs that they get involved with once they enter the medical field.

What makes it so difficult for many people with fertility problems to say no to (further) treatment, to jump off the roller coaster? What makes them go from one treatment to another? What makes them so inclined to continue treatment, so 'eager for medicalization' (Becker and Nachtigall 1991: 456)? The simple answer, of course, is that these couples dearly wish to have a child. If not, they would not have gone to the clinic. And this wish for a child certainly in part explains their determination. Several (ethnographic) studies have illustrated the importance of childbearing for many people worldwide, and the resulting suffering and social consequences when people do not succeed in this; this makes them eager to search for a solution (see for example Inhorn and Van Balen 2002; Greil et al. 2010). But there is more, and that is what this book is about.

Critiques of ARTs

Since the advent of ARTs at the end of the 1970s, many scholars from different perspectives have addressed the above questions and examined and critiqued the continuing medicalization of infertility and childlessness and couples' (persistent) use of ARTs.[3] Criticism has been directed at the limited success rates;[4] the physical and emotional burdens of treatment;[5] ethical issues; the high costs; and the medical risks involved. These risks, in particular for the women and/or the children to be conceived, and the effectiveness of (newly introduced) treatments have been said to be insufficiently known (Buitendijk 2000; Heesterbeek and Ten Have 2001), prompting alarms about women's bodies becoming sites of medical experimentation (Klein and Rowland 1989). In this context, female risk taking has been perceived as particularly problematic when male infertility is treated by intracytoplasmic sperm injection (ICSI), whereby the healthy woman becomes the 'patient' who has to bear the risks of medical reproduction (Kirejczyk 1996).[6]

In particular, and especially in the early days of IVF, criticism focused on how ARTs were offered and the involvement of potential users in decision-making. Above all, doctors and clinics have been criticized for being paternalistic, for their reluctance to inform women (and men) about the possible adverse effects of the hormonal drugs used in IVF treatments, and for their tendency to raise success rates by selecting only promising candidates for treatment as well as manipulating the data presented to them by presenting biased, incomplete and sometimes altered information. All of which was suggested to raise unrealistic expectations and distort informed decision-making (Sandelowski 1993; Gupta 1996; Van Balen and Inhorn 2002; Thompson 2005). Overall, (radical) feminist and other critical scholars have particularly criticized the role played by doctors and the medical system in the ever increasing medicalization of fertility problems, as the summary of these critiques below shows:

[Doctors] actively participate in women's medical risk taking by encouraging their repetitive and often extreme use of the latest technologies . . . rather than by developing low-tech solutions, giving 'nature' more time, advocating adoption or fostering, suggesting that treatments be stopped altogether and childlessness accepted, or searching for ways to prevent infertility. (Van Balen and Inhorn 2002: 14)

Patient-Centred Medicine

The past two decades have witnessed significant changes in the provision of ARTs, both at the level of policy and within clinics, partially addressing these critiques. Many fertility clinics, particularly
in Western countries, have introduced patient-centred practices to
reduce the paternalism that previously infused medical encounters and guarantee patient autonomy and informed decision-
making. The way in which ARTs are being provided has changed
enormously; indeed, in Western countries, the field of ARTs has
even become known for its patient-centred services and for its
accountability to stakeholders (e.g., Thompson 2005).[7] The focus
of this book is on how such new forms of ART provision, which
are more patient-centred and accountable, affect the use of these
technologies.

Patient-centred medicine can be said to be comprised of medical
practices that give due attention to the interpersonal aspects of
care and the need to fully inform patients and involve them in
decision-making.[8] Such aspects of care have been recognized as
key determinants of patient satisfaction in healthcare more generally (Mead and Bower 2000) and have been found to be particularly important for how people experience infertility treatment,
for a number of reasons (Dancet et al. 2010).[9] First, as both the
experiences of infertility and treatment (which generally entails
numerous procedures over an extended period) are emotionally
demanding, empathic treatment and psycho-social support are
considered key to making treatment more bearable, minimizing
stress and (supposedly) limiting drop-out rates (Alper et al. 2002;
Smeenk et al. 2004). Stress reduction has even been referred to
as a 'non-invasive way of improving infertility' (Campagne 2006:
1656), and it has been suggested that psycho-social interventions –
in particular when directed at a 'pre-treatment clinically depressed
group' – can increase pregnancy rates (Smeenk et al. 2004: 267).
Second, as infertility care is personal and intimate, people value
being treated by personally engaged clinical staff in ways that
respect their privacy (Inhorn 2003; Blonk, Kremer and Ten Haaf
2006). Third, the provision of adequate and repeated information
is thought to be crucial to empower patients to enable them to be
fully involved in decision-making (Kremer et al. 2007). This is particularly so as women and men undergoing fertility examinations
and treatments must make decisions about complex medical issues

at various points along their treatment trajectory.[10] A recent study underlined the importance of patient-centredness in infertility care: women and men undergoing IVF were found to be willing to trade off a proportion of the pregnancy success rate per cycle in order to receive more patient-centred care (Van Empel et al. 2011). In addition, 'lack of patient-centredness' was the most often mentioned non-medical reason for changing fertility clinics.

Another View on Patient-Centredness

Scholars who focus on the empowering effects of patient-centred practices generally do not pay attention to the unintended effects that these practices may also have. These other effects have been examined by a number of medical anthropologists, science and technology scholars and ethicists who, inspired by Foucauldian ideas of biopower and disciplinary power, have critiqued concepts such as patient empowerment, autonomy and informed consent.[11] From this perspective, practices designed to better inform lay populations so that they can wrest control away from doctors – such as patient empowerment and health education (Gastaldo 1997) – are thought to further the medicalization of people's lives as they encourage them to acquire medical knowledge for themselves more actively (Lupton 1997). The 'disciplinary power of biomedicine' is said to operate through patients' internalizing of appropriate discourses on 'how they should know and experience, behave, monitor and regulate themselves' (Jaye et al. 2006: 141). In addition, these practices may 'involve the imposition of "truths" about health, in which the patient loses control of her or his own body' (Gastaldo 1997: 129–130).

Finally, as Mayes (2009) argues, the literature on the patient-centred approach generally conceives of power as something that an individual or group (doctors) possesses and uses as a repressive force, from which the patient has to be liberated. But from a Foucauldian perspective, power is 'a relational and productive force that constructs each actor to act, think and expect certain responses from themselves and others' (Mayes 2009: 484). Thus, Mayes argues, although patient-centred medicine may liberate the medical encounter from paternalistic power, it nevertheless introduces a new complexity of power relations between doctors and patients that may have other – disciplining and normalizing – consequences, which in turn may increase medicalization. Hardon and Moyer (2014: 107) point to such unexpected and complex dynamics of health care constellations when they propose that social scientists should inquire into the 'micro dynamics of power' surrounding medical technologies in order to understand the full complexity of responses to (new) forms of health care or new medical technologies. This is exactly what I intend to do in this book.

The Aim of this Book

In the first place, this book provides an extended ethnographic portrait and analysis of the daily practices in a Dutch fertility clinic – the Radboud Clinic – which strongly profiles itself as being patient-centred. It also presents in-depth insight into the situated accounts of the women and men visiting the clinic. The main question I address is how visiting such a patient-centred clinic – in all its different dimensions – affects people with fertility problems. What do all the empowering and supporting practices and expressions of concern, empathy and commitment do to these women and men? How do the patient-centred practices affect the way they experience treatment and make decisions about using ARTs?

Throughout the book, I will show and discuss the various – intended and unintended – effects that these practices have, and argue that at times they may (and do) actually conflict with the aims of patient-centredness. For instance, such practices may interfere with processes of autonomous decision-making, one of the cornerstones of patient-centredness. This complex dynamic I have labelled the 'paradox of patient-centredness', and it lies at the heart of my analysis of infertile couples' journeys through the intricate and ambiguous process of medically achieving a child of their own. Both clinic practices and the couples' journeys are placed in the context of 'Dutch IVF' – referring to ART legislation and regulations in the Netherlands – and trends in contemporary Dutch society.

Outline of the Book

In Chapter 1, I first discuss the theoretical and empirical insights within social science studies of ARTs that have informed the current book, addressing an important turn in social science scholarship: from a focus mainly on dominant discourses to a more nuanced understanding of the medicalization of fertility problems. Next, I picture some relevant features and trends of Dutch society, the Radboud Clinic and the study design (a hospital ethnography) and methods.

Chapter 2 depicts the main aspects of Dutch ART legislation, national professional guidelines and current health insurance coverage, which strongly inform the actual practice and use of ARTs in Dutch fertility clinics.

In Chapter 3, I introduce the main players in this study: the couples whom I followed intensively over the course of their treatment trajectories. I first describe their socio-demographic backgrounds, and then use case studies to picture the diversity of their situations at the moment they found themselves confronted with fertility problems. Following this, I describe the ways in which they acted from that point on, including their quest for a child, in the biomedical health system and from complementary and alternative healers, and the ways in which they approached – and predominantly refused – adoption as an option.

In the next four chapters, different aspects of the daily practices in the Radboud Clinic are described and couples are followed throughout their treatment trajectories in the clinic. Each chapter shows the fertility treatment trajectory and the couples' experiences from a different angle.

Thus in Chapter 4, I sketch out the daily patient-centred practices in the Radboud Clinic, and couples' appreciation and – occasional – discontentment with these practices. The chapter focuses particularly on four themes that stood out in couples' stories and my own observations: interpersonal aspects of care; privacy; the provision of information; and psycho-social support. Subsequently, I discuss the empowering impact of these daily practices, but also point to 'missed opportunities' in the practice of patient-centredness. In the chapter's conclusion, I assert that some of these patient practices may render couples more inclined to continue with treatment. These practices and their effects are further described and scrutinized in the following chapters.

In Chapter 5, I consider the abundant information that couples receive about the risks and success rates of fertility treatments, and the way in which they interpret and handle this information. I will show that, as expected, this information increases their capacity to make well-informed decisions, but I also reveal how many find it difficult to apply the information to their own situation. Trust in health staff appears to be of crucial importance in decision-making, which challenges one of the core principles of patient-centred medicine.

In Chapter 6, the treatment process is analysed from the angle of technology. I first describe couples' initiation into the medical world of infertility, which increases their 'medical gaze' towards their fertility problem and possible solutions. In the second part of the chapter, I follow the couples through all of the distinct steps in an IVF cycle and examine how the visualization of all these steps and the ample ways in which couples are informed about their in-between results affect their insights, experiences, hopes and decision-making. An extended case study, consisting of excerpts of a diary of one of the study participants, illustrates the meaning and impact of visualizing technologies.

Chapter 7 first provides a detailed account of the way in which women and men experience the unequal burdens of IVF in the different treatment stages, reflecting gender dynamics in current-day Dutch conjugal relationships. I also describe cases of loss and grief as a result of a late miscarriage and the death of a prematurely born child following IVF. The chapter also portrays the intensive support that the clinic offers women and men, intended to decrease the treatment burden, which may also have the ambiguous effect of keeping most couples on the treatment track.

Chapter 8 discusses the requests for medical assisted conception that Radboud Clinic staff perceive as ethically sensitive and thus bring for discussion at their multidisciplinary ethics meetings, and the practices they employ to address and resolve their concerns. It places staff concerns, practices and decisions in the context of 'Dutch IVF' and the clinic's Catholic roots.

Finally, in Chapter 9, I wrap up the key insights and arguments of the book and present some after-thoughts and reflections about the future of IVF services in the Netherlands and internationally.

Notes

1. Aspects to do with permission for doing the study and anonymity of study respondents are dealt with in Appendix 1.
2. For research in the Netherlands, see Koomen (1997), Verdurmen (1997) and Smeenk et al. (2004). Smeenk et al. (2004) found that about one-tenth of couples undergoing IVF treatments decided on their own to refrain from further treatments after a failed first IVF treatment, even though their prognosis was still good, and about one-fifth did so after a second failed treatment. In the same period, two other studies (in Australia and Sweden) found 'high dropout rates' among people undergoing fertility treatments, showing that several couples

voluntarily discontinued subsidized IVF treatments (Hammarberg et al. 2001; Olivius et al. 2004).

3. See, e.g., Corea (1985); Tijmstra (1987); Klein (1989); Greil (1991); Sandelowski (1991, 1993); Franklin (1997); Cussins (1998); Becker (2000); Kahn (2000); Inhorn (2003); Thompson (2005); Franklin and Roberts (2006); Birenbaum-Carmeli and Dirnfeld (2008).

4. Average success rates per IVF treatment cycle in Dutch fertility clinics are currently around 25 per cent. Success rates of fertility clinics in the Netherlands are published per clinic on a yearly basis (http://www. lirinfo.nl).

5. See, e.g., Franklin (1997); Koomen (1997); Pasveer and Heesterbeek (2001); Verhaak et al. (2001, 2002, 2005).

6. Throughout the book, I consciously avoid the use of the word 'patients' to refer to women and men with fertility problems, as I do not consider them as such. Only occasionally, when presenting the views of other authors, do I use the term patients.

7. In the introduction to her book 'Making Parents', Charis Thompson explains her personal stance towards ARTs, in the midst of 'feminist, academic, and lay criticisms of these technologies', in the following way: 'I argue that these [assisted reproductive] technologies began as anything but a model for other areas of practice (there were few clinics, which had astonishing low success rates, imposed gruelling treatment regimens, and excluded most would-be patients because they were unable to pay or were judged to be suitable (sic) as parents) but have become unusually accountable to various stakeholders and have been established as a site of activism within medicine' (Thompson 2005: 25).

8. Different views and definitions of patient-centred medicine exist (see Mead and Bower 2000 for an overview).

9. Dancet et al. (2010) provide a systematic overview of studies on patients' perspectives on infertility care, in which they describe the dimensions of patient-centred practices to which patients attach importance. Overall, they found that people with fertility problems 'want to be treated like human beings with a need for: medical skills, respect, coordination, accessibility, information, comfort, support, partner involvement and a good attitude of, and relationship with, fertility clinic staff' (ibid: 467). See also Becker and Nachtigall (1991); Greil (1991); Halman, Abbey and Andrews (1993); Hojgaard, Ingerslev and Dinesen (2001); Inhorn (2003).

10. In addition, Schmidt et al. (2003) have pointed out that private clinics, especially, need to cater to the multiple needs of patients in order to attract and retain 'consumers'.

11. See e.g. Cussins (1998); Gastaldo (1997); Mayes (2009); Pasveer and Heesterbeek (2001); Sawicki (1991); Thompson (2005).

References

Alper, M.M. Brinsden, P.R., Fischer, R., & Wikland, M. 2002. 'Is your IVF programme good?', *Human Reproduction* 17(1): 8–10.

Becker, G. 2000. *The Elusive Embryo: How women and men approach new reproductive technologies*. Berkeley: University of California Press.

Becker, G. and R.D. Nachtigall. 1991. 'Ambiguous responsibility in the doctor–patient relationship: The case of infertility', *Social Science and Medicine* 32(8): 875–85.

Birenbaum-Carmeli, D. and M. Dirnfeld. 2008. 'In Vitro Fertilisation policy in Israel and women's perspectives: The more the better?', *Reproductive Health Matters* 16(31):182–191.

Blonk, L., J.A.M. Kremer and T. ten Haaf. 2006. 'Het ontwikkelen van een patiënttevredenheid vragenlijst', *Tijdschrift voor Verpleegkundigen* (7–8): 54–57.

Buitendijk S.E. 2000. 'IVF Pregnancies: Outcome and follow-up', Ph.D. dissertation. Leiden: University of Leiden.

Campagne, D.M. 2006. 'Should fertilization treatment start with reducing stress?', *Human Reproduction* 21(7): 1651–58.

Corea, G. 1985. *The mother machine: Reproductive technologies from artificial insemination to artificial wombs*. New York: Harper and Row.

Cussins, C.M. 1998. 'Ontological choreography: agency for women patients in an infertility clinic', in Berg, M. & A. Mol (eds), *Differences in medicine. Unraveling practices, techniques, and bodies*. Durham and London: Duke University Press.

Dancet, E.A.F., W.L.D.M. Nelen, W. Sermeus, L. De Leeuw, J.A.M Kremer and T.M. D'Hooghe, 2010. 'The patients' perspective on fertility care: A systematic review', *Human Reproduction Update* 16: 467–87.

Franklin, S. 1997. *Embodied Progress: A cultural account of assisted conception*. London: Routledge.

Franklin, S. and C. Roberts. 2006. *Born and Made: An ethnography of preimplantation genetic diagnosis*. Princeton: Princeton University Press.

Gastaldo, D. 1997. 'Is health education good for you? Re-thinking health education through the concept of bio-power', in A. Petersen and R. Burton (eds), *Foucault, Health and Medicine*. London and New York: Routledge, pp. 113–33.

Greil, A.L. 1991. *Not yet pregnant. Infertile couples in contemporary America*. New Brunswick and London: Rutger University Press.

Greil, A.L., K. Slauson-Blevins and J. McQuillan. 2010. 'The experience of infertility: A review of recent literature', *Sociology of Health and Illness* 32(1): 140–62.

Gupta, Y. 1996. 'New Freedoms, New Dependencies: New reproductive technologies, women's health and autonomy', Ph.D. dissertation. Leiden: University of Leiden.

Hammarberg, K., J. Astbury and H.W.G. Baker. 2001. 'Women's experience of IVF: A follow-up study', *Human Reproduction* 16: 374–83.

Hardon, A. and E. Moyer. 2014. 'Medical technologies: Flows, frictions and new socialities', *Anthropology and Medicine* 21(2): 107–112.

Heesterbeek, S. and H. Ten Have. 2001. 'Het normatieve spanningsveld tussen autonomie en paternalisme', in S. de Joode (ed.), *Zwanger van de kinderwens: Visies, feiten en vragen over voortplantingstechnologie*. The Hague: Rathenau Instituut, pp. 138–54.

Hojgaard A., H. Ingerslev and J. Dinesen. 2001. 'Friendly IVF: Patient opinions', *Human Reproduction* 16(7): 1391–1396.

Inhorn, M.C. 1994. *Quest for Conception: Gender, infertility, and Egyptian medical traditions*. Philadelphia: University of Pennsylvania Press.

⎯⎯⎯ 2003. *Local Babies, Global Science: Gender, religion and in vitro fertilization in Egypt*. New York: Routledge.

Inhorn, M.C. and F. Van Balen. 2002. *Infertility around the Globe: New thinking on childlessness, gender and reproductive technologies*. Berkeley: University of California Press.

Jaye, C., T. Egan and S. Parker. 2006. '"Do as I say, not as I do": Medical education and Foucault's normalizing technologies of self', *Anthropology and Medicine* 13(2): 141–55.

Kahn, S.M. 2000. *Reproducing Jews: A cultural account of assisted conception in Israel*. Durham, NC: Duke University Press.

Klein, R. (ed.) 1989. *Infertility: Women speak out about their experiences of reproductive technologies*. London: Pandora Press.

Kirejczyk, M. 1996. *Met technologie gezegend? Gender en de omstreden invoering van in vitro fertilisatie in de Nederlandse Gezondheidszorg*. Utrecht: Uitgeverij Jan van Arkel.

Klein, R. and R. Rowland. 1989. 'Hormone cocktails: Women as test-sites for fertility drugs', *Women's Studies International Forum* 12: 333–48.

Koomen, C. 1997. 'IVF? Nee, dan maar geen kind', in van Balen, F., D. van Berkel and J. Verdurmen (eds.). *Het kind van morgen. Consequenties van voortplantingstechnologie*. Groningen: Van Brug, pp. 61–73.

Kremer, J., M.J.A. van Eijndhoven, J. van der Avoort, B. Cohlen, D. Braat 2007. 'Zorg over de grens. Geen grip op kwaliteit van buitenlandse fertiliteitsbehandelingen', *Medisch Contact* 62(33/34): 1342–46.

Lupton, D. 1997 'Foucault and the medicalisation critique', in A. Petersen and R. Burton (eds), *Foucault, Health and Medicine*. London: Routledge, pp. 94–110.

Mayes, C. 2009. 'Pastoral power and the confessing subject in patient-centred communication', *Bioethical Inquiry* 6(4): 483–93.

Mead, N. and P. Bower. 2000. 'Patient-centeredness: A conceptual framework and review of the empirical literature', *Social Science and Medicine* 51(7): 1087–110.

Olivius, K., B. Friden, K. Lundin and C. Bergh. 2004. 'Why do couples discontinue in vitro fertilization treatment? A cohort study', *Fertility and Sterility* 81: 289–93.

Pasveer, B. and S. Heesterbeek. 2001. *De voortplanting verdeeld. De praktijk van de voortplantingsgeneeskunde doorgelicht vanuit het perspectief van patienten.* The Hague: Rathenau Instituut.

Sandelowski, M. 1991. 'Compelled to try: The never enough quality of conceptive technology', *Medical Anthropological Quarterly* 5: 29–47.

_____ 1993. *With Child in Mind: Studies of the personal encounter with infertility.* Philadelphia: University of Pennsylvania Press.

Schmidt, L., B.E. Holstein, J. Boivin, T. Tjornhoj-Thomsen, J. Blaabjerg, F. Hals, P.E. Rasmussen and A. Nyboe Andersen. 2003. 'High ratings of satisfaction with fertility treatment are common: Findings from the Copenhagen Multi-centre Psychosocial Infertility (COMPI) Research Programme', *Human Reproduction* 18(12): 2638–2646.

Smeenk, J.M.J., C.M. Verhaak, A.M. Stolwijk, J.A. Kremer, and D.D. Braat, 2004. 'Reasons for dropout in an in vitro fertilization/intracytoplasmic sperm injection program', *Fertility and Sterility* 81(2): 262–68.

Tijmstra, T. 1987. 'Het imperatieve karakter van de medische technologie en de betekenis van geanticipeerde beslissingsspijt', *Nederlands Tijdschrift voor Geneeskunde* 131(26): 1128–1131.

Thompson, C. 2005. *Making Parents: The ontological choreography of reproductive technologies.* Cambridge, MA: The MIT Press.

Van Balen, F. and M.C. Inhorn. 2002. 'Introduction: Interpreting infertility: A view from the social sciences', in M.C. Inhorn and F. Van Balen (eds), *Infertility around the Globe: New thinking on childlessness, gender and reproductive technology.*: University of California Press, pp. 3–32.

Van Empel, I.W., E.A. Dancet, X.H. Koolman, W.L. Nelen, E.A. Stolk, W. Sermeus, T.M. D'Hooghe and J.A.M. Kremer. 2011. 'Physicians underestimate the importance of patient-centredness to patients: A discrete choice experiment in fertility care', *Human Reproduction* 26(3): 584–93.

Verdurmen, J. 1997. 'Keuzes bij onvruchtbaarheid. Besluitvorming bij onvruchtbare paren', Ph.D. dissertation. Amsterdam: University of Amsterdam.

Verhaak, C.M., Smeenk, J.M.J., Kremer, J.A.M., Braat, D.D.M., and Kraaimaat, F.W. 2002. 'De emotionele belasting van kunstmatige voortplanting: Meer angst en depressie na mislukte eerste behandeling', *Nederlands Tijdschrift voor Geneeskunde* 146(49): 2363–66.

Verhaak, C.M., Smeenk, J.M.J., Van Minnen, A., Kremer, J.A.M., and Kraaimaat, F. W. 2005. 'A longitudinal, prospective study on emotional adjustment before, during and after consecutive fertility treatment cycles', *Human Reproduction* 20(8): 2253–60.

Chapter 1

STUDYING ARTS

THEORY, CONTEXT, THE CLINIC AND METHODS

Understanding the Use of ARTs

This book, while focusing on the workings and effects of a patient-centred fertility clinic, strongly builds on previous work in this area and in particular on social science studies regarding the medicalization of infertility and the use of ARTs. Over the last three decades, many social science scholars, including feminist and medical anthropologists, have studied ARTs and their manifold ramifications for social life, such as in the domains of marriage, kinship, gender, medicine and religion (Inhorn and Birenbaum-Carmeli 2008).[1] In her seminal overview of feminist scholarship on ARTs, Charis Thompson (2002, 2005) distinguishes two different phases/generations of social science scholars and points out differences among radical and more liberal feminist critiques. Below, following Thompson to a certain extent, I briefly sketch an important turn in ART social science scholarship: from being focused mainly on dominant discourses to, as I see it, a more nuanced understanding of women's (and men's) views and experiences.[2]

Pronatalist and Patriarchal Imperatives

Radical feminists (in the 1970s and 1980s) tended to explain and critique women's persistent use of ARTs by pointing to the pronatalist and patriarchal imperatives that informed the 'development, deployment and use' of these technologies (Sandelowski 1991: 34).

As Sandelowski phrased it, radical feminists depicted women with fertility problems as (ibid.):

> [C]ompelled by their male doctors and their male partners to undergo medical treatments for infertility because of the strong cultural pressure for married couples to have children of their own and for women, in particular, to demonstrate their normality as women by reproducing.

This view should be understood in the light of second wave feminism, where (radical) feminist scholars strongly criticized the ongoing medicalization of childbirth, as this placed motherhood at the centre of women's lives and transferred reproductive control from women to (male) medical professionals (e.g., Corea 1985; Klein 1989; Strickler 1992; Thompson 2002, 2005). These scholars saw the expansion of reproductive technologies as part of a continuous process whereby the patriarchal medical system was gaining control over women's procreative bodies and reducing them to passive objects of medical surveillance and management (Sawicki 1991: 76–77). Furthermore, they were strongly critical of the pushing and forcing role that the medical system and doctors played in the medicalization of fertility problems (Van Balen and Inhorn 2002: 14).

Infertile women's despair – and thus their eagerness to use reproductive technologies – was presented by scholars in this field as 'a by-product of largely anti-woman pronatalist and patriarchal norms' (Sandelowski and De Lacey 2002: 42); or alternately, infertile women were depicted as 'not-truly-desperate at all, or as not having to be desperate, but rather made to appear, or encouraged to be, desperate by physicians, drugs companies, and other marketers of infertility services and products' (ibid.).

Turn to Pragmatism: A More Nuanced Understanding

Medical anthropologists and other social science scholars have critiqued radical feminist scholars – and I share these critiques – because their insights were rarely based on empirical studies, and their analyses focused almost exclusively on the dominant discourses governing reproduction.[3] Without denying the impact of such discourses, these later scholars argued that women (and men) should not be perceived as 'passive vessels, simply acting in culturally determined ways' (Lock and Kaufert 1998: 2), nor as people docilely following hegemonic biomedical discourses and practices (Lupton 1997), but instead as pragmatic users of (reproductive) medicine:

> The response of women to medicalization is often mixed. They rarely react to the specific technology, or simply to the manipulation of their bodies, but rather on the basis of their perceptions as to how medical surveillance and interventions might enhance or worsen their daily lives. (Lock and Kaufert 1998: 16)

Lock and Kaufert identified pragmatism as a notion firmly guiding people's behaviour in the medical realm, as people do not act solely based on a series of fixed and stable principles or standpoints, but rather they weigh the pros and cons given their needs and their situation at a certain moment. To understand people's responses to (reproductive) medicine, a voice should be given to (infertile) women themselves, 'as real and living individuals with varying responses to infertility' (Sandelowski and De Lacey 2002: 42). This requires ethnographic investigation, studying how people perceive and use reproductive technologies in their daily life contexts.[4]

From the 1990s[5] onwards, a large number of nuanced ethnographic studies – in both Western and non-Western countries – have been completed, providing insight into the meaning and experiences of fertility problems and childlessness for the women (and sometimes men) involved in various social, cultural, religious and economic contexts, and the ways in which they have acted upon their infertility, seeking medical and non-medical solutions. Other studies have focused on the ways in which people in these different contexts experience (biomedical) fertility treatments and ARTs (when offered) and/or have examined how people's use of ARTs affects their views on and further use of these technologies.[6] In the Netherlands, a number of empirical studies have also been conducted (none of them ethnographic) that provide valuable insights into people's experiences of and responses to infertility and reproductive technologies.[7]

Below, I discuss some of the empirical and theoretical insights gained from these studies that are particularly relevant for the current book, and which contribute to the understanding of the medicalization of fertility problems and of people's (persistent) use of ARTs or their resistance to them.[8]

Compelling Reproductive Technologies

Medical technologies play a powerful role in processes of medicalization.[9] More and more lay people have come to see the body as a machine consisting of parts, which – when damaged or failing – can be repaired or replaced (Shilling 1993). This has created high expectations of the potential solutions biomedicine has to offer, and therefore it has been argued that the mere existence of medical technologies renders people eager to use them. The very availability of ART treatments thus makes most people want to fully exploit them, in order to avoid the potential regret of not having tried everything possible; a notion coined as anticipatory regret (Tijmstra 1987). Women find it hard to say no to further treatment, as they are surrounded by evidence that IVF and other techniques do result in babies (Sandelowski 1991).

Aside from the impact of its mere availability, reproductive technologies have other effects as well. Sandelowski (ibid.: 31) has looked at the 'nature' of reproductive technology and 'how it operates' to grasp why it is so compelling for many couples with fertility problems. In so doing, she argues against locating the compelling character of such technologies exclusively in pronatalist values and patriarchal agendas, as radical feminists have previously done. Rather, she starts from the position that in order to understand persistence in the use of reproductive technologies, these technologies should be looked at both from the inside and the outside. Viewed from the outside, cultural values may indeed push couples and doctors to use these technologies. Viewed from the inside, reproductive technologies also have their own pull. Sandelowski found, for instance, that one of the aspects that makes these technologies so compelling is their fragmenting character. By means of these technologies, 'hidden' aspects of conception become exposed to the eye and to the consciousness, which permits couples 'to live each step of getting pregnant' (Sandelowski 1993: 123). Achievement at one stage in the process compels couples to move on to the next.[10] Increasing visualization of the body's interior and bodily processes influences the way in which people perceive their own – ill, infertile or pregnant – bodies and how they act upon them (Van der Geest 1994; Layne 2003).

Sandelowski and other scholars have further identified a number of other features of ARTs that make them so compelling and hard to resist. They have pointed to the repetitive character of these technologies: hormonal stimulation, artificial insemination and IVF are not simply expected to be immediately successful; they must be repeated in order to achieve success. This repetitive feature in a way parallels the natural process of getting pregnant, since in general people do not conceive after the first try.[11] Women thus come to see these technologies as natural, which makes it easier to carry on with treatments and facilitates the acceptance – and obscuring – of their relative ineffectiveness.[12] In addition, as infertility treatments often serve diagnostic purposes, each treatment gives additional insight into what is going wrong in the conception process, and thus offers new chances to resolve or circumvent this particular problem in subsequent treatment (Franklin 1997). Finally, the fact that many (hormonal) treatment variations exist and reproductive technologies are constantly in development and being made known to the public – and may thus potentially offer new chances again and again – make it more difficult to stop treatments completely (Verdurmen 1997; Thompson 2005).

In sum, the mere existence and particular features of ARTs turn them into technologies with a strong 'pull' effect, which explains – to a certain extent – their persistent use by infertile couples/individuals. However, this persistence also draws people onto an 'emotional roller coaster', where they oscillate between hope and despair.[13] This book firmly builds on the above insights, and addresses the question of how, in a context of the increasing availability and use of visualizing technologies and ample provision of information by health professionals, such factors construct people's ideas and experiences of ARTs.

The Impact of Entering the Biomedical Domain

Social science scholars have examined how entering the biomedical domain of fertility clinics – with its disciplinary and normalizing practices – affects the way in which people come to see themselves, the treatments they undergo and their use of reproductive technologies (Sawicki 1991; Cussins 1998; Pasveer and Heesterbeek 2001; Thompson 2005). It is because of these practices, these scholars argue, that women (they rarely speak of men) undergoing fertility treatments are more and more inclined to look at themselves and their bodies with a 'medical gaze', to see themselves as 'patients', a shift that also enables them to behave as patients (Lupton 1997). Disciplinary power, Sawicki (1991) further argues, does not force these medicalized views upon people in treatment (as orthodox medicalization critiques would have it), but rather these medicalized views simply result from the disciplining that takes place and is embedded in clinical encounters. In addition, these clinical encounters and the reproductive technologies offered are strongly appealing to women as they incite desires, address their real needs and come up with concrete solutions, and therefore women willingly subject themselves to them (ibid.: 85). Women's and men's ideas, wishes and choices are thus seen as being co-produced through their contacts with biomedicine and the clinic. The hegemony of biomedicine is 'achieved through consent rather than by force' (Gramsci 1971).

Two studies, conducted in the USA and the Netherlands, examined in detail what happens when women (and men) enter fertility clinics and actively engage in 'disciplinary work'; what the researchers refer to as the 'objectification of the body' (Cussins 1996, 1998; Pasveer and Heesterbeek 2001; Thompson 2005).[14] These authors argue that when visiting a fertility clinic, women have to objectify their body, as it is only through this disciplinary work that they can achieve their goal: becoming pregnant and thus becoming a parent. They show how this disciplinary work accustoms women to the clinic's bureaucratic routines and encourages them to follow medical instructions, embrace medical knowledge and undergo painful medical examinations and treatments (Pasveer and Heesterbeek 2001). Furthermore, being good in 'bureaucratic work' may facilitate their flow through the clinic and being well-informed may enhance their active participation in their own care. This disciplinary work may be looked upon as potentially threatening to women's individuality, as they have to conform to the clinic's rules. It may also be seen as rendering them as 'obedient patients' – as the provided information allows them to better understand and follow up on what doctors propose, rather than criticise or debunk the doctors' expertise – or as 'medical objects' – as their bodies have to be disciplined to become examinable and treatable.

Nevertheless, the authors argue that these women (and men) are not passively undergoing this objectification. They are constantly required to play an active role in objectifying their bodies, and therefore should not be seen as (mere) victims of biomedicine, but rather as autonomous persons who are able to exert agency. Thompson (2005) explicitly speaks about 'agency through objectification', instead of placing the two in opposition to one another (as radical feminists would do). As she puts it, 'The patients do not so much let themselves be treated like objects to comply with the physician as they comply with the physician to be treated like objects' (ibid.: 191).

The authors further state, however, that there is a risk attached to this: if women (and men) are not good (enough) at playing an active role (which happens to some, for example when confronted with repeat failures), they risk being taken over by the technology and treatment and losing their agency.[15] In addition, Pasveer and Heesterbeek (2001) argue that because of the treatments they

have gone through, and because of the various forms of objectification that they have been involved in, infertile women change
over the course of the treatment trajectory. They are no longer the
same – stable and rational – people they were when they first visited
their general practitioner with their fertility problem; they often
become more ambivalent, simultaneously wanting to continue and
yet discontinue treatments. Treatment trajectories, Pasveer and
Heesterbeek assert, do not take into account these changing person-
alities or people's ambivalence; they are designed for the continuation of treatment, without pauses or stops. Consequently, infertility
patients only stop if they are desperate or on the explicit advice of
the medical doctors. From this perspective, continuing or not continuing treatment is not (only) about conscious agency and informed
decision-making by autonomous individuals, since women whose
views have been shaped by disciplinary work in infertility clinics
become more and more inclined to just go on (ibid.: 69–70).[16] These
insights, which are mainly based on interview accounts, constitute an important inspiration for the study presented in this book,
since they underline the importance of observing what is actually
going on in the clinics and of following couples throughout their
treatment trajectories.

Agency and Resistance

Compelling reproductive technologies and long-term involvement in treatments in fertility clinics may thus render people more
inclined to continue using ARTs. Yet other authors have emphasized that the hegemonic biomedical discourse and health system do
not fully or solely determine how women (and men) with fertility
problems act. These women and men do possess and exert some
form of agency, and are actively engaged in choosing the way in
which they deal with their fertility problems.[17] Infertile people consciously decide about entering, not entering or withdrawing from
the medical field, and – once having entered the clinic – they decide
on what treatments they want to undergo. However, the extent
to which they perceive themselves as in control may differ greatly
(Verdurmen 1997).

   Infertile women may also exert their agency by attempting to
'work' the medical system and medical doctors in order to get
what they want (Greil 2002: 103). Greil firmly rejects a limited,
dichotomous view of women's responses to reproductive medicine,
which depicts women as 'either acquiescing to medical metaphors
and interpretations or resisting them' (ibid.). He lists a number of

strategies that infertile women employ to work with the system in the way they wish, such as reading as much information as possible to become more knowledgeable about infertility, making suggestions to their doctors to influence the course of their medical treatments and switching doctors if they feel they cannot persuade him/her to modify the treatment regimen. Greil further argues that while women may certainly experience their infertility as a 'failure of body and self', and infertility treatments as frustrating, the women in his study did not present themselves as 'passive victims content to be treated as objects' (ibid.: 113). He depicts them as 'active strategists and negotiators', attempting to maximize control over their treatment by working the system.

In a similar vein, Sandelowski (1993) speaks of the 'calculus of pursuit' that she saw as characteristic of the behaviour of infertile couples:

> They weighed the options known and accessible to them and then constructed their own calculus of pursuit, involving four domains of venture capital: time, money, and physical and psychic energy. Couples used this matrix of resources to determine which route in the maze of routes to parenthood to pursue. (Sandelowski 1993: 95)

Sandelowski found that women and men with fertility problems, when faced with decisions at different moments, were not guided by one dominant view or principle on the acceptability of reproductive technologies. Rather, they pragmatically considered numerous pros and cons, taking into account, for example, the perceived risks or side-effects of (hormonal) treatment, the experienced or foreseen impact of the treatment on the quality of their marriage, the costs and possible success rates of different fertility treatments versus adoption, and so on (ibid.: 91–104). This process of weighing pros and cons before making decisions may also render people ambivalent about the choices they ultimately make, as no decision is ever fully ideal (Pasveer and Heesterbeek 2001).

Lupton further argues that going along with and accepting medical advice or treatments should not necessarily be viewed as passive acceptance of the medical gaze (1997: 105).[18] Accepting medical advice might be seen as engaging in particular 'practices of self' that people see as the most adequate at that particular moment for their own well-being, in order to become free of pain and suffering, or – as in the case of this book – to overcome their infertility. To achieve this, Lupton continues, people may relate to doctors in different ways: the same person may behave as an autonomous, reflexive and non-passive individual, or as a 'good patient' who follows doctors' orders; but s/he may also behave in both ways varyingly or even simultaneously.

Resistance, sometimes defined as 'oppositional agency' (Ahearn 2001:116), is another notion frequently debated in contemporary studies on people's responses to (reproductive) medicine. In the resistance debate, intentionality and the level of consciousness is a recurring theme: how intentional should acts of resistance be in order to be considered genuine (Fegan 1986, in Lock and Kaufert 1998: 12)? Some researchers have argued that feminists, in their eagerness to depict women as active agents rather than passive followers or victims, have gone a step too far and have been inclined to over-emphasize – or romanticize (Abu-Lughod 1990) – resistance at the expense of depicting constraints (Inhorn 2003: 17). Nevertheless, several authors agree that the meaning of practices of resistance can only be assessed and understood in the context in which they take place.[19]

Resistance in the field of infertility and ARTs may come in various forms, either on an individual level or collectively, and can be located within or outside the clinic. Resistance can, for example, be found against 'the power of cultural norms' regarding womanhood, manhood and biological parenthood that infertile and childless women are confronted with (Becker 2000: 30), and against the stigma, discrimination and blaming that childless women face in many countries (Riesmann 2000; Todorova and Kotzeva 2003). Women and men with fertility problems may also resist any form of medicalization of their fertility problems and consciously choose not to visit a doctor (Koomen 1997). Resistance in the context of reproductive technologies, however, does not necessarily imply an attack on the medical system or a withdrawal from medical control and treatments (Lock and Kaufert 1998). On the contrary, resistance can exist against policies and practices that exclude certain groups of people from particular treatments or from reimbursement from health insurance – for example, lesbian or homosexual couples or single parents – and thus lead to a plea in favour of the extension of medicalization.

Elaborating on the above insights, this book examines the diversity of positions and choices that women and men with fertility problems take towards ARTs. Their positioning, as I will show, partly depends on their specific physical conditions, circumstances and biographies (which are presented in Chapter 3). These circumstances and biographies, however, can only be understood in the context of present day Dutch society, some features and trends of which I present below.

The Dutch Context:
Families, Children and Childlessness

Since the 1970s, Dutch society has undergone huge transformations, and this is particularly the case for the composition of Dutch families, partner relations and the role of children (Van Balen and Gerrits 2001; Van den Troost 2005). While in the 1960s more than half of Dutch households consisted of a (working) father, a (caring) mother and two or more children, four decades later this applies to barely one third of households. Having or not having children in the Netherlands is more and more an individual and conscious choice (Beets 1999; Gerrits and Van Balen 2001). Through the introduction and wide acceptance of the contraceptive pill, sexuality and pregnancy have become disconnected. Present day Dutch women (couples) can – to a large extent – decide whether, when and how many children to have. In case a woman does become pregnant against her will, she can have a legal abortion. The number of unwanted children in the Netherlands is low, demonstrated, for example, by the fact that in the last decade, only twenty-six children became available for adoption each year.

Late Parenthood, Part-Time Work and Gender Inequality

Currently, a Dutch woman has on average 1.8 children (in the 1960s, the average was 3.1), which is slightly higher than the European Union average.[20] However, Dutch women start rather late: since the 1970s, the average age of Dutch women having their first child has increased from twenty-four to around twenty-nine in 2002 (Beets 1999; De Graaf 2004a). Subsequently, the age at which women have a second or third child – the latter is the wish of one-fifth of Dutch women (De Graaf 2004b) – has also increased. In the period between 2000 and 2002, only 40 per cent of children born in the Netherlands had a mother younger than thirty (De Graaf 2004a). While a similar trend of delayed first childbirth has been observed in many Western countries, the Netherlands has been referred to as the 'world champion' of late parenthood, for no other country is known to have an older average age for first-time mothers (ibid.: 4). Compared to women, men are on average three years older when they have their first child.[21]

Dutch women's increasing delay of childbirth is first of all explained by their increasing levels of education and subsequent employment rates (Beets 1999). The number of working women was very low in the 1960s (only 7 per cent), but since then it has been steadily increasing, from 53 per cent in 1995 to almost 70 per cent in 2011 (Niphuis-Nell and de Beer 1997). Nevertheless, many women work part-time: two out of three working women are employed on a part-time basis, compared to 16 per cent of men, and for mothers with young children this figure is even higher.[22] This figure is also higher than in any other Western country and partly explains the inequality in income between women and men.[23]

Since 2000, the right to work part-time has been established in law, and the option to work part-time has also been suggested as a way to resolve 'the compatibility problem between a paid job and childcare' (Van den Troost 2005: 11). While study results show that most women and men working part-time do so out of free choice, these preferences should be understood in the context of prevailing 'cultural norms and traditions, collective pressures and gender identities' (Plantenga 2002: 63). In the Netherlands, there is a strong cultural tradition that expects women (and men to a certain extent) to undertake a large part of childcare tasks themselves (Brinkgreve and Te Velde 2006). The Dutch government was rather late in establishing formal subsidized childcare, only doing so in the 1990s, which did lead to more women entering the workforce (though more recently these subsidies have decreased enormously, which has led to some women withdrawing from their jobs).[24] While overall the number of working women has increased significantly in recent times, when children arrive most Dutch families become a 'one earning family' or adopt a 'one and a half earner model' with the man as the main income provider (Van den Troost 2005). This is particularly the case for lower-educated pairs, but also applies to middle- and higher-educated couples. Despite the progressive and emancipated image that the Netherlands generally holds, mothers still spend considerably more time on household and childrearing tasks than fathers, and many are not financially independent, which increases gender inequality (Van der Lippe 1997).[25] Nevertheless, while most fathers do not forego work time to raise their children (though some do), Dutch men do increasingly consider it important to have an affective relationship with their children; according to Van den Troost, this is because 'Society expects them to do so' (2005: 33).

Changing Marriage Patterns and Secularization

From the 1970s onwards, the popularity of marriage in the Netherlands has waned (Van den Troost 2005).[26] This should not be seen as a signal of a decreased interest in relationships; rather, formal marriage has been replaced by informal partnerships, with many young people cohabiting. Indeed, cohabitation has nowadays been normalized in most social circles (though it is less accepted among those who adhere to Orthodox Christian churches and also less common among young people from for example Turkish or Moroccan background).[27]

The institution of formal marriage has further decreased in importance due to increasing divorce rates: this figure increased from 5.5 per cent in the 1960s to 38 per cent in 2013 (Van den Troost 2005).[28] Lower-educated women in the Netherlands are less likely to leave their partner than highly educated women, which might be related to the higher economic dependence of the former group or because the latter group is less likely to have children. The high divorce rate has an impact on the family life of children. One in six children are confronted with parental divorce and many grow up in so-called patchwork or blended families (Bos 2013; Van Balen and Gerrits 2001a).

The increase in divorce and changes in family composition since the 1970s have been associated with 'a more individualistic partnership model, directed towards self-fulfilment and equality of partnership' (Van den Troost 2005: 14). The aforementioned economic emancipation of women in part explains these changes: women gain less from being married. At the same time, a shift in dominant values has taken place: economic security and growing welfare have resulted in increased attention to the goals of achieving quality of life and self-expression, a process that is accompanied by the emergence of individual autonomy and the erosion of normative prescriptions.

In addition, secularization has been very pervasive in many parts of the Netherlands. In 2013, only around half of the Dutch population belonged to a church, with Catholicism and Protestantism the most dominant religions. The number of people belonging to a church has decreased enormously in the last three to four decades. For example, the percentage of registered Catholics decreased from 40 per cent in 1980 to 26 per cent in 2013, and their active church participation (such as church visits on Sundays, child baptism and church marriages) has decreased even more.[29] Similar tendencies have been observed in some of the Protestant churches; only members of the Orthodox Protestant churches (a small minority) continue to be highly active church members.

Secularization and individualization have also led to different expectations about the quality of marital and intimate relationships, partnership and romantic love. The survival of partnership is now increasingly dependent on the preparedness of partners to take the well-being and emotional needs of the other into account, and good communication between partners is highly valued (Van den Troost 2005).

Same-Sex Families

Another major change in Dutch society is the increased number of cohabiting same-sex couples: from 35,000 in 1995 to 56,000 in 2009, a quarter of which are formally married – in 2001, the Netherlands became the first country to make same-sex marriages possible (Keuzenkamp 2010).[30] The number of male couples is higher than the number of female couples (31,000 and 25,000 respectively), though more female couples live with children than male couples (20 per cent and 3 per cent respectively); some of these children were born in previous heterosexual relationships. The Netherlands has a relatively positive climate regarding lesbian and gay people and same-sex marriage compared to other Western countries (Bos 2013; Keuzenkamp 2010). However, when children are involved, support for the principle of equal rights dwindles. For example, more than 20 per cent of the Dutch population rejects the idea of equal adoption rights for same-sex couples. Recent research shows that around one third of same-sex couples have a wish for a child; for young girls and boys with a homosexual or bisexual preference, these percentages are even higher (Bos and Van Gelderen 2010). To fulfil this wish, same-sex couples can adopt a child, opt for co-parenthood, or use third party material (lesbian couples) and/or surrogacy options (male homosexual couples). Formally, according to Dutch legislation (as I will discuss in Chapter 2), lesbian couples and single women do have equal access to medically assisted reproduction in fertility clinics, though in practice this does not always work out so easily.

Voluntary Childlessness

Notwithstanding the fact that motherhood continues to be a central feature of the Dutch feminine identity, having children is no longer obvious for all women. Motherhood competes with other roles and interests (Van Troost 2005: 31). The last decades have seen an increase in voluntary childlessness: a study showed that 20 per cent of women aged 36 to 45 years are expected to remain childless, of whom 55 per cent consider it voluntary (De Graaf and Loozen 2005). It should be noted, however, that the line between voluntary and involuntary childlessness cannot always be clearly drawn. Some people may have always assumed that they would have children, but at a later stage decide not to go for it, or never find themselves in a position that would enable them to have children (for example, because they do not encounter a partner with whom they want to have children, or their partner does not want children). Other women (and men) consciously postpone having children until a later age and then find that they are no longer able to (Gerrits and Van Balen 2001; Brinkgreve and Te Velde 2006).

Women mentioned several reasons behind their choice to remain childless: they felt that children would restrict their liberty and that raising children was a huge time investment; their partners did not want to have children; and the combination of work and children was thought to be difficult. In addition, some women felt too old to have children, or considered children too expensive or organizing childcare too problematic (Gerrits and Van Balen 2001: 42–43). Interestingly, these motivations for voluntary childlessness diverge strongly from the motivations that women mentioned in the 1970s. At that time, resistance to the traditional motherhood and housewife roles and politically inspired motivations (such as concerns about overpopulation, the nuclear bomb and third world problems) were more frequently referred to (Van Balen and Gerrits 2001). Nobis (2007: 78), who conducted a study among voluntarily childless women in the Netherlands, observed that the general acceptance of voluntary childlessness in Dutch society has increased over the past three decades, though on a personal level voluntarily childless women still find that they have to justify their choice. Parenthood is still the norm.

Infertility and Involuntary Childlessness

Despite the many changes that have taken place in partner relationships and the composition of families in contemporary Dutch society, having children is still the dominant norm and the desire of most Dutch women and men. But not all manage to fulfil that desire. The National Study of Behaviour during Infertility (NOGO), carried out in 1992, showed a primary national infertility rate of 14 per cent after twelve months of trying to conceive, and an 8.4 per cent infertility rate after twenty-four months (Van Balen et al. 1995, 1997).[31] The prevalence of childlessness (voluntary and involuntary) in the Netherlands is 17 and 11 per cent among Dutch women aged forty and sixty respectively. Women's educational level is strongly correlated with childlessness: a quarter of highly educated women over forty-five remain childless, while only nine per cent of lower-educated women of the same age group are childless. Highly educated women have fewer permanent relationships than lower-educated women, and are more likely to live on their own, delay having children or decide not to have children at all. The increasing age of Dutch women when trying for their first child is generally considered to contribute to the increase in involuntary childlessness (Te Velde 1991; Beets 1999).[32]

While the postponement of childbearing certainly enhances the infertility rate, women's age is not the sole factor explaining current Dutch infertility rates. Hospital based studies show that male factors are implicated in up to 60 per cent of couples' infertility problems (NVOG 1998), with male fertility also showing a gradual decline with increasing age, though this decline affects men at a later age (from 40 to 50 onwards) than women (from 30 onwards).[33] Roughly half of the infertility problems of the couples participating in the study upon which this book is based were caused – solely or partly – by a physical problem of the male partner (see Chapter 3). The fact that population-based infertility rates only refer to female infertility and not to male infertility may overemphasize the impact of a woman's age on (increasing) infertility levels.

In studies conducted in the 1990s, involuntarily childless people in the Netherlands, when asked why they wanted to have children, mentioned motives related to personal happiness, parenthood and being able to give and receive love and affection (Van Balen 1991; Van Balen and Trimbos-Kemper 1993). When confronted with fertility problems and involuntary childlessness, this is often experienced as distressing (Van Balen 1991), even though Dutch society and culture is less harsh and stigmatizing towards infertile and childless women (and men) than has been reported elsewhere, particularly in non-Western countries.[34] Still, Dutch long-term infertile women show a significantly lower level of well-being compared to women in general (Van Balen and Trimbos-Kemper 1993: 53). Manifold illustrations of women's (and men's) sorrow and grief in case of childlessness can be found, for example, in the testimonies on the website of Freya, the Dutch association for childless couples, and a compilation of letters written by Dutch childless women and men (Van Walbeek 1995).

Most Dutch women and men confronted with fertility problems attempt to resolve these problems by seeking medical assistance: 84 per cent of couples confronted with fertility problems (between 1965 and 1992) consulted their general practitioner, and 72 per cent visited a specialist in a hospital (Van Balen et al. 1995). Only five per cent of couples opted for adoption and two per cent for fostering. Another later study showed that overall, one in five women (born between 1945 and 1979) visited the doctor because they had not managed to become pregnant with their first child; of those women who already had one child – and thus suffered from secondary infertility – one in ten visited the doctor for the same reason (De Graaf 2004b). It should be noted that in both of the above-mentioned studies, some of the couples referred to encountered fertility problems in a period when ARTs, including IVF, were not yet or hardly available. With the increasing availability of ARTs in the Netherlands, the percentages for medical help seeking may be expected to have increased as well.

In the next chapter, I provide an overview of current Dutch ART legislation, professional guidelines and health insurances policy – all of which I refer to as 'Dutch IVF' – which constitutes the framework within which ARTs can be offered in the Netherlands. Below, I introduce the Radboud Clinic, which is one of the fourteen Dutch clinics licensed to provide ARTs and was the field site of the study on which this book is based.

The Radboud Clinic

The Radboud Clinic in the city of Nijmegen serves a rather wide mixed urban and rural area in the southeast of the Netherlands. This area covers parts of the provinces of Noord-Brabant and Limburg, which was traditionally predominantly Catholic, and a large part of the province of Gelderland, which was originally mainly Protestant. Secularization has taken place among large sections of the population in this region, as in the rest of the Netherlands. At the time of fieldwork the Radboud Clinic refered to its Catholic origins on its website, and claimed to perform its task with particular attention to this religious inheritance, which had – as we will see in Chapter 8 – an impact on some of the ethical stances the clinic took.[35]

The Radboud Clinic has a long history of delivering fertility services: the first artificial inseminations were carried out in the 1950s and the first IVF treatment in 1984. Over the last decades, the clinic has gradually expanded; at the time of fieldwork, around six hundred artificial inseminations and twelve hundred IVF and related treatments were being carried out on a yearly basis. Various regional hospitals refer their patients in need of advanced reproductive medicine to the Radboud Clinic. The clinic has an agreement of collaboration with the fertility departments of two regional hospitals. Moreover, at the time of fieldwork, patients from all over the country came to Nijmegen for IVF-ICSI-PESA treatment, since the Radboud Clinic was one of only three clinics in the Netherlands permitted to provide this specialized treatment as part of a clinical trial. When the study was conducted, the Radboud Clinic did not make use of donor material, which implied that single women and lesbian and homosexual couples could not be treated (see Chapter 8).

Patient Care

Over the course of the years, the clinic has developed a comprehensive policy – including a large set of working procedures, norms and guidelines – regarding medical-technical and laboratory procedures, quality of care, patient information, psycho-social support and ethical issues. The clinic sees 'the provision of high quality services in a patient friendly ambience' as its main task.[36] Improving the quality of care is a focal point of the clinic, for which the NIAZ (Netherlands Institute for the Accreditation of Hospitals) quality system is applied.[37] Yearly, a patient satisfaction study is conducted considering issues such as patient information, privacy, waiting times, attendance by doctors, etc. Furthermore, based on a survey held among users of fertility centres nationwide, the clinic has received the Dutch Infertility Award (DIA) from Freya four times, being chosen as the most patient-friendly fertility clinic in the Netherlands.

Offering 'adequate and modern patient information' is another focal point of the Radboud Clinic. The clinic has set up extensive guidelines about what information should be given at what moment, by whom and how, and over the course of the years several materials have been developed to support this. In 2004 – about the same time as the fieldwork for this book began – the clinic initiated the Digitale Poli, an online platform to increase communication between clinic staff and patients. Couples undergoing IVF treatment can access their personal medical records via the Internet, and can have the opportunity to chat with fellow couples in treatment and health professionals about their experiences and concerns. The Digitale Poli is founded on the principle of patient empowerment:

better-informed patients are expected to be more actively involved in the treatment process and in decision-making over the course of treatment (see Chapter 4 for more details). This innovative project was at the time unique in the Netherlands, and received attention from the media and policy makers.[38] Furthermore, couples visiting the Radboud Clinic who are in need of psycho-social support have access to a social worker, psychologist and sexologist, all of which is covered by health insurance. On a monthly basis, a social work meeting is held, during which doctors and nurses talk with the social worker and psychologist about the women and men they are seeing, and discuss how they can best support them. All of these patient-centred practices, the way in which women and men experience them, and their impact will be considered in the chapters that follow.

Bimonthly, the clinic staff also holds a multidisciplinary ethics meeting, in which couples' requests for medical assistance that raise ethical concerns or 'feelings of uneasiness' among them are discussed. The way in which the clinic addresses these concerns, the principles and practices involved – that is, the clinic's 'bio-ethics in practice' – and the impact these may have on couples' autonomy and decision-making, will be specifically discussed in Chapter 8.

Research and External Engagement

While patient care is the clinic's core task, most of the clinic staff is also involved in academic research. Their studies cover a wide-ranging area of topics and reflect the broad interests of the health staff, and not only in clinical-technical aspects. Study topics, for example, have included: the psycho-emotional impact of IVF treatment (Verhaak 2003); Internet use by IVF patients (Haagen et al. 2003); the effects of the introduction of the Digitale Poli (Tuil et al. 2009); IVF patients' satisfaction (Blonk et al. 2006); a follow-up of IVF/ICSI children (Woldringh et al. 2011a, 2011b); and the cost-efficiency of IVF (Bouwmans et al. 2008a, 2008b). At the time of research, one of the staff members was chairing a national 'umbrella study' to assess the efficiency of fertility treatments. Aside from disseminating study results through academic journals and conferences, insights gained from the studies also inform clinical practices and national level policy and practice. Results from the umbrella study, for example, were proactively used by NVOG to lobby for the re-introduction of health insurance covering the payment of initial IVF treatments (see Chapter 2).

Senior clinic staff are also actively engaged in NVOG activities, such as the development of guidelines and setting up a national IVF registration system. They also play an active role in other nation-wide activities in the field of infertility and ARTs in the Netherlands, including the development of the Model Protocol for the Embryowet 2003 and the Model Protocol in case of 'moral contraindications in infertility treatments' (NVOG 2010). At times, they can also be heard and seen in the Dutch mass media, often as representatives of NVOG, commenting on issues related to the use of ARTs in the Netherlands. The clinic staff members' explicit involvement in the national ART arena, and their public appearances, underline the fact that their concerns and interests are not limited to purely medical-technical issues.

The Study

The Radboud Clinic was the study site of the ethnographic research on which this book is based. I collected data by means of extensive observations in the clinic (constituting hospital ethnography) and by prospectively following couples with fertility problems visiting the clinic. In addition, I widely read and consulted relevant litera-ture (social science and medical), policy documents, professional guidelines and patient information materials.

The main reason I had for approaching the Radboud Clinic with the request to carry out this study was – as I have sketched above – the clinic staff's strong engagement in public, political and profes-sional debates on fertility issues and ARTs, thus showing an interest beyond medical-technical issues, including issues that I intended to address in my study.

For a study of this type to be feasible, gatekeepers interested in the study topic, and their willingness to permit researchers entrance to their field, are crucial (Inhorn 2004), not only to get initial formal permission, but also to be assured of continuing collaboration and access to relevant persons, places and events throughout the course of the study. In an overview of hospital ethnographies, Van der Geest and Finkler suggest that the 'defensiveness of hospital authorities and their hesitation to allow observers to their workplace' might be one possible explanation for the limited number of ethnographic studies carried out in hospital settings, in particular in Western countries (2004: 1996). In my study, I was not confronted with such defensiveness; on the contrary, after having discussed the study proposal – in particular, I had to 'defend' some methodological concerns related to the qualitative nature of the study[39] – it did not take long for the head of the clinic to grant me permission to proceed. In addition, ethical clearance to conduct the study was requested from and granted by the regional medical-ethical commission (CMO Regio Arnhem-Nijmegen).

Hospital Ethnography

Hospital ethnography is a valuable approach to assessing patients' experiences of ill health and care delivery. Yet it is also valued as a means of enhancing understanding of a range of (complex) social phenomena and processes within clinics, such as the organization and culture of clinics (Savage 2000: 1401), the impact of changing health policies (Gibson 2004), the production of expert knowledge (Atkinson 1995), ethical decision-making (Vermeulen 2001, 2004), and the way in which biomedical information is communicated to patients and how this affects them (Rapp 1999; The 1999, 2002). In addition, hospital ethnographies have the potential to point to local variations in biomedical views and practices, and can show how sociocultural values and societal structures and relations are reflected in the medical setting.[40]

Ethnographic observation provides access to what people do and what they say about it, instead of only listening to what people say that they themselves or others do (Green and Thorogood 2004: 131). Observations also provide a researcher with insight into aspects that study participants may forget to tell or purposely do not want to tell, as well as aspects that participants simply do not notice (because of their seeming obviousness) or do not realize might be relevant for the researcher. When observing, new questions may also be raised, which provide input for further conversations and interviews with study participants. Finally, sharing time and events in a real context with patients/care seekers and clinic staff enhances a researcher's empathic understanding of their experiences and the interactions between the two, as Annemei The (1999) underlines: 'The ambience in the waiting room, the sinking silence in the bad news consultations, the desperate and hopeful glances of patients . . . can hardly be repeated in interviews' (The 1999: 332, author's translation). It is not only the patients' positions and experiences – or in the case of this book, those of women and men with fertility problems – that are better understood when the ethnographic researcher shares part of them, but s/he also obtains in-depth insight into the dilemmas that clinical staff are confronted with, for example when dealing with issues of hope or regarding informed consent (ibid.: 330).

Ethnographic observations in the clinic allowed me to gain insight into what people – both women and men visiting the clinic, and clinic staff – actually do, undergo and say when encountering each other and the reproductive technologies. As women's and men's experiences in the clinic are not only shaped through contact with the doctors in consultation and treatment rooms, but also by encounters and interactions in other spaces and on other occasions in the clinic, I also conducted observations in other places, such as waiting rooms and at the reception desk. In addition, I was allowed to attend staff meetings, which contributed enormously to my insights into how staff members talked about the women and men with fertility problems and considered and decided upon clinical, social and ethical issues.

Following Couples

In addition to doing extended observations, I followed prospectively and intensively twenty-three couples with fertility problems visiting the clinic, through which I acquired insight into these couples' situated and lived accounts, their experiences and views, and the changes therein over time. Two distinct groups of couples were approached by sending them a patient information letter: the first group consisted of couples who were visiting the clinic for the very first time with their fertility problem; the second group was made up of couples who were starting their first IVF treatment (either for the very first time or the first time for a second child). As the treatment trajectories for people with fertility problems may take several years – much longer than I would be able to follow couples as part of the study – selecting couples at different stages of their treatment trajectories allowed me coverage of all stages, though not the entire trajectory of each and every couple. In addition, a number of inclusion criteria for participants were defined.[41]

The couples were followed over a period of one to two years by means of in-depth interviews at their homes (two or three per couple; fifty-seven in total; each interview lasted 2–4 hours); observations of couples' consultation hours and treatment sessions at the clinic (sixty-two); and extensive phone calls (thirty-two) and e-mails (thirty-four); in addition, six women kept an individual diary on behalf of the study. During the interviews, aside from asking questions and following up on the answers given, I used two so-called projective techniques. First, I asked the couples to construct a 'timeline', which helped to elaborate their reproductive life histories. Second, I asked them to 'sort cards' as a means to facilitate and stimulate them to talk about the sources of information that they used related to their fertility problem and about their concerns and what made them feel stressed.[42]

Following people in such an intensive way offers a number of advantages compared to only listening to one retrospective account. First of all, I was present at several important moments/occasions and could therefore build up a relationship and 'share' their experiences to a certain extent, which meant that I could probably better understand them in their context. It also gave people the opportunity to talk about 'fresh' experiences, less hindered by the limitations of human memory; and by following women and men over time, changing and contradictory experiences and perceptions could be addressed. Following the couples and visiting them at home also allowed me to gain more insight into their background and living situation, into the interactions and communication between the two partners of a couple, and to view how these changed over time.

Data collection took place during the period between September 2003 and August 2006. In the first period (up to April 2005), fieldwork was carried out both in the clinic and at couples' homes; in the period thereafter, I maintained contact with the couples still in treatment by phone and email.

Throughout the thesis I quote from the interviews and/or conversations I had with study participants and clinic staff, from conversations observed amongst themselves, and from phone calls, e-mails, and diaries. I personally translated these quotes from Dutch to English and – when needed – I edited them slightly to improve their readability. I use fictitious first names to refer to the study participants. In addition, for the sake of anonymity I refer to all doctors as female. (More detailed information about the study methods can be found in Appendix 1.)

Reflections on the Position of the Anthropologist

The personal experiences of social scientists may influence the manner in which they conduct their studies and may have implications for knowledge production.[43] It has become good practice among qualitative researchers to adopt a critical attitude towards their data, 'to be reflexive and identify – honestly – some of the social, practical and biographical contingencies that helped to produce the data' (Brewer 2000: 5). In so doing, instead of denying or trying to eliminate the effects of these contingencies, researchers add credibility to their analysis and increase faith in its reliability and validity.[44] While I share Thompson's reluctance 'to put myself in my academic writing and thereby lose some of my own and family's privacy' (Thompson 2005: 22), I concede that some accounting of personal and professional connections and experiences with the topic is proper for the sake of transparency and validity.

I have been 'involved' with infertility since the early 1990s. In 1993, I conducted a study on infertility and childlessness in Mozambique; in 1994, I became the mother of twins by means of IVF; and from 2003 to 2006, I conducted the fieldwork for the current book. Clearly, important themes in my academic and personal life are closely related and have mutually affected one other. This of course raises a number of questions. Here I will focus on two of them (see also Gerrits 2012).[45]

First, how did this shared experience affect the interactions between me and the research participants, and thus the production of data? Aware of the fact that the way in which I introduced myself to the study participants might make a difference in terms of how they reacted to me, I deliberately decided that I would present myself simply as a researcher and not as an 'experiential expert', as someone who had been infertile and a user of ARTs herself. I could easily do this, as the 'condition' I shared with the study participants was invisible. Later on, if it felt appropriate, I could always tell them about my personal experience.

The reasons I had for not wanting to immediately share my own ART experience differed for health staff and couples. When seeking permission to carry out the study from the heads of the department, I did not introduce myself as an experiential expert because I wanted to prevent anyone – including myself – from thinking that I had been granted permission mainly or solely because of my personal experience or that I would be 'uncritical' of the technologies. Only after being granted permission, when we were talking about the practicalities related to the study and one of the gynaecologists asked me what I actually knew about the daily practice of fertility treatments, did I reveal that I had undergone an IVF treatment myself.[46]

With regard to the couples participating in the study, I had two major reasons for not wanting to introduce myself as an experiential expert. In the first place, as my own first IVF treatment had been successful, my story could have become one of those success stories that would give hope and inspire couples to start or continue IVF treatment; or conversely, my informants could find it more difficult to express their doubts about or arguments against treatment if they knew that I was a former user of infertility services. Secondly, if they did not know that I had undergone IVF treatment, I thought that it would be easier to ask them in detail about their treatment experiences, without their assuming that I already knew what they meant (as I had gone through it myself) or asking me about my experiences and wishing to compare their experiences and opinions with mine.

Though I was firmly decided against introducing myself as an experiential expert, I also realized that given the informal interviewing technique and frequent contacts with informants (including in their homes), it would not take long before some of them started to question me about my own situation. And indeed, about half of the couples asked me if I myself had children; a few of them wondered in the very first interview, though most posed questions only at a later stage of the study. I always replied that I had children, often adding that I had twins; and as twins in this context always raise 'suspicion', in general I said that I also had my own treatment story. Only when couples asked me directly did I give more details about my treatment trajectory, but I never went into great detail about how I had experienced treatments or how I had made my decisions. When people heard that I had my own experience in the field, their first reaction was often that it might explain my interest in the topic, or they commented that it might help me to understand what they were going through. Sometimes they also referred to it when telling me about their own experiences, using expressions such as 'You have gone through it yourself, so you know how it is'.

Some qualitative researchers who have shared, or came to share, personal characteristics with their respondents that were central to their research have mentioned that their informants opened up or started to share different stories once they became aware of their common experiences (Cassel 1987; Krumeich 1994). I did not get the impression that this was the case in my study. Most of the study participants had been eager to share their stories anyway, and were quite open and informative right from the beginning. I did not employ the method of sharing experiences as a means to come to a more experience-near anthropology, an interview technique suggested by Sjaak van der Geest (2007).

This does not mean that I did not share similar experiences with several of my study participants, and this raises the second question that I want to address: how did this shared experience affect my involvement in the study and the way in which I made sense of what I saw and heard? Given the fact that I had been a successful user of IVF treatment myself, one may question whether and to what extent I would be willing and able to take a critical stance towards the medicalization of fertility problems and the use of ARTs. This question was at the front of my mind throughout the research process, and I did discuss this many times with my supervisors and other audiences. I am fully aware that my own well-considered 'submission' to IVF treatment (despite a period of ambivalence and reluctance) and the subsequent successful outcome made me, in some way, loyal to ARTs, and this indeed complicates my ability to take a critical position. Yet in all study phases I attempted to approach the topic both critically and in a nuanced way, which is reflected in the presentation and interpretation of the data in the various publications based on this study, including the current book.

Furthermore, I find it worth considering the difference between hearing stories and experiences that I recognized and could easily relate to, compared to those that were less recognizable or far removed from my own experiences and views. At times during the fieldwork, when I was listening to the stories of the couples or observing them in the clinic, I could very well imagine what they wanted to tell me or what they were experiencing, and I was sometimes reminded of events, conversations and emotions from the time that I had gone through fertility treatment myself. For example, when attending foetal ultrasounds – *the* moment of truth at the end of an extended and often stressful period of IVF treatment – I clearly recalled this moment from my own experience and the meaning it had for me. In Chapter 6, I write about the tension that couples experience when undergoing this pregnancy ultrasound. Would a researcher who had not lived through this him/herself have noticed, experienced, interpreted and written about such an event in a similar way? I could come up with a number of other comparable situations and ask the same question. In these cases, to be sure that I was not making up a point or argument that reflected my own experience and emotions, and to guarantee that it was not subjectively driven and biased by my own experience, I always double-checked my empirical data and looked for 'deviant cases' (cf. Hesebeck 2012). Hesebeck – who conducted a study among adolescents living with the same congenital heart disease as herself – states that because she had experienced situations and bodily sensations that were very similar to what her informants told her about, her own 'embodied knowledge' enabled her to phrase some of the experiences of her participants and her interpretations thereof as confidently as she did (Hesebeck 2012). Following this remark, I cautiously suggest that this observation may also apply to me: having similar experiences may have led to a more grounded, embodied interpretation and presentation of the research findings.

However, I was, as expected, also confronted with many embodied experiences, emotions and viewpoints that I did not share or recognize (cf. Van Dongen 1996: 343).[47] In addition, as I had been fortunate to have experienced a successful first IVF treatment, I was never in the difficult position of having to decide whether to do another IVF treatment, and thus I did not share this experience with my informants at all. Consequently, even though I had been in a comparable situation and had definitely shared comparable experiences, there was much dissimilarity – in many aspects – with many of my informants as well. Though many times I was emotionally touched by my informants' stories, I did not experience it as personally confronting or painful to hear them; it did not emotionally unbalance me, as Hesebeck (2012) had noticed. In retrospect, I would say that only in a few exceptional cases was I emotionally 'caught up' when handling my data. This observation raises the question of whether the fact that by the time of my research I had overcome my infertility problem (it was conducted almost ten years after my own treatment) had turned me into a partial outsider, even when I had once been a full insider. This is also the reason why I am hesitant to overstate the impact of my comparable condition on my knowledge production, and on the interpretation and presentation of my data. Ultimately, I leave it to the reader to judge.

Notes

1. Inhorn and Birenbaum-Carmeli (2008) state that at the time, over fifty anthropologists were conducting ART studies all over the world.
2. This sketch by no means intends to give a comprehensive overview of ART scholarship. For such overviews, I refer to Van Balen and Inhorn (2002); Thompson (2002, 2005); Inhorn and Birenbaum-Carmeli (2008).
3. See e.g. Sawicki (1991: 70); Sandelowski (1993: 38); Sandelowski and De Lacey (2002); Van Balen and Inhorn (2002); Thompson (2005).
4. Sawicki (1991); Lock and Kaufert (1998); Rapp (1999); Inhorn (2003).
5. Some authors have observed that (medical) anthropologists have been studying many aspects of the human reproductive life cycle over the past two to three decades, but that they were rather late in studying the 'lived world of infertility and reproductive medicine' (Thompson 2002:

63; Van Balen and Inhorn 2002: 4). Van Balen and Inhorn suggest that this may be partly attributed to the fact that social science investigators, as feminist scholars themselves, may not have wanted to appear committed to 'the essentializing notion that motherhood, and quests to achieve it, should be a woman's sole purpose in life' (2002: 6).

6. These ethnographic studies have been conducted in several countries worldwide, such as Bangladesh (Nahar 2007), Bulgaria (Todorova and Kotzeva 2003), Cameroon (Feldman-Savelsberg 1994), China (Handwerker 1998), Ecuador (Roberts 2006, 2012), Egypt (Inhorn 1994, 1996, 2003), Israel (Kahn 2000), Mozambique (Gerrits 1997, 2002), Tanzania (Kielman 1998), Gambia (Sundby 1997, 2002), the UK (Franklin 1997; Franklin and Roberts 2006), the USA (Becker 2000; Greil 1991; Sandelowski 1993; Thompson 2005) and Zimbabwe (Sundby 2002). See also Greil et al. (2010), Inhorn and Birenbaum-Carmeli (2008) and Van Balen and Inhorn (2002) for overviews of (ethnographic) studies in this area.

7. These studies include Tijmstra (1987); Van Balen (1991); Koomen (1997); Van Balen et al. (1995); Verdurmen (1997); Pasveer and Heesterbeek (2001); Verhaak et al. (2001, 2002, 2005); CvZ (2002); Verhaak (2003); Van Rooij et al. (2009); Van Rooij and Korfker (2009). None of these studies in the Netherlands were ethnographic and hardly any attention has been paid to context. These studies were predominantly based on retrospective accounts, often after a single interview or questionnaire; most often, only women were interviewed, with men rarely included – with the exception of Verdurmen (1997), Verhaak et al. (2001, 2002, 2005) and Verhaak (2003) – and the views of medical doctors were only presented in one study on ethical questions (Bolt et al. 2004; Hunfeld et al. 2004).

8. By no means do I intend to present an exhaustive overview of the ART literature.

9. See, e.g., Berg and Mol (2001); Blume (2006); Rapp (1999); Van der Geest (1994).

10. See also Sandelowski (1991, 1993); Williams (1988).

11. See Modell (1989); Sandelowski (1991); Thompson (2005).

12. Franklin (1997); Sandelowski (1991); Thompson (2005).

13. Becker (2000); Franklin (1997); Sandelowski (1991, 1993).

14. It should be noted that Cussins and Thompson are one and the same author. Pasveer and Heesterbeek's (2001) analysis was inspired by Cussins' (1998) early work, and their findings and argumentation on the objectification of the body show remarkable similarities. The authors distinguish four different ways of objectifying the body, namely through becoming 'bureaucratic objects' and 'medical objects' and through 'epistemic disciplining' and 'naturalization'.

15. Cussins (1996, 1998); Pasveer and Heesterbeek (2001); Thompson (2005).

16. It should be noted that this argument is based on the accounts of a limited number of women interviewed; the authors did not conduct any observations, nor did they interview staff members. The authors themselves also point to this limitation in their study and plea for more ethnographic research on the impact of daily clinical practices (Pasveer and Heesterbeek 2001).

17. See, e.g., Sandelowski (1993); Verdurmen (1997); Lock and Kaufert (1998); Greil (2002).

18. Lupton does not speak about fertility treatments in particular.

19. Riesmann (2000); Todorova and Kotzeva (2003); Nahar (2007).

20. See: http://www.indexmundi.com.

21. In 2012, the average age of men at the birth of their first child was 32.4 years, while women were 29.4 years (www.nationaaalkompas.nl).

22. 75 per cent of women in the Netherlands in the age group 25–54 with dependent children work part-time. In France, for example, this is only 26 per cent (www.nationaaalkompas.nl).

23. Female part-time employment in the Netherlands is 68.6 per cent, compared to 33.5 per cent in European Community countries on average; for men, this is 17.9 and 6.1 percent respectively (Plantenga 2002: 60). At median earnings, the gender pay gap in the Netherlands is 17 per cent, and more than half of this pay gap is related to gender differences in working hours (www.nationaaalkompas.nl).

24. From the 1990s Dutch policies started to focus on increasing the labor participation of women, resulting from economic crises and European Union policy regarding equal treatment of women and men (Brinkgreve and Te Velde 2006: 146). From that moment onwards (young) women have been supposed to be able to be financially self-supplying/independent.

25. It has been argued that this is also related to the half-hearted regulations for pregnancy and parental leave, which give limited space for women to stay at home after the birth of a child and even less for men. This is particular so compared to regulations and childcare services in Scandinavian countries. On the other hand, Dutch women (and men) are envied – by women (and men) from Scandinavian countries – as they have more possibilities to work part-time and spend time with their children (Brinkgreve and Te Velde 2006: 154–55).

26. For women, the mean age at first marriage increased from 24.5 in 1960 to 27.3 in 1995. For men, these figures are respectively 26.8 and 29.7 years.

27. De Graaf and Distelbrink (2005); Stephan Bol and Gerald Bruins, 'Gereformeerden wonen vaker samen', *Nederlands Dagblad*, 17 November 2012. Retrieved 15 February 2015 from http://www.nd.nl/artikelen/2012/november/17/samenwonen-sluipt-binnen-in-kerken-van-orthodox-gemeenten.

28. CBS Statline, 'Huwelijksontbindingen; door echtscheiding en door overlijden'. Retrieved 12 December 2014 from http://statline.cbs.nl/.
29. From 1980 to 2013, the number of Catholics going to church on Sundays decreased from 24 per cent to 8 per cent; Catholics having their child baptized decreased from 31 per cent to 18 per cent; and Catholics marrying in church decreased from 31 per cent to 9 per cent (Becker et al. 2006).
30. Despite this substantial increase, cohabiting same-sex couples only constitute one per cent of the total number of Dutch cohabiting and/or married couples. (See http://www.cbs.nl/nl-NL/menu/themas/bevolk ing/publicaties/artikelen/archief/2005/2005 -1823-wm.htm).
31. This is the only nationwide study that has been conducted on the prevalence of infertility in the Netherlands.
32. Women who tried to become pregnant with their first child between the ages of 20 and 28 years had a 10–15 per cent chance of being confronted with fertility problems; this percentage increased to 25 per cent when women reached the age of 35 (Beets 1999: 12).
33. Kühnert and Nieschlag (2004); Raad voor de Volksgezondheid en Zorg (2005).
34. See, e.g., Gerrits (1997); Inhorn and Van Balen (2002); Inhorn (2003); Nahar (2007).
35. Since then the way the clinic profiles itself (on the website) has changed. See: UMCN website, https://www.radboudumc.nl.
36. UMCN website, https://www.radboudumc.nl.
37. On a four year basis, internal (RUMC) and external (NIAZ) audits are performed to assess whether the department fulfils certain quality norms.
38. Since then, the Digitale Poli has been expanded and is accessible to all IVF patients.
39. These concerns included the – from their point of view – relatively small sample size of couples whom I would prospectively follow, the use of non-validated data collection instruments and issues of objectivity versus subjectivity.
40. See, e.g., Inhorn (1994); Andersen (2004); Van der Geest and Finkler (2004); Zaman (2004).
41. Inclusion criteria included: couples had to reside in the 'region for fertility care', i.e., southeast Netherlands (for practical reasons, as I intended to travel to their homes for interviews); at least one of the partners within a couple had to be 'autochthon' Dutch (to limit the number of variables); both had to speak fluent Dutch (to enable intensive communication); and those who were visiting the clinic for the very first time with their fertility problem had to have been referred by a general practitioner (in order to avoid the inclusion of medically complicated 'cases' referred by other hospital specialists).
42. Both projective techniques are described in more depth in Appendix 1.

43. See, e.g., special issues of the journal *Medische Antropologie* on 'Intersubjectivity' 2007, 19(2) and on 'Ethnography and Self-Exploration' 2012, 24(1).
44. See, e.g., Hammersley and Atkinson (1983:17); Green and Thorogood (2004: 19).
45. Elsewhere I have addressed these questions more extensively (Gerrits 2012). In that article, I also refer to other examples in the literature that show the close connection between the personal biography of researchers and the choice of their research topic, which is particularly striking in the area of 'failed reproduction'. Well-known researchers, including for example Gay Becker (2000), Arthur Greil (1991), Marcia Inhorn (1994), Linda Layne (2003), Rayna Rapp (1999), Johanne Sundby (1999), Charis Thompson (2005) and Frank Van Balen (1991), have all been very explicit about the linkage between their personal experience with some form of 'failed reproduction' and their academic interest in the area. They all had various reasons for choosing the topic, which I discuss in the above mentioned article.
46. In addition, in my contacts with the health staff and other personnel during the first months of the study, when we were getting to know each other and talking about professional and personal issues, I sometimes brought up my own experience with fertility treatments. This was never planned; it fully depended on the moment and the specific situation, and whether I felt it was appropriate or relevant to the conversation. At the end of the fieldwork period, about half of the health staff knew that I had undergone fertility treatments, and occasionally, after having shared my own experience, they or I sometimes referred to it in conversations.
47. Views and emotions that I did not recognize included, for example: women who said that they would rather not have been informed about the potential risks or side-effects of hormonal treatments and the limited success rates of IVF, as they felt that this was discouraging and frightening; women who appeared extremely focused on having a child and felt that their dreams for the future would be fully destroyed if they did not succeed in conceiving; men and women who 'glorified' doctors and medical technology as performing miracles.

References

Abu-Lughod, L. 1990. 'The romance of resistance: Tracing transformations of power through Bedouin women', *American Ethnologist* 17: 41–55.
Ahearn, M.L. 2001. 'Language and agency', *Annual Review of Anthropology* 30: 109–37.
Andersen, H.M. 2004. '"Villagers": Differential treatment in a Ghanaian hospital', *Social Science and Medicine* 59: 2003–12.

Atkinson, P. 1995. *Medical Talk, Medical Work*. London: Sage Publications.

Becker, G. 2000. *The Elusive Embryo: How women and men approach new reproductive technologies*. Berkeley: University of California Press.

Becker, J., J.J.M. Hart and L. Arnts. 2006. *Godsdienstige veranderingen in Nederland: Verschuivingen in de binding met de kerken en de christelijke traditie*. The Hague: Sociaal en Cultureel Planbureau.

Beets, G.C.N. 1999. 'Education and age at first birth', Special Issue, *Demos* 15: n.p.

Berg, A. and A. Mol. 2001. *Ingebouwde normen. Medische technieken doorgelicht*. Utrecht: Van der Wees.

Birenbaum-Carmeli, D. and M. Dirnfeld. 2008. 'In Vitro Fertilisation policy in Israel and women's perspectives: The more the better?', *Reproductive Health Matters* 16(31): 182–91.

Blonk, L., J.A.M. Kremer and T. ten Haaf. 2006. 'Het ontwikkelen van een patiënttevredenheid vragenlijst', *Tijdschrift voor Verpleegkundigen* (7–8): 54–57.

Blume, S.S. 2006. *Grenzen aan Genezen: Over wetenschap, technologie en de doofheid van een kind*. Amsterdam: Bert Bakker.

Bolt, L.L.E., M.A.J.M. Buijsen and J.A.M. Hunfeld. 2004. *Morele contra-indicaties voor ouderschap? Een psychologisch, ethisch en juridisch onderzoek naar de selectie van hulpvragers voor een IVF-behandeling*. Ethiek en Beleid NWO. Budel: Uitgeverij Damon.

Bos, H. 2013. 'Lesbian-mother families formed through donor insemination', in A.E. Goldberg and K.R. Allen (eds), *LGBT-Parent Families*. New York: Springer Science and Business Media, pp. 21–37.

Bos, H., and L. Van Gelderen. 2010. 'Homo en lesbisch ouderschap in Nederland', in S. Keuzenkamp (ed.), *Steeds gewoner, nooit gewoon: Acceptatie van homoseksualiteit in Nederland*. The Hague: Sociaal en Cultureel Planbureau, pp. 104–118.

Bouwmans, C. A., Lintsen, B. A., Al, M., Verhaak, C. M., Eijkemans, R. J., Habbema, J. D. F., and Hakkaart-Van Roijen, L. 2008a. 'Absence from work and emotional stress in women undergoing IVF or ICSI: an analysis of IVF-related absence from work in women and the contribution of general and emotional factors', *Acta Obstetricia et Gynecologica Scandinavica* 87(11): 1169–1175.

Bouwmans, C.A., Lintsen, B.M., Eijkemans, M.J., Habbema, J.D.F., Braat, D.D., and Hakkaart, L. 2008b. 'A detailed cost analysis of in vitro fertilization and intracytoplasmic sperm injection treatment', *Fertility and sterility*, 89(2): 331–341.

Brewer, J.D. 2000. *Ethnography*. Buckingham: Open University Press.

Brinkgreve, C. and E. Te Velde. 2006. *Wie wil er nog moeder worden?* Amsterdam: Uitgeverij Augustus.

Cassel. J. 1987. *Children in the field: Anthropological experiences*. Philadelphia: Temple University Press.

CvZ (College voor Zorgverzekeraars). 2002. *IVF/ICSI: Aanbevelingen voor wijziging van de regeling op basis van de resultaten van effect- en evaluatieonderzoek.* Amstelveen: College voor Zorgverzekeringen.

Corea, G. 1985. *The Mother Machine: Reproductive technologies from artificial insemination to artificial wombs.* New York: Harper and Row.

Cussins, C.M. 1996. Ontological choreography: Agency through objectification in infertility clinics. *Social Studies of Science* 26(3): 575–610.

_____ 1998. 'Ontological choreography: Agency for women patients in an infertility clinic', in M. Berg, and A. Mol (eds), *Differences in Medicine: Unraveling practices, techniques, and bodies.* Durham, NC: Duke University Press, pp. 166–200.

De Graaf, A. 2004a. *Geboorteregeling in 2003. Bevolkingstrends, 1ᵉ kwartaal 2004.* The Hague: CBS.

_____ 2004b. 'Kinderloosheid en opleidingsniveau', CBS Webmagazine 24 May. Retrieved 23 March 2016 from www.cbs.nl.

De Graaf, A. and M. Distelbrink. 2005. *De demografische levensloop van jonge Turken en Marokkanen. Enquêteonderzoek onder allochtonen.* Den Haag: CBS.

De Graaf, A. and S. Loozen. 2005. *Door omstandigheden vaak geen of één kind. Bevolkingstrends, 1ᵉ kwartaal 2005.* The Hague: CBS.

Fegan, B. 1986. Tenants' non-violent resistance to landowner claims in a central Luzon. *The Journal of Peasant Studies, 13*(2), 87-106.

Feldman-Savelsberg, P. 1994. 'Plundered kitchens and empty wombs: Fear of infertility in the Cameroonian grassfields', *Social Science and Medicine* 39(4): 463–74.

Franklin, S. 1997. *Embodied Progress: A cultural account of assisted conception.* London: Routledge.

Franklin, S. and C. Roberts. 2006. *Born and Made: An ethnography of preimplantation genetic diagnosis.* Princeton University Press.

Gastaldo, D. 1997. 'Is health education good for you? Re-thinking health education through the concept of bio-power', in A. Petersen and R. Burton (eds), *Foucault, Health and Medicine.* London: Routledge, pp. 113–33.

Gerrits, T. 1997. 'Social and cultural aspects of infertility in Mozambique', *Patient Education and Counselling* 31: 39–48.

_____ 2002. 'Infertility and matrilineality. The exceptional case of the Macua', in M.C. Inhorn and F. Van Balen (eds), *Infertility around the Globe: New thinking on childlessness, gender and reproductive technology.* Berkeley: University of California Press, pp. 233–46.

_____2012. 'Interweaving personal biography and academic work: Studying infertility among "others" and "at home"', *Medische Antropologie* 24(1): 73–95.

Gerrits, T. and F. Van Balen. 2001. '(On)gewenste kinderloosheid: Twijfel, uitstel en afstel', in S. De Joode (ed.), *Zwanger van de kinderwens: Visies, feiten en vragen over voortplantingstechnologie.* The Hague: Rathenau Instituut, pp. 38–47.

Gibson, D. 2004. 'The gaps in the gaze in South African hospitals', *Social Science and Medicine* 59: 2013–24.

Gramsci, A. 1971. *Selections from the Prison Notebooks*. London: Lawrence and Wishart.

Green, J. and N. Thorogood. 2004. *Qualitative methods for health research*. London: Sage Publications.

Greil, A.L. 1991. *Not Yet Pregnant: Infertile couples in contemporary America*. New Brunswick: Rutgers University Press.

_____. 2002. 'Infertile bodies: Medicalization, metaphor and agency', in M.C. Inhorn and F. Van Balen (eds), *Infertility around the Globe: New thinking on childlessness, gender and reproductive technology*. Berkeley: University of California Press, pp.101–18.

Greil, A.L., K. Slauson-Blevins and J. McQuillan. 2010. 'The experience of infertility: A review of recent literature', *Sociology of Health and Illness* 32(1): 140–62.

Haagen, E.C., Tuil, W., Hendriks, J., de Bruijn, R. P. J., Braat, D. D. M., and Kremer, J. A. M. 2003. 'Current Internet use and preferences of IVF and ICSI patients', *Human Reproduction* 18(10): 2073–78.

Hammersley, M. and P. Atkinson. 1983. *Ethnography: Principles in practice*. London: Routledge.

Handwerker, L. 1998. 'The consequences of modernity for childless women in China: Medicalization and resistance', in M. Lock and P.A. Kaufert (eds), *Pragmatic Women and Body Politics*. Cambridge: Cambridge University Press, pp. 178–205.

Hesebeck, K.I. 2012. 'The anthropologist as an expatriate native: Anthropological research on and with congenital heart disease(s)', *Medische Antropologie* 24(1): 115-129.

Hunfeld, J.A.M., Passchier, J., Bolt, L.L.E., and Buijsen, M.A.J.M. 2004. 'Protect the child from being born: Arguments against IVF from heads of the 13 licensed Dutch fertility centres, ethical and legal perspectives', *Journal of Reproductive and Infant Psychology* 22(4): 279–89.

Inhorn, M.C. 1994. *Quest for Conception: Gender, infertility, and Egyptian medical traditions*. Philadelphia: University of Pennsylvania Press.

_____ 1996. *Infertility and Patriarchy: The cultural politics of gender and family life in Egypt*. Philadelphia: University of Pennsylvania Press.

_____ 2003. *Local Babies, Global Science: Gender, religion and in vitro fertilization in Egypt*. New York: Routledge.

_____ 2004. 'Privacy, privatization, and the politics of patronage: ethnographic challenges to penetrating the secret world of Middle Eastern, hospital-based in vitro fertilization', *Social Science and Medicine*, 59(10), 2095–2108.

Inhorn, M.C. and D. Birenbaum-Carmeli. 2008. 'Assisted reproductive technologies and culture change', *Annual Review of Anthropology* 37: 177–96.

Inhorn, M.C. and F. Van Balen. 2002. *Infertility around the Globe: New thinking on childlessness, gender and reproductive technologies.* Berkeley: University of California Press.

Kahn, S.M. 2000. *Reproducing Jews: A cultural account of assisted conception in Israel.* Durham, NC: Duke University Press.

Keuzenkamp, S. (ed.). 2010. *Steeds gewoner, nooit gewoon: Acceptatie van homoseksualiteit in Nederland.* The Hague: Sociaal en Cultureel Planbureau.

Kielman, K. 1998. 'Barren ground: contesting identities of infertile women in Pemba, Tanzania', in M. Lock, and P.A. Kaufert (eds), *Pragmatic Women and Body Politics.* Cambridge: Cambridge University Press, pp. 127–63.

Klein, R. (ed.). 1989. *Infertility: Women speak out about their experiences of reproductive technologies.* London: Pandora Press.

Koomen, C. 1997. 'IVF? Nee, dan maar geen kind', in F. Van Balen, D. van Berkel and J. Verdurmen (eds), *Het kind van morgen. Consequenties van voortplantingstechnologie.* Groningen: Van Brug, pp. 61–73.

Krumeich, A. 1994. *The Blessings of Motherhood: Health, pregnancy and child care in Dominica.* Amsterdam: Het Spinhuis.

Kühnert, B. and E. Nieschlag. 2004. 'Reproductive functions of the ageing male', *Human Reproduction Update* 10(4): 327–39.

Layne, L. 2003. *Motherhood Lost: A feminist account of pregnancy loss in America.* New York: Routledge.

Lock, M. and P.A. Kaufert. 1998. *Pragmatic Women and Body Politics.* Cambridge: Cambridge University Press.

Lupton, D. 1997 'Foucault and the medicalisation critique', in A. Petersen and R. Burton (eds), *Foucault, Health and Medicine.* London: Routledge, pp. 94–110.

Modell, J. 1989. 'Last chance babies: Interpretations of parenthood in an in vitro fertilization program', *Medical Anthropology Quarterly* 3(2): 124–38.

Nahar, P. 2007. 'Childless in Bangladesh. Suffering and resilience among rural and urban women', Ph.D. dissertation. Amsterdam: University of Amsterdam.

Niphuis-Nell and de Beer (eds). 1997. *Sociale atlas van de vrouw, Deel 4, Veranderingen in de primaire leefsfeer.* Rijswijk: SCP.Nobis, E. 2007. *Geen kinderen geen bezwaar. Waarom niet alle vrouwen moeder willen zijn.* Amsterdam: Uitgeverij Contact.

NVOG. 1998. *Patiëntenvoorlichting. Vruchtbaarheidsproblemen bij mannen.* Retrieved 1 March 2015 from www.nvog.nl.

NVOG. 2010. *Model protocol in geval van mogelijke morele contra-indicaties bij vruchtbaarheidsbehandelingen.* Retrieved 1 March 2015 from www.nvog.nl.

Pasveer, B. and S. Heesterbeek. 2001. *De voortplanting verdeeld. De praktijk van de voortplantingsgeneeskunde doorgelicht vanuit het perspectief van patiënten.* The Hague: Rathenau Instituut.

Plantenga, J. 2002. 'Combining work and care in the polder model: An assessment of the Dutch part-time strategy', *Critical Social Policy* 22(1): 53–71.

Raad voor de Volksgezondheid en Zorg [Board for Public Health and Care]. 2005. *Prijsverschillen voor IVF behandelingen. Grote verschillen in prijzen IVF behandelingen.* Nieuwsberichten, 21 June 2005. Retrieved 23 March 2016 from www.rvz.net.

Rapp, R. 1999. *Testing Women, Testing the Fetus: The social impact of Amniocentesis in America.* New York: Routledge.

Riesman, C.K. 2000. 'Stigma and everyday resistance practices: Childless women in South India', *Gender and Society* 14(1): 111–35.

Roberts, E.F. 2006. 'God's laboratory: Religious rationalities and modernity in Ecuadorian in vitro fertilization', *Culture, Medicine and Psychiatry* 30(4): 507–36.

_____ 2012. *God's laboratory: assisted reproduction in the Andes.* University of California Press.

Sandelowski, M. 1991. 'Compelled to try: The never enough quality of conceptive technology', *Medical Anthropological Quarterly* 5: 29–47.

_____ 1993. *With Child in Mind: Studies of the personal encounter with infertility.* Philadelphia: University of Pennsylvania Press.

Sandelowski, M. and S. De Lacey. 2002. 'The use of a "disease": Infertility as a rhetorical vehicle', in M.C. Inhorn and F. Van Balen (eds), *Infertility around the Globe: New thinking on childlessness, gender and reproductive technology.* Berkeley: University of California Press, pp. 33–51.

Savage, J. 2000. 'Ethnography and health care', *British Medical Journal* 321: 1400–02.

Sawicki, J. 1991. *Disciplining Foucault: Feminism, power and the body.* New York: Routledge.

Schmidt, L., Holstein, B.E., Boivin, J., Tjørnhøj-Thomsen, T., Blaabjerg, J., Hald, F. and Andersen, A.N. 2003. 'High ratings of satisfaction with fertility treatment are common: Findings from the Copenhagen Multicentre Psychosocial Infertility (COMPI) Research Programme', *Human Reproduction* 18(12): 2638–46.

Shilling, C. 1993. *The Body and Social Theory.* London: Sage Publications.

Smeenk, J.M.J., C.M. Verhaak, A.M. Stolwijk, J.A. Kremer, and D.D. Braat. 2004. 'Reasons for dropout in an in vitro fertilization/intracytoplasmic sperm injection program', *Fertility and Sterility* 81(2): 262–68.

Strickler, J. 1992. 'Editorial: The new reproductive technology: Problem or solution?', *Sociology of Health and Illness* 14(1): 111–32.

Sundby, J. 1997. 'Infertility in The Gambia: Traditional and modern health care', *Patient Education and Counseling* 31: 29–37.

_____ 1999. 'Sad not to have children, happy to be childless: a personal and professional experience of infertility', *Reproductive Health Matters,* 7(13), 13-19.

_____ 2002. 'Infertility and health care in countries with less resources', in M.C. Inhorn, and F. Van Balen, (eds), *Infertility around the Globe: New thinking on childlessness, gender and reproductive technology.* Berkeley: University of California Press, pp. 247–59.

Te Velde, E.R. 1991. *Zwanger worden in de 21ste eeuw: Steeds later, steeds kunstmatiger.* Utrecht: Oratie, Rijksuniversiteit Utrecht.

The, A. 1999. 'Emotie en inzicht: eigen onderzoekservaringen als data', *Medische Antropologie* 11(2): 323–34.

_____ 2002. *Facing Death: Palliative care and communication: Experiences in the clinic.* Buckingham: Open University Press.

Tijmstra, T. 1987. 'Het imperatieve karakter van de medische technologie en de betekenis van geanticipeerde beslissingsspijt', *Nederlands Tijdschrift voor Geneeskunde* 131(26): 1128–31.

Thompson, C. 2002. 'Fertile ground: Feminists theorize infertility', in M.C. Inhorn and F. Van Balen (eds), *Infertility around the Globe: New thinking on childlessness, gender and reproductive technology.* Berkeley: University of California Press, pp. 52–78.

_____ 2005. *Making Parents: The ontological choreography of reproductive technologies.* Cambridge, MA: The MIT Press.

Todorova, I.L.G. and T. Kotzeva. 2003. 'Women's resistive voices: Facing involuntary childlessness in Bulgaria', *Women's Studies International Forum* 26(2): 139–51.

Tuil, W.S., M. van Selm, C.M. Verhaak, P.F. de Vries Robbé, and J.A.M. Kremer. 2009. 'Dynamics of Internet usage during the stages of in vitro fertilization', *Fertility and Sterility* 91(3): 953–56.

Van Balen, F. 1991. *Een leven zonder kinderen: Ongewilde kinderloosheid: beleving, stress en aanpassing.* Assen: Dekker and Van de Vegt.

Van Balen, F. and T. Gerrits. 2001. 'Kinderwens in context', in S. de Joode (ed.), *Zwanger van de kinderwens: Visies, feiten en vragen over voortplantingstechnologie.* The Hague: Rathenau Instituut, pp. 28–37.

Van Balen, F. and M. Inhorn. 2002. 'Introduction: Interpreting infertility: A view from the social sciences', in M.C. Inhorn and F. Van Balen (eds), *Infertility around the Globe: New thinking on childlessness, gender and reproductive technology.* Berkeley: University of California Press, pp. 3–32.

Van Balen, F., E. Ketting and J. Verdurmen. 1995. *Zorgen rond onvruchtbaarheid: Voornaamste bevindingen van het Nationaal Onderzoek naar Gedrag bij Onvruchtbaarheid.* Delft: Eburon.

_____ 1997. 'Choices and motivations of infertile couples', *Patient Education and Counselling* 31: 19–27.

Van Balen, F. and T.C.M. Trimbos-Kemper. 1993. 'Long-term infertile couples: A study of their well-being', *Journal of Psychosomatic Obstetrics and Gynecology* (Special Issue) 14: 53–60.

_____ 1995. 'Involuntary childless couples: Their desire to have children and their motives', *Journal of Psychosomatic Obstetrics and Gynecology.* 16: 137–44.

Van den Troost, A. 2005. *Marriage in Motion: A study on the social context and processes of marital satisfaction.* Leuven: Leuven University Press.

Van der Geest, S. 1994. 'Medische technologie in cultureel perspectief. Inleiding', in S. Van der Geest, P. Ten Have, G. Nijhof and P. Verbeek-heida

(eds), *De Macht der dingen. Medische technologie in cultureel perspectief.*
Amsterdam: Het Spinhuis, pp. 1–19.

_____ 2007. 'Is it possible to understand illness and suffering?', *Medische Antropologie* 19(1): 9–21.

Van der Geest, S. and K. Finkler. 2004. 'Hospital ethnography: Introduction', *Social Science and Medicine* 59: 1995–2001.

Van der Lippe, T. 1997. 'Verdeling van onbetaalde arbeid, 1975–1995', in M. Niphuis-Nell (ed.), *Sociale atlas van de vrouw, Deel 4,Veranderingen in de primaire leefsfeer.* Rijswijk: SCP, pp. 117–57.

Van Dongen, E. 1996. 'De 'native' als vreemdeling. Medisch-antropologisch onderzoek in Nederland', *Medische Antropologie* 8(2): 340–49

Van Rooij, F.B., F. Van Balen and J.M. Hermanns. 2009. 'The experiences of involuntarily childless Turkish immigrants in the Netherlands', *Qualitative Health Research* 19(5): 621–32.

Van Rooij, F. and D. Korfker. 2009. 'Infertile Turkish and Moroccan minority groups in the Netherlands: Patients' views on problems within infertility care', In L. Culley, N. Hudson and F. Van Rooij (eds), *Marginalized Reproduction: Ethnicity, infertility and reproductive technologies.* Routledge, pp. 134–50.

Van Walbeek, R. 1995. *Ongewenst kinderloos. Brieven over een leven zonder kinderen.* Hoogezand: Van Brug.

Verdurmen, J. 1997. 'Keuzes bij onvruchtbaarheid. Besluitvorming bij onvruchtbare paren', Ph.D. dissertation. Amsterdam: University of Amsterdam.

Verhaak, C. 2003. 'Emotional Impact of Unsuccessful Fertility Treatment in Women', Ph.D. dissertation. Nijmegen: Radboud University Nijmegen.

Verhaak, C.M., Smeenk, J. M., Eugster, A., van Minnen, A., Kremer, J. A., and Kraaimaat, F. W. 2001. 'Stress and marital satisfaction among women before and after their first cycle of in vitro fertilization and intracycloplasmic sperm injection', *Fertility and Sterility* 76(3): 521–31.

Verhaak, C.M., Smeenk, J.M.J., Kremer, J.A.M., Braat, D.D.M., and Kraaimaat, F.W. 2002. 'De emotionele belasting van kunstmatige voortplanting: Meer angst en depressie na mislukte eerste behandeling' *Nederlands Tijdschrift voor Geneeskunde* 146(49): 2363–66.

Verhaak, C.M., Smeenk, J.M.J., Van Minnen, A., Kremer, J.A.M., and Kraaimaat, F.W. 2005. 'A longitudinal, prospective study on emotional adjustment before, during and after consecutive fertility treatment cycles', *Human Reproduction* 20(8): 2253–60.

Vermeulen, H.E. 2001. *Een proeve van leven. Praten en beslissen over extreem te vroeg geboren kinderen.* Amsterdam: Aksant.

_____ 2004. 'Dealing with doubt: Making decisions in a neonatal ward in The Netherlands', *Social Science and Medicine* 59: 2071–85.

Williams, L. 1988. '"It is going to work for me": Responses to failure of IVF', *Birth* 15: 153-156.

Woldringh, G.H., Horvers, M., Janssen, A. J. W. M., Reuser, J. J. C. M., de Groot, S. A. F., Steiner, K., and Kremer, J. A. M. 2011a. 'Follow-up of children born after ICSI with epididymal spermatozoa', *Human Reproduction* 26(7): 1759–67.

Woldringh, G.H., Hendriks, J.C., van Klingeren, J., van Buuren, S., Kollée, L.A., Zielhuis, G. A., and Kremer, J.A. et al. 2011b. 'Weight of in vitro fertilization and intracytoplasmic sperm injection singletons in early childhood', *Fertility and Sterility* 95(8): 2775–77.

Zaman, S. 2004. 'Poverty and violence, frustration and inventiveness: Hospital ward life in Bangladesh', *Social Science and Medicine* 59: 2025–36.

Chapter 2

'DUTCH IVF'

LEGISLATION, GUIDELINES AND HEALTH INSURANCE

S ince the introduction of artificial insemination (AI) in the Netherlands at the end of the 1940s, more and more medical interventions and technologies have become available for people who are in need of medically assisted conception. In the 1960s hormonal treatments began, and from the 1970s microsurgery enabled the correction of deviations of the reproductive organs (Van Balen et al. 1995). The first IVF baby in the Netherlands was born in 1983, resulting from a treatment at the Dijkzigt Academic Hospital in Rotterdam. In the following years a number of variations of IVF developed, such as ICSI, PESA, TESE, cryopreservation, egg donation and surrogacy. The mere development of new treatments and technologies, however, did not immediately imply that they were made readily available for all Dutch women and men who might need them (from their own and/or from a medical point of view). The same applies for newly developed technologies to screen embryos before implantation in the uterus (PGD and PGS).

While initially hardly any legislation or guidelines existed to accompany the introduction and use of these new technologies (Kirejczyck 1996), over the course of the years legislation and professional guidelines have been framed, specifically detailing what treatments are available, for whom and under which conditions (Modelreglement Embryowet 2003; see also NVOG 1998b, 1999a and 2000). Current legislation and guidelines regulating reproductive medicine have developed through a complex process of societal, political and professional interactions, debates and negotiations, in which several institutions and actors have played a role. The main actors include the Dutch government, political parties, health insurance companies and professional and patient organizations, while at times various interest and critical groups, such as lesbians, single people, 'women with gynaecological cancer' (Dermout 2001), ethicists, feminists and Christians have also been involved.

These debates are highly dominated by ethical concerns. Across society, people differ in the extent to which they feel medicine should interfere in human life and human reproduction; they have, for example, different views on the status of the foetal person (cf. Rapp 1999). People also have different views on, and engage in disputes about, whether all individuals/couples should be eligible for fertility treatments (raising issues about responsible/fit parenthood and acceptable kinship relations), and about who should make such decisions (addressing issues of patient autonomy versus doctors' authority/responsibility versus state interference) (Ten Have 1995; De Joode and Fauser 2001; Stern et al. 2002, 2003; Bolt et al. 2004). Major ethical concerns are also expressed about the use of ART treatments involving so-called third parties (sperm and egg donors and surrogates), mainly given their potential to exploit those third parties (Braat 2000). Finally, unequal access to ARTs is another issue of concern. Given limited resources for medical services, critics have questioned the spending of public (and personal) resources on high-tech fertility treatments. Questions about whether not being able to have a child should be considered a medical problem or an unful-filled social desire, whether fertility treatments should be considered a basic health right, and whether (all) available fertility treatments should be paid for by governments or health insurance, continue to be debated by politicians at the national level (CvZ 2002).

Medical, ethical, juridical and financial issues were and continue to be debated and negotiated among all these groups. It is beyond the scope of this book to provide a full and detailed historical overview or critical analysis of the processes and debates regarding the introduction and applications of reproductive technologies in the Netherlands. Yet I want to draw attention to some features of these debates and negotiations that have been observed as particular for Dutch society.

First, in a critical analysis of the societal and political debate on IVF in the 1980s, Kirejczyck (1996) underlines the crucial role the NVOG (Dutch professional organization for gynaecologists and obstetricians) and the patient association for people with fertility problems (which is now called Freya) played in these debates, part of which took place in the mass media. At that time the main aim of Freya was lobbying to get IVF treatments paid for by Dutch health insurance. Soon after its creation policymakers recognized this association as the formal representative for people with fertility problems in the Netherlands (ibid.: 121). According to Kirejczyck's analysis, in their lobbying for the expansion of Dutch IVF capacity the patient association emphasized the tremendous suffering of childless people, and argued that this suffering had recently increased – in particular among women who were nearing the age of forty – due to the then-restrictive Dutch policies which withheld IVF treatments from women who otherwise might have been able to have a child of their own. In addition, Kirejczyck observed an 'alliance' between these women and medical specialists who were willing and able to help these women. In the media most medical specialists were portrayed as positive about increasing success rates and were shown to want to calm the public's fears about the risk of 'distortions' in children born from these treatments. Over the years NVOG and Freya continue to be extremely important and influential players at the policy level concerning ARTs and they continue to be involved in activities such as the formulation and evaluation of legislation, subsidiary regulations and insurance schemes.

Secondly, in a recent publication two Dutch ethicists (Dondorp and de Wert 2012) point to a recurrent pattern in the debates and negotiation processes on ARTs, every time a new technological option becomes available. Again and again, they assert, the different actors (groups) take their positions in favour of or against expansion of ARTs and their use, based on the specific principles they adhere to. These principles are (logically) different for each of the different actors (groups) and therefor they will never be able to convince each other. As a result, the authors argue, these principles have never been determinant for decision-making. Agreement can more easily be reached about the conditions under which the ARTs can be applied, including safety and quality criteria. Once these conditions are established, the principal objections do not hold and rejection of the implementation of the technique can no longer be justified. Therefore, they claim, thus far all new reproductive technologies have been accepted. The authors refer to this repetitive pattern of negotiating, debating and finally approving of ARTs in the Netherlands as a 'ritual dance' (ibid.: 5).

In this chapter I will show where this ritual dance has led. I provide an overview of current Dutch ART legislation, professional guidelines and health insurance policy – which I refer to as 'Dutch

IVF' – which constitutes the framework within which ARTs can be offered in the Netherlands. These national policies and guidelines, as we will see repeatedly in this book, affect to a large extent actual treatment practices in Dutch fertility clinics – how infertility care is provided, where it is provided and to whom.

Legislation and Guidelines

Restricting the Number of Licensed Clinics

In the Netherlands, as in many other countries, the government has established regulations and guidelines to regulate the practice of ARTs, including the restriction of clinics which are licensed to carry out IVF and related treatments (Jones and Cohen 2004).[1] IVF and related treatments in the Netherlands can only be carried out in a restricted number of licensed clinics (Ministerie van VWS 1998). These clinics are obliged to follow strict professional guidelines (NVOG 1998a, 1998b, 1999b) and each started IVF cycle has to have a minimum success rate of fifteen per cent. A number of criteria have been formulated to ensure the quality of the performance of these clinics. The Planningsbesluit IVF (1998) emphasizes – next to medical-technical, laboratory and organizational aspects – the importance of giving due attention to providing adequate information and psycho-social support to couples undergoing treatment; to the way embryos are handled; and to the (future) interest of the child. Moreover, clinics are obliged to collaborate in reporting results and in countrywide registration of IVF treatments. Surveillance of the correct application of quality criteria consists of periodic reports and on-site visits. If a clinic does not work to conform to the set regulations, their license may be withdrawn (NVOG 1998a; Jones et al. 2004: S15). In 2015, in the Netherlands, IVF and related treatments are conducted in fourteen licensed clinics (eight academic clinics, five peripheral public clinics, and one private clinic).[2] These licensed clinics are allowed to collaborate with 'satellite' or 'transport' clinics, which are smaller clinics that can only do part of the IVF treatment. Satellite clinics only do hormonal stimulation, and in transport clinics egg retrieval takes place as well (CvZ 2002: 12). The remaining parts of the IVF treatment are carried out at a licensed clinic. On a yearly basis Dutch clinics carry out around 16,000 IVF and related treatments.[3]

Contrary to the explicit regulations for IVF treatments, Dutch clinics do not need a special license to carry out low-tech treatments (like artificial insemination). In principle, all clinics and doctors may perform these treatments, though of course they also have to abide by quality guidelines and legal regulations concerning, for example, the use of gametes and embryos. The NVOG has, for example, stipulated that clinics and laboratories offering these treatments should be opened minimally five, and preferably six or seven days a week for maximal timing of the insemination (NVOG 2000), and patients should be informed of any local logistical limitations of this kind before starting the treatment in a clinic. The exact number of IUI cycles performed in the Netherlands is not known (as no central registration exists), but for 2003 it was estimated at around 28,500 IUI cycles (Steures et al. 2007).

Low Tech Treatments, 'Expectative Policy' and Maximum Two Embryos

Medically assisted conception involves health risks for the woman undergoing the treatment and for the children to be born (NVOG 2001),[4] and in the past decade risk reduction has received more explicit attention than before (see, e.g., Ten Have 1995). NVOG guidelines recommend starting with low-tech treatments (depending on a couple's diagnosis) before heading for more risky – and more burdensome and expensive – IVF treatments (NVOG 1998b, 2000). Moreover, NVOG guidelines suggest encouraging couples, in particular when the woman is still young and depending on a couple's specific diagnosis, to wait a substantial period of time before starting any type of treatment, in the hope that a spontaneous pregnancy occurs (known as an expectative policy) (NVOG 1998b). As the efficiency of IVF and related treatments – compared to not intervening at all or to low-tech treatments – has only been proven for bilateral tubal pathology (and not for other indications mentioned in the 'Indications for IVF' (NVOG 1998b), a nationwide cost-efficiency study has been undertaken. This study showed that the chance of an ongoing pregnancy without any treatment – while on the waiting list for an IVF or ICSI – was below 10 per cent, but might be as high as 25 per cent within one year for selected patient groups (Bouwmans et al. 2008; Eijkemans et al. 2008).

The major health concerns with medically assisted conception are the risks of ovarian hyperstimulation syndrome (OHSS),[5] and multiple pregnancies (twins, triplets or more),[6] which may occur due to ovarian stimulation (in combination with AID, IUI or IVF) or when more than one embryo is transferred in IVF procedures. Intensive monitoring of follicle growth is therefore mandated for all infertility treatments involving hormonal ovarian stimulation.

Guidelines for AID and IUI further stipulate that these treatments should be cancelled if more than three follicles (>16 millimetre) are produced (NVOG 2000). Moreover, as women's experiences of using these hormones may differ widely, guidelines explicitly emphasize taking into account the burden of ovarian stimulation *as perceived* by the individual patient when deciding on insemination with or without ovarian stimulation, and on the type of stimulation.

With regard to IVF and related treatments the Modelreglement Embryo Law recommends transferring a maximum of two embryos per IVF cycle (Modelreglement Embryowet 2003; Braat and Kaandorp 2004), which has been common practice in all Dutch clinics since 2003. Since 2006, the NVOG recommends single embryo transfer (SET) in many cases as being more appropriate than dual embryo transfer (DET), in order to diminish the chance of more risky twins pregnancies (NVOG 2006). From 2013 onwards, only one embryo has been transferred in the first two IVF cycles when women are younger than thirty-eight (Freya 2013b).Worldwide, a trend to transfer fewer embryos has been noticed, though in some countries – as for example in the USA – up to five embryos are still transferred per IVF cycle (Jones and Cohen 2004). On the contrary, in some European countries, for example, Belgium and Sweden, SET is nowadays common practice, in particular for the first treatment cycle (ibid.).[7]

Restricting PESA and TESE (and Cross-Border Reproductive Care)

The introduction of IVF and ICSI – in the Netherlands and elsewhere – without proper scientific assessment of the effectiveness, safety, costs, risks and benefits of these technologies has been strongly criticised (see, e.g., Buitendijk 1995; Ten Have 1995). In 1996 the NVOG and the professional association for clinical embryologists (KLEM) were concerned that ICSI treatments involving micromanipulation of sperm and/or ova, as occurs in PESA and TESE, might imply more risks for the future child than regular ICSI (NVOG 2001). For that reason, the professional organizations fully prohibited the performance of percutaneous or microsurgical epididymal sperm aspiration (PESA/MESA)[8] and testicular sperm extraction (TESE), treatments that are used when the man does not have any sperm in the ejaculate.[9] As a result, until 2000, PESA and TESE were not permitted in the Netherlands, due to uncertainty about risks involved for the offspring. The Netherlands – together with Norway – was one of the few countries in the world that legally restricted the application of PESA and TESE (Heida 2001).

Since 2000, PESA has been permitted and performed in three Dutch clinics – including the Radboud Clinic – as part of a clinical trial (with follow-up of the children). During the period in which the fieldwork for the current study took place, TESE was still completely 'under moratorium' in the Netherlands: animal proofs first had to give clarity about potential risks for the offspring, as sperm that was damaged or not fully ripened might be used in this technique (Heida 2001: 115). Since January 2007 (after the fieldwork period), TESE has also been permitted as part of a clinical trial (Kremer and Visser 2008). As the results of both the clinical trials were positive – both PESA and TESE did not increase the percentage of children born with distortions compared to children born in regular ICSI – the moratorium was ended and treatments can now be offered more widely. Yet a number of quality-control criteria have been set to guarantee that 'this high complex low-volume care will be conducted in IVF-centres with the required expertise' (NVOG 2013: 4).[10]

In the period when TESE was not allowed in the Netherlands, a number of Dutch IVF clinics (not the Radboud Clinic) offered TESE in collaboration with clinics in neighbouring countries (Belgium and Germany), where part of the IVF treatment was done in the Netherlands and part – the actual TESE microsurgery – was done abroad. Two couples participating in this study were taking part in such a bi-country treatment: after they unsuccessfully tried PESA treatment at the Radboud Clinic they decided to visit another Dutch clinic that worked with a German clinic offering TESE. As has been argued elsewhere, restrictions set by national legislation may lead to 'reproductive tourism' or 'cross-border reproductive care'.[11] Dutch couples were found to travel to Belgium for several sorts of fertility treatments – which change over time and reflect policy developments and treatment capacity in the Netherlands – including couples in need of ICSI, women over forty years, women who had already received three reimbursed cycles, couples undergoing PESA and TESE, and those in need of donor semen and PGD (Pennings et al. 2009).[12]

Access to ARTs: Medical and Non-medical Contraindications

The Modelreglement Embryowet 2003 and NVOG guidelines formulated a series of medical indications and contraindications for IVF treatments (see NVOG 1998b). Medical contraindications for IVF included being HIV positive, and – although not formulated in guidelines – being a couple who had an increased chance of having a child with serious congenital defects (Bolt et al. 2004; Hunfeld et al. 2004). At the time of fieldwork, the contraindication for HIV+ patients only applied to IVF-ICSI treatments.[13]

Further, IVF – initially – was not recommended for women of forty-one years or older (as this was rarely found to be success-ful), though this was not formulated as a hard condition (NVOG 1998b). In 2000, 14.8 per cent of all IVF and ICSI treatments in the Netherlands were performed for women of forty years and older, a percentage similar to that found on a worldwide scale (Adamson et al. 2006). More recently, as the 'ovarian age' of women can now be better predicted individually, it is recommended that the maximum age of women using IVF should be individualized (Bansci et al. 2002). In 2010 NVOG advised that IVF after the age of forty-one should be assessed individually and would depend on the woman's ovarian reserve (NVOG 2010a).

In the Netherlands, psycho-social contraindications for IVF treat-ment, which refer to the welfare of the child, include the situation that a woman or her partner has formerly maltreated or neglected her/his child(ren), or when the woman is psychologically unstable (Bolt et al. 2004). It is emphasized, however, that the medical doctor should be very cautious and avoid subjective judgments in the application of psycho-social contraindications. To support clinic staff decision-making in cases of ethically sensitive requests for medical assisted reproduction, NVOG – on the request of the Dutch Ministry of Health – has composed a so-called 'model protocol for possible moral contraindications' (NVOG 2010b).

Further, neither marriage nor being in a stable relationship are formal requirements for eligibility for IVF (or for any other infer-tility treatment), and in principle single and lesbian women have equal access to these treatments (Jones and Cohen 2004) (see page 60 for a discussion of current practice). An overview of ART leg-islation worldwide shows that marriage is also not a requirement in other Western countries, though some (e.g., France, Denmark, Italy, Norway, Portugal and Switzerland) request a stable relation-ship. Lesbian and single women can only be treated in a limited number of (mainly Western) countries (e.g., Belgium, Finland and the United Kingdom) (Jones and Cohen 2004: S19). In Chapter 8, I shall discuss how the Radboud Clinic dealt in practice with these medical and non-medical contraindications for treatment.

The Use of Stored Sperm, Ova and Embryos

When medically assisted conception takes place, ova, sperm or embryos may be left over. Nowadays, sperm, ova and embryos can be frozen for later use, such as for a further attempt to conceive a child (at the time of fieldwork mature ova could not yet be safely frozen).[14] Major advantages of cryopreservation of spare embryos are that it allows the transfer of fewer embryos per cycle and therefore diminishes the risk of multiple pregnancies. It also diminishes the risk of OHSS, as a so-called fresh transfer can be cancelled if indications of a threatening OHSS are present (Jones and Cohen 2004: S23). Cryopreservation of embryos is common practice in all Dutch fertility clinics. Remaining materials, however, are not always used by the men and women who provided them. The Embryowet stipulates the conditions under which the Dutch government permits the use of human gametes and embryos, and regulates the use of remaining materials (Modelreglement Embryowet 2003).[15] Theoretically, frozen gametes and the cryopreservation of embryos enables one partner to create offspring after the other partner's death.[16] Dutch law allows post mortal use of stored sperm or embryos, under the condition that the partner who passed away has given explicit permission for its use before he died. In addition, the surviving partner has to undergo an obligatory two-year period for reflection, and intensive psychotherapeutic counselling has to be part of the decision-making process (Modelreglement Embryowet 2003; Braat and Kaandorp 2004).[17] In practice, four IVF clinics in the Netherlands allow (future) widows to make use of medically assisted conception with the stored sperms of their deceased or terminally ill husbands (Bolt et al. 2004; Hunfeld et al. 2004). Bolt et al. found that doctors' considerations for not offering treatment to (future) widows included the well-being of the child (being/becoming a half orphan at a very young age), and the well-being of the would-be parent(s) (the doctors thought that the couples could better spend their time saying a proper farewell than undergoing treatment, and that the process of IVF treatment would hinder a widow's mourning process). In the Radboud Clinic, post mortal use of sperms and embryos is not allowed (see Chapter 8).

The Embryowet also stipulates that sperm, ova and embryos that will no longer be used for a pregnancy of the couple that provided them may be handed over to others, either to achieve a pregnancy (i.e., third party involvement in conception), for medical treatment or for certain types of scientific research. In all cases, the condition is that the woman and man who supplied the materials should explicitly agree to its further use (Modelreglement Embryowet 2003). The Embryowet explicitly forbids creating embryos for the sake of scientific research, as well as for cloning.

Third Party Involvement in Conception: Donors and Surrogacy

The use of donor sperms and eggs in fertility treatments opens possibilities for a heterosexual couple to conceive a child that is genetically related to only one of them.[18] It also enables single women and
lesbian couples to conceive. In 2000 the Dutch Minister of Health
– in line with the Law on Equal Treatment – stated that lesbian
and single women should have the same access to AI and IVF with
donor semen as heterosexual couples (Borst 2000). In practice,
however, while eleven of the thirteen licensed IVF clinics offer IVF
treatment to lesbian couples, only four clinics offer this treatment to
single women (Bolt et al. 2004). Some clinics refuse to treat single
women and/or lesbian couples because they argue that this may
negatively impact on the psycho-social well-being of the child (Bolt
et al. 2004: 29).[19] It is estimated that on a yearly basis around 1,100
heterosexual couples, 250 lesbian couples and 100 single women in
the Netherlands request donor semen; while annually an estimated
700 children are conceived by donor semen (Janssens et al. 2006).

The preferred status of the gamete donor – anonymous versus
identifiable – has been a highly debated issue in the Netherlands,
as well as in many countries worldwide (Heida 2001: 113; Jones
and Cohen 2004; Janssens et al. 2006). Until 2004 women and
men who intended to use donor semen for any type of fertility
treatment could choose either an anonymous or a known donor.
In practice, one third of the inseminations took place with sperm
of a known donor, and two-thirds with sperm of an anonymous
donor. Since 2004 a new law regarding the anonymity of donors in
the case of artificial fertilization (Wet Donorgegevens Kunstmatige
Bevruchting) has been accepted. This law prevents anonymous
donation of sperm, ova or embryos. At the age of twelve, children
that have been conceived with donor material can avail themselves
of data that do not allow the donor to be identified, such as medical
and other characteristics, and from sixteen years onwards they also
have the opportunity to access identifying data, as long as the donor
does not pose any objection (and – of course – only in cases where
the child knows s/he is conceived by donor gametes). In cases where
the donor objects, the child can only get access to the data if their
interests weigh heavier than the donor's interests, for example if a
child seriously suffers from the anonymity.[20] It has been observed
that the abolition of donor anonymity has had an enormous impact
on the availability of donor sperm:[21] in the period when this was
still under debate, and being covered in the media, the number of

donors had already decreased by more than seventy per cent, and the number of semen banks has been halved from twenty-one in 1990 to twelve in 2005 (Janssens et al. 2006).

When comparing Dutch legislation regarding semen donation with that of other Western countries, it is evident that different countries have taken completely different positions: a number of countries also explicitly forbid the use of anonymous donors (e.g., Sweden, the United Kingdom and Switzerland), while other countries allow or even require it (e.g., France, Norway and Belgium) (Janssens et al. 2006).[22]

The use of donated ova is – medically and technically – more complicated than the use of donor semen because it involves more medical interventions, both for the acceptor as well as for the donor (Braat 2000). Initially, most of the egg donation in the Netherlands was anonymous: women who had undergone IVF treatment themselves and produced many eggs (>15) were asked if they would be prepared to donate four of their eggs to somebody else. With the improved possibilities for conserving embryos through cryopreservation, according to Braat (2000), all couples in IVF treatment now have all their ova fertilized and their embryos – if they are of good quality – frozen. This implies that IVF patients no longer donate their ova; thus at present the only way to make use of egg donation is by bringing your own donor. The donor – often a friend or a sister of the potential mother-to-be – has to undergo the first part of an IVF treatment, namely the hormonal stimulation and ova pick-up, which implies that the female donor is exposed to the same risks as a woman in a normal IVF procedure (see Chapter 5 about risks). Braat (2000) estimated that – at that time – egg donation in the Netherlands took place around 150 to 200 times a year.

The Embryo Law also regulates egg donation: the protocol defines the medical indications for egg donation (such as premature ovarian failure), the minimum and maximum age of the donating woman (respectively eighteen[23] and forty years), the maximum age of the accepting woman (forty-five years) and strictly forbids commercial egg donation (Modelreglement Embryowet 2003). Currently (2015), eight Dutch clinics offer the option of egg donation. In most of these clinics would-be parents have to bring their own egg donor; in 2012 two clinics started recruiting egg donors for their own 'egg banks' (yet huge waiting lists exist). One other clinic introduced the system of 'cooperative' or fair reciprocity' (Pennings 2005): couples coming for egg donation are – on a voluntary basis – being asked to donate sperm to help other couples who are in need of donated sperm; and the other way round, couples that come for donor insemination are being asked to donate eggs (Freya 2013a).[24] This method has led to a huge ethical debate in the Dutch media and within NVOG. To date NVOG does not approve the system of 'fair reciprocity', as there are no procedural guarantees that the people involved can take a deliberate and independent decision (NVOG 2011). The possibility of egg freezing for non-medical reasons (which has been allowed in the Netherlands since 2011), enabling women to prolong the possibility of conceiving with their own genetic material, can be expected to diminish the demand for egg donation (De Groot et al. 2013).

Surrogacy, the situation where a woman becomes pregnant with a child that is meant to grow up with another couple, is another way to involve a third party in conception. Surrogacy is an option if the wish-mother does not have a (functioning) uterus (often resulting from gynaecological cancer), or if a pregnancy might be life threatening for her. Theoretically, it can also be an option for two men who want to fulfil their wish for a child, using the sperm of one partner (Heida 2001), an option that is more and more pursued by Dutch homosexual couples (Bos and Van Gelderen 2010).

Two types of treatment are available to achieve surrogacy, referred to as gestational (high-tech) and traditional (low-tech) surrogacy. The gestational option involves IVF treatment, where the wish-mother provides the ova that are fertilized with the sperm of her own partner, and subsequently one or two embryos are implanted in the 'surrogate' woman's uterus. In the traditional variation, the 'surrogate' woman becomes pregnant, either through coitus or self-insemination (both not involving any clinical intervention) or through artificial insemination using the sperm of the wish-father. Thus, in the gestational variation the child is the genetic off-spring of both the would-be parents, and in the traditional variation the wish-father is the genetic father and the 'surrogate' woman is the genetic mother. In both cases – according to Dutch law – the 'surrogate' mother is the legal mother, as the woman who delivers a child is always the legal mother (and if she is married her husband is the legal father). Thus, while the wish-father is the genetic father in both situations, in neither of the two variations is he the legal father (Heida 2001).

Since 1997 gestational surrogacy has been permitted in the Netherlands as long as it is non-commercial, and (preferably) it should be offered as part of (clinical) research (Dermout 2001). Following the decision by the Ministry of Health to allow non-commercial surrogacy, NVOG has formulated guidelines for this type of treatment (NVOG 1999). According to this guideline surrogacy should be considered an *ultimum remedium*; the surrogate mother has to have one or more children herself and she should not be older than forty-four years; she may receive a compensation for the costs involved in the treatment and the pregnancy, but this compensation should not be a substantial amount of money, as commercial surrogacy is strictly forbidden. Counselling of all partners involved is an obligatory part of the gestational surrogacy procedures. Before starting the medical procedures the surrogate mother and the would-be parents have to settle a contract in which they, among other things, agree that the surrogate mother resigns the child immediately after its birth. Legally, however, this agreement is void, and it is impossible for any of the partners in the contract to force its compliance. After the birth of a child conceived by surrogacy, a number of legal procedures have to be accomplished through which the would-be parents first foster the child. After one year of actually caring for the child the would-be parents may start adoption procedures (Dermout 2001: 16).[25]

In practice, gestational surrogacy has mainly been practiced in the Netherlands as part of a study that – predominantly – took place in one fertility clinic in the Netherlands (in Voorburg), where twenty-two couples were treated (Dermout 2001). In most cases a sister or sister-in-law acted as the 'surrogate' mother. In 2004, the existing surrogacy programme stopped due to lack of financial means to cover the extra expenses for the intensive screening and counselling of the couples (De Visser 2006). In 2006, the clinic for reproductive medicine of the Free University in Amsterdam started a new programme enabling surrogacy; they are treating approximately ten couples a year (Boele-Woelki et al. 2011).

Pre-Implantation Genetic Diagnosis and Screening (PGD and PGS)

Over the last decades two methods for genetically screening embryos have been developed, namely pre-implantation genetic diagnosis (PGD) and pre-implantation genetic screening (PGS). These two techniques serve different ends, and – at the time of the fieldwork – both were only permitted in the Netherlands as part of clinical trials, which have to be approved by the central medical-ethical committee (CCMO). Neither of these screening methods were conducted at the Radboud Clinic, though clinic staff sometimes referred their patients to a clinic where PGD was conducted.

PGD is a diagnostic method used to detect a genetic defect in the embryo before it is transferred into the woman's uterus

(Gezondheidsraad 2003). PGD is not an infertility treatment, though IVF or ICSI are a necessary part of the PGD procedure. Couples at risk of having a child with certain known genetic defects can have their embryos screened, and the woman undergoes all steps of a 'normal' IVF treatment (although these couples do not have fertility problems). On the third day after the fertilization of the ova with the semen in the lab – at which point the embryo consists of about six to eight cells – one or two of the cells of the embryo are biopsied and their genetic constitution examined. In the case of sex-bound genetic defects, the sex of the pre-embryos is defined and only embryos of the sex that cannot be affected with the particular disease are implanted. For a restricted number of genetic diseases (such as cystic fibrosis) a more specific test can be done. Only unaffected embryos will be transferred to the woman; the affected embryos are 'discarded'. A PGD procedure examines only the defect for which an increased risk in one or both partners is known.

A potential advantage of PGD above prenatal diagnosis (PND), like amniocentesis or chorionic villus sampling, is that the PND tests take place *after* the woman has become pregnant.[26] With PGD, embryos are tested *before* implantation, and therefore – in principal – an induced abortion can be avoided. Nevertheless, as the PGD procedure is relatively new, couples are still offered PND in case a pregnancy evolves. Though this far children conceived after PGD do not seem to have more defects than children born after 'normal' IVF, researchers stress the importance of long-term follow-up to allow for more certainty in this regard (De Wert 2003: 14).

Until 2007 PGD was only conducted in the Netherlands in one academic hospital (University of Maastricht), as part of a clinical trial. In 2007 'transport' PGD was initiated, in which three academic medical centres started to collaborate with the Maastricht Academic Hospital in 'PGD-Nederland'.[27] It has been observed that the Netherlands has a restricted attitude towards PGD (Pennings et al. 2009). In 2008, for example, there was an emotional public debate on PGD for genetic breast cancer (BRCA). As said before, the limited availability of PGD is one of the reasons that Dutch couples travel to Belgium for treatment.

In PGS, the embryo is also screened before it is implanted into the woman's uterus. Yet, in contrast to PGD, the aim of PGS is to increase the success rate of IVF treatments (Mastenbroek et al. 2007). IVF success rates decrease substantially when women get older: among women over thirty-five years, this decrease might be caused by an incorrect constitution of the hereditary genetic material (there might be too few or too many chromosomes). PGS, in combination with IVF, permits the definition of part of the genetic make-up of an embryo. Three days after fertilization, one cell of each embryo is biopsied and examined, and only those embryos that are shown to have a normal number of chromosomes are transferred. Worldwide this type of screening has taken place for a number of years. Recently, a randomised controlled study – conducted by a Dutch clinic – showed that PGS declined IVF success rates rather than increased them (Mastenbroek et al. 2007) and for this reason PGS is no longer offered in the Netherlands.

Health Insurance Coverage

In principle, it is the availability and legal allowance of ARTs which enable or limit their use or non-use in the Netherlands. Its actual usage, however, is further determined by the extent to which these treatments are covered by health insurance. This coverage has changed over time, and continues to do so. In the course of the field-work (2003–6) some major changes took place in the Netherlands with regard to the health insurance system in general, and the financing of fertility treatments in particular.

Until January 2004 public health insurance (Ziekenfonds) – accessible for people up to a certain maximum income[28] – paid for all fertility treatments, including most of the medication used and three complete IVF treatments.[29] After a pregnancy of twelve weeks, or after the birth of a child, a further three treatment cycles would be paid for. Private health insurance policies also covered most low-tech fertility treatments and medications, though IVF and related treatments were generally not covered by the 'standard packages'; to have the expenses for IVF covered, people needed additional insurance. The conditions for reimbursement by private insurance were generally stricter than those of the Ziekenfonds: in some instances people had to pay a financial contribution for each treatment or a maximum of three treatments were covered (instead of three IVF treatments per pregnancy) (Freya 2002).

These regulations changed substantially in January 2004, as part of new Dutch political thinking that people ought to bear more of their 'own responsibility', in combination with the budgetary urge to cut down expenses in healthcare. From then onwards all medication used in low-tech treatments, such as IUI and hormonal stimulation, plus the first IVF treatment (including medication) had to be paid for by patients themselves. A second and third IVF treatment – including the medication – would continue to be covered by health insurance. This measure applied for both the Ziekenfonds and private insurance policies. With both types of insurance, people could take additional insurance, which (partly) covered low-tech fertility medications and the first IVF treatment as well. In 2005, the expenses of one IVF cycle (excluding medication) in the Netherlands varied from approximately 1,900 to 2,300 Euros (Raad voor de Volksgezondheid in Zorg 2005).[30]

The deterioration of insurance coverage for fertility treatments raised concern and resistance among professional and patient organizations. Representatives of both organizations – NVOG and Freya – actively lobbied to convince policy makers to withdraw this measure, relying on two major arguments, one medical and one more political. Firstly, they argued, if people had to pay for the treatments themselves they would be inclined to maximize their success rates, and therefore, for example, would want to go for high-tech treatments even if low-tech treatments were still an option, would opt for more intensive ovarian stimulation or for the transfer of more embryos – all of which might lead to increasing medical risks, including a higher chance of multiple pregnancies. Secondly, the organizations claimed that such measures would lead to unacceptable inequity in the Dutch healthcare system, as people who were unable to pay for a first round of IVF treatment would not have access to any IVF treatment at all, and as such would be denied the right to proper medically assisted conception. When presenting the IVF results for 2004, NVOG underlined that for the first time the annual number of IVF treatments in the Netherlands had decreased by 3 per cent. NVOG suggested that this decline was related to the cut-backs in coverage of IVF treatments, and in particular migrants and people with low incomes were thought to be restricted in their use of these treatments (NVOG 2005).

The cut-backs on medications for fertility treatments had another side effect – the sudden expansion of a 'black market' of leftover hormonal medicines. As the exact amount of hormonal medicines to be used in fertility treatments cannot be precisely defined when starting the treatment, people often have their medicines prescribed in surplus. From the moment people had to pay for their medications, these leftover medicines were being actively offered – for sale and for free – and demanded. Both Freya and medical professionals objected to this practice and pointed to the risks of such an uncontrolled market (see Freya 2004).

While the struggle over the coverage of fertility treatments was still ongoing, the health insurance system in the Netherlands underwent a drastic change in 2006 when the division between the Ziekenfonds and private insurance was abolished. From then onwards, all Dutch inhabitants had to hold an obligatory basic health insurance, which they could expand with additional insurance. The basic insurance covered the same expenses for fertility treatments as described above (i.e., excluding the expenses for medication in low-tech fertility treatments and excluding the first IVF treatment). When taking additional insurance, (part of) these latter expenses could be covered.

As the coverage of fertility treatments did not improve with the introduction of the new health insurance system, professional and patient organizations (NVOG and Freya respectively) continued to be dissatisfied and went on lobbying for change. In June 2006 this lobbying proved to be somewhat effective: the Dutch Minister of Health decided that from January 2007 onwards three IVF treatments would be covered by the basic health insurance, though the medication for low-tech treatments continued to be excluded from the insurance package. This might, as for example Pennings and Ombelet (2007) argued, push people to prefer to start with high-tech treatments – which are more burdensome and involve more risks – instead of first trying low-tech treatments. In January 2013 another change was introduced to health insurance coverage: now IVF is covered until the woman is forty-three years old (and cryopreservation until forty-five); and costs for low-tech treatments (ovulation induction and IUI) are fully covered (Freya 2013).[31]

Couples participating in this study were thus confronted with changes in health insurance policies – and the consequent confusions – over the course of their treatment trajectories. In Chapter 4 we will see how financial matters, and in particular the health insurance regulation to pay for three IVF treatments, affected their views on (further) treatment.

Conclusion

This overview of contemporary Dutch ART policy shows, on the one hand, its aims to enable the use of (high quality) IVF and related technologies to its citizens in need of assisted reproduction: it requests clinics to be transparent about risks and success rates, and it has made IVF and related treatments accessible and affordable for all (up to three IVF treatments 'per child'), including for lesbian and single women, though in practice – given the limited availability of donor sperm – this does not always work out. On the other hand, a number of strict boundaries are set at the supply side, based on ethical, medical-technical, cost-efficiency and juridical considerations, which have implications for the way people with fertility problems can and do make use of these technologies.

First, these restrictions include limiting the number of clinics that are licensed to offer treatments and requiring these clinics to adhere to strict quality criteria and other requirements. This restricts the uncontrolled growth of private fertility clinics as is currently taking place in many countries worldwide (e.g., in the USA, in the Middle East and India), where clinic success rates may be used for marketing purposes and where doctors' incomes may directly depend on the number of treatments their centre performs (see, e.g., Becker and Nachtigall 1994: 515). Under such circumstances, the wish to reach large numbers of patients and to make a profit may steer clinical practices more than the intention to provide safe and high quality treatments to people with fertility problems.

Second, not all technically possible treatments, such as PESA, TESE, PGS and PGD, have readily been made available and/or allowed in the Netherlands based on their effectiveness – and fairly strict criteria are set on their use. This is in sharp contrast to the early introduction of 'normal' IVF and ICSI in the Netherlands, practices that have been strongly criticised.

Third, recently introduced legislation stipulates – and clearly restricts – the conditions under which the Dutch government permits the use of human gametes and embryos, and regulates the use of (remaining) materials for self and others (Modelrelglement Embryowet 2003).

Fourth, in the case of assumed medical contraindications for medically assisted procreation, additional examinations are indicated and the attending doctor has the right to withhold treatment when s/he thinks the outcome of these examination(s) is worrisome (Gezondheidsraad 1997). Doctors also have the right to withhold treatment on grounds of psycho-social contraindications. In Chapter 8 we will see how staff members at the Radboud Clinic dealt with these regulations when confronted with couples whose medical or psycho-social situation concerned them.

Fifth, NVOG has recommended a number of medical measures aiming to increase cost-efficiency and to decrease risks and the burden of treatment for the women involved. These measures include encouraging couples to wait a substantial period of time before starting any type of fertility treatment; promoting single embryo transfer instead of transferring two or more embryos; starting with low-tech fertility treatments before initiating high-tech treatments (though strangely enough, as has been discussed, until recently health insurance policy did *not* allow for reimbursement of the hormonal medicines used in low-tech fertility treatments).[32] In a way these NVOG recommendations can be considered to be de-medicalizing, as they intend to postpone the actual medicalization of fertility problems in some cases or diminish the intensity of medicalization. Some other (in particular Western) countries also have restrictive guidelines, policies or legislation on part of the above-mentioned issues and treatments (see Jones and Cohen 2004; Janssens et al. 2006). In particular the trend to transfer fewer embryos has been noticed in various countries, though in some countries – as for example in the USA – up to five embryos are still transferred per IVF cycle (Jones and Cohen 2004). Yet, overall, the Netherlands is internationally known for its restrictive ART policy.[33]

Finally, the fact that Dutch health insurance pays for up to three IVF treatments (per child born) restricts the number of IVF treatments couples undergo, as we will see later in this book. Thus, while on the one hand the current health insurance policy to pay for three IVF treatments is enabling, on the other it also sets boundaries to its use.

Dutch legislation and professional guidelines address some of the issues that were debated in the period when IVF was first introduced (see Van Balen and Inhorn 2002: 14). In particular, the increased transparency about potential risks and limited success rates, the measures to postpone or diminish the intensity of medicalization, and the fact that a number of new reproductive technologies are now introduced with proper clinical trials can be considered important steps in reducing the risks and burden for women and/or children born from these treatments. How these policies actually affect clinical practices and couples' experiences will be discussed in the chapters that follow.

Notes

1. Jones and Cohen (2004) provide an overview of ART legislation and guidelines including forty-seven countries worldwide, which shows that twenty-six (including most Western) countries do have some form

of ART legislation. Ireland, Portugal, Poland, and the USA, however, only have professional guidelines for ARTs (and no legislation), and Canada has neither legislation nor guidelines. Of the twenty-six countries with ART legislation mentioned in the overview, almost all – with the exception of four countries – have licensing bodies as well. These four exceptions include two European countries (Denmark and Greece).

2. See: www.zorgkaartnederland.nl/ivf-kliniek. At the time of fieldwork fourteen clinics were licensed to offer the full IVF cycle.

3. See statistical information for all registered clinics (www.lirinfo.nl). At the time of fieldwork the total number of annual treatments was around fifteen thousand.

4. For a full discussion of risks involved see Chapter 5.

5. Symptoms of OHSS syndrome may include ovarian enlargement, gastrointestinal symptoms, abdominal distension and weight gain. Severe cases can be complicated with cardiovascular, pulmonary, and electronic disturbances, which can require hospitalization and in some documented cases have even led to death (Thompson 2005: 312).

6. Risks of multiple pregnancies include premature birth (which may lead to retarded development); in addition the chance of twins dying is ten times higher compared to singletons.

7. If the criteria for the number of embryos to transfer are respected, the new Belgium legislation allows for payment of a maximum of six IVF cycles (Jones and Cohen 2004: S16).

8. Further referred to as PESA.

9. PESA refers to the treatment in which sperm cells are directly retrieved from the epididymis, and TESE involves the retrieval of sperm cells from the testicles.

10. One of these quality requirements is that a clinic performs a minimum number of PESA and TESE treatments per year (NVOG 2013).

11. See, e.g., Inhorn and Birenbaum-Carmeli 2008; and Special Issue on cross border reproductive care in Reproductive BioMedicine Online (Inhorn and Gürtin 2011).

12. In total 1,763 Dutch couples/women used ARTs in Belgium in the period from 2005–7, which constituted 29 per cent of all foreign ART users in that period (Pennings et al. 2009).

13. Personal information Prof. Dr J. Kremer.

14. Lately, the technology of fast freezing of ova (ova vitrification) has been further developed and is now also allowed and used in several Dutch clinics, both for so-called medical reasons (for example in cases of early menopause or cancer treatments) and for non-medical reasons (for women who wish to postpone their pregnancy, often because they do not yet have a partner with whom they want to conceive a child) (De Groot et al. 2013).

15. The Embryowet (2002) obliges institutions who are involved in the creation of embryos out of the human body to develop a protocol with regard to acts involving human gametes and embryos. The Modelreglement Embryowet (2003) serves as a guideline for the protocols to be developed by the institutions. The commission developing the Modelreglement consisted of representatives of NVOG and other professionals and professional organizations in this area. The patient organization Freya has also commented on a draft version of the Modelreglement.

16. Theoretically, it is also possible that if the woman has died one or more embryos can be transferred to the uterus of a surrogate mother (gestational surrogacy – see below) on behalf of the surviving man. As limited experience exists with both gestational surrogacy and with post mortal reproduction, the commission formulating the *Modelreglement* was not in favour of this option (Modelreglement Embryowet 2003: 43).

17. Worldwide criteria for post mortal use of sperms and/or embryos differ. In Spain, for example, the time period for use of the material is set at six months after the death of the partner, and in Israel one year after the storage (and only after the explicit permission of the court) (Jones and Cohen 2004: S23).

18. It should be noted that third party donations did not take place at the Radboud Clinic during the period when the fieldwork took place. If couples at the Radboud Clinic opted for any form of third party involvement in conception, they had to visit another clinic. To my knowledge none of the participants in my study opted for this.

19. A literature study showed that the psycho-social development of children growing up with lesbian couples does not differ from that of children growing up with heterosexual parents. Due to a lack of studies nothing was said about the development of *older* children growing up with lesbian parents, or about the development of children growing up with singles (Bolt et al. 2004: 30). The report of the Commission for Equal Treatment concluded that study results about the psychological development of children in single parent families is not unequivocally clear, and that therefore 'not treating' could be justified, based on the principle of 'not treating in case of doubts' (Veerman 2000).

20. This will be decided by the Stichting Donorgegevens Nederland (Foundation Donor Data Netherlands).

21. Recent data from England, though, showed that the donor being identifiable did not negatively affect the availability of donor semen. (Prof. Dr D. Braat – personal information).

22. This is a point that needs further research, as such different ART policies reflect the particular 'local moral worlds' of the religion and culture in which they are embedded (Kleinman 1995; Inhorn and Birenbaum-Carmelli 2008). Interestingly, the ethicist Guido Pennings remarked

that most northern European countries forbid anonymous gamete
donation, while several southern European countries prescribe anonymous donation. He hypothesizes that in northern European countries
genetic connections seem to be more valued (Pennings, quoted in Van
der Burg 2010: 149).

23. However, the Commission developing the Modelreglement advised
clinics to be reticent regarding ova donors younger than thirty years.

24. This clinic performs around 1,500 IVF cycles a year, of which circa 40
per cent include egg donation (Van der Burg 2010).

25. Initially, the wish-parents could only adopt their child after having fos-
tered it for a period of four years; as a result of the study accompanying
the introduction of gestational surrogacy in the Netherlands this period
of four years was reduced to one year.

26. Whether one sees this as an advantage or not has to do with the
moral status one attaches to a pre-embryo and a foetus respectively.
Moreover, PGD is heavily criticised for a number of reasons, such as
its implications for the societal position of handicapped people (the
eugenic argument) and concerns about a 'slippery slope' in the direction of undesired forms of embryo selection (e.g., on sex for other than
medical grounds or to create the 'perfect child') (De Wert 2003). A full
discussion of these criticisms is beyond the scope of this chapter. For
an in-depth – anthropological – discussion of the use of PGD see *Born
and Made*, an ethnography about PGD in the United Kingdom (Franklin
and Roberts 2006).

27. For more information see: www.pgdnederland.nl.

28. In 2002 the maximum gross yearly income that permitted inclusion in
the Ziekenfonds was 30,700 Euros.

29. Though these treatments were covered by the Ziekenfonds, they were
not a regular part of insurance, but depended on a special subsidiary
regulation.

30. This is substantially less than the costs involved for one IVF cycle in
the USA. A study of 266 American IVF centres found that the average
charge for an IVF cycle in 1993 was 6,233 USD (this amount was
adjusted for the fact that some cycles were never completed).

31. Another recent change is that under the age of thirty-eight only one
embryo is transferred in the first two IVF cycle: retrieved 5 March 2015
from http://www.nvog.nl/voorlichting/Nieuws-+en+persberichten/
Persbericht.

32. The applicability of these guidelines depends on couples' specific diagnosis and situation.

33. Personal information Prof. Dr D. Braat and Prof. Dr J. Kremer. Guido
Penning (a Belgium ethicist in this field) also pointed to the pioneering
role of the Netherlands in diminishing the risks and stress for women
undergoing IVF by giving less hormones (quoted in Van der Burg 2010:
109).

References

Adamson, G., J. de Mouzon, P. Lancaster, K.G. Nygren, E. Sullivan, F. Zegers-Hochschild and International Committee for Monitoring Assisted Reproductive Technology. (2006. 'World collaborative report on in vitro fertilization', *Fertility and Sterility* 85(6): 1586–622.

Bansci L.F., F.J. Broekmans, M.J. Eijkemans, F.H. de Jong, J.D.F. Habbema, and E.R. te Velde. 2002. 'Predictors of poor ovarian response in in vitro fertilization: A prospective study comparing basal markers of ovarian reserve', *Fertility and Sterility* 77(2): 328–36.

Becker G. and R.D. Nachtigall. 1994. "Born to be a mother': The cultural construction of risk in infertility treatment in the U.S.', *Social Science and Medicine* 39(4): 507–18.

Boele-Woelki, K., I. Curry-Sumner, W. Schrama and M. Vonk. 2011. *Draagmoederschap en illegale opneming van kinderen.* Utrecht: Universiteit Utrecht-Molengraaff Instituut voor Privaatrecht.

Bolt, L.L.E., M.A.J.M. Buijsen and J.A.M. Hunfeld. 2004. *Morele contra-indicaties voor ouderschap? Een psychologisch, ethisch en juridisch onderzoek naar de selectie van hulpvragers voor een IVF-behandeling.* Ethiek en Beleid NWO. Budel: Uitgeverij Damon.

Borst, E. 2000. *Standpunt op oordeel CGB inzake toelatingsbeleid IVF-klinieken.* Brief van Minister van VWS aan de Commissie Gelijke Behandeling, 10 Februarie 2000. The Hague: Ministerie van VWS.

Bos, H. and L. Van Gelderen. 2010. 'Homo en lesbisch ouderschap in Nederland', in S. Keuzenkamp (ed.), *Steeds gewoner, nooit gewoon: Acceptatie van homoseksualiteit in Nederland.* The Hague: Sociaal en Cultureel Planbureau, pp. 104–18.

Bouwmans, C.A., Lintsen, B.M., Eijkemans, M.J., Habbema, J.D.F., Braat, D.D., and Hakkaart, L. 2008. 'A detailed cost analysis of in vitro fertilization and intracytoplasmic sperm injection treatment', *Fertility and sterility*, 89(2): 331–341.

Braat, D.D.M. 2000. 'Donor-eicellen: Wanneer en bij wie?', in W.C.M. Weijmar-Schultz (ed.), *Fertiliteit en ethiek, een kind tot (w)elke prijs?* Symposium WPOG, 10 November 2000. Groningen: Instituut Wenckebach.

Braat, D.D.M. and C.J.E. Kaandorp. 2004. 'Modelreglement Embryowet.', *Nederlands Tijdschrift voor Geneeskunde* 148: 1030–33.

Buitendijk, S.E. 1995. 'Evidence-based in-vitro fertilisation', *The Lancet* 346: 901.

CvZ (College voor Zorgverzekeraars). 2002. *IVF/ICSI: Aanbevelingen voor wijziging van de regeling op basis van de resultaten van effect- en evaluatieonderzoek.* Amstelveen: College voor Zorgverzekeringen.

De Groot, M., E.A.F. Dancet, S.Repping, D. Stoop, M. Goddijn, F. Van der Veen and T. Gerrits, T. 2013. 'Abstract: The voice of Dutch women with anticipated gamete exhaustion who consider oocyte freezing to increase their chances on shared parenthood', *Human Reproduction* 28: 66.

De Joode, S. and B. Fauser. 2001. 'Keuzes, verantwoordelijkheden en dilemma's van een gynaecoloog', in S. De Joode (ed.), *Zwanger van de kinderwens: Visies, feiten en vragen over voortplantingstechnologie*. The Hague: Rathenau Instituut, pp. 84–102.

Dermout, S.M. 2001. 'De eerste logeerpartij: Hoogtechnologisch draagmoederschap in Nederland'. Ph.D. dissertation. Groningen: Rijksuniversiteit Groningen.

De Visser, E. 2006. 'VU begint centrum voor draagmoeders.', *Volkskrant* 6 April.

Dondorp W, and G. de Wert. 2012. Reageerbuisdebat; over de maakbaarheid van de voortplanting. Den Haag: ZonMw. Retrieved 23 March 2016 from www.zonmw.nl.

Eijkemans, M.J.C., A.M.E. Lintsen, C.C. Hunault, C.A.M. Bouwmans, L. Hakkaart, D.D.M. Braat and J.D.F. Habbema. 2008. 'Pregnancy chances on an IVF/ICSI waiting list: A national prospective cohort study', *Human Reproduction* 23: 1627–32.

Franklin, S. and C. Roberts. 2006. *Born and Made: An ethnography of preimplantation genetic diagnosis*. Princeton: Princeton University Press.

Freya. 2002. *Brochure nr. 14. Vergoeding van vruchtbaarheidsbehandelingen*. Retrieved 1 March 2015 from www.freya.nl.

―――― 2004. *Doorgeven/doorverkopen van hormoonpreparaten*. Retrieved 1 March 2015 from www.freya.nl.

―――― 2013a. *Brochure nr. 8. Eiceldonatie*. Retrieved 1 March 2015 from www.freya.nl.

―――― 2013b. Drie IVF-pogingen vergoed in 2013. Retrieved 5 March 2015 from www.freya.nl/web_politiek/regels2013.

Gezondheidsraad. Signalering Ethiek en Gezondheid. 2003. Gezondheidsraad. Den Haag: Gezondheidsraad, 2003; publicatie nr 2003/08. Retrieved 23 March 2016 from www.gezondheidsraad.nl .

Heida, A. 2001. 'Juridische aspecten van reproductieve technieken', in S. de Joode (ed.), *Zwanger van de kinderwens: Visies, feiten en vragen over voortplantingstechnologie*. The Hague: Rathenau Instituut, pp. 108–21.

Hunfeld, J.A.M., J. Passchier, L.L.E. Bolt and M.A.J.M. Buijsen. 2004. 'Protect the child from being born: Arguments against IVF from heads of the 13 licensed Dutch fertility centres, ethical and legal perspectives', *Journal of Reproductive and Infant Psychology* 22(4): 279–89.

Inhorn, M.C. and D. Birenbaum-Carmeli. 2008. 'Assisted reproductive technologies and culture change', *Annual Review of Anthropology* 37: 177–96.

Inhorn, M.C., and Z.B. Gürtin. 2011. Cross-border reproductive care: a future research agenda. *Reproductive Biomedicine Online* 23(5): 665-676.

Janssens, P.M.W., A.H.M. Simons, R.J. Van Kooij, E. Blokzijl, and G.A.J. Dunselman. 2006. 'A new Dutch law regulating provision of identifying information of donors to offspring: Background, content and impact', *Human Reproduction* 21(4): 852–56.

Jones, H.W. and J. Cohen. 2004. 'IFFS Surveillance 04', *Fertility and Sterility* 81(5), Suppl. 4: S1–S54.

Kirejczyk, M. 1996. *Met technologie gezegend? Gender en de omstreden invoering van in vitro fertilisatie in de Nederlandse Gezondheidszorg.* Utrecht: Uitgeverij Jan van Arkel.

Kleinman, A. 1995. *Writing at the Margin: Discourse between anthropology and medicine.* Berkeley: University of California Press.

Kremer, J.A.M. and A.P. Visser. 2008. 'Testicular sperm extraction (TESE) with intracytoplasmic sperm injection (ICSI) now allowed in the Netherlands', *Nederlands Tijdschrift Geneeskunde* 152(3): 164–66.

Mastenbroek, S., M. Twisk, J. van Echten-Arends, B. Sikkema-Raddatz, J.C. Korevaar, H.R. Verhoeve, and C.H. Buys, 2007. 'In Vitro Fertilization with Preimplantation Genetic Screening', *The New England Journal of Medicine* 357(1): 9–17.

Ministerie van VWS 1998. Planningsbesluit IVF. *Staatscourant* 95: 14.

Modelreglement Embryowet. 2003. *Modelreglement Embryowet.* Utrecht: Kwaliteitsinstituut voor de Gezondheidszorg CBO.

NVOG. 1998a. *Kwaliteitsnorm In vitro fertilisatie.* Retrieved 1 March 2015 from www.nvog.nl.

_____ 1998b. *Richtlijn indicaties voor IVF.* Retrieved 1 March 2015 from www. nvog.nl.

_____ 1999. *Richtlijn Hoog-technologisch Draagmoederschap.* Retrieved 1 March 2015 from www.nvog.nl.

_____ 2000. *IUI Richtlijnen.* Retrieved 1 March 2015 from www.nvog.nl.

_____ 2001. *Patiëntenvoorlichting. Afwegingen bij de keuze voor ICSI.* Retrieved 1 March 2015 from www.nvog.nl.

_____ 2005. *Persbericht 8.11.2005.* Retrieved 1 March 2015 from www.nvog. nl.

_____ 2006. *Standpunt definitie IVF behandeling.* Retrieved 1 March 2015 from www.nvog.nl.

_____ 2010a. *Richtlijnen voortplantingsgeneeskunde. Onverklaarde subfertiliteit.* Retrieved 1 March 2015 from www.nvog.nl.

_____ 2010b. *Model protocol in geval van mogelijke morele contra-indicaties bij vruchtbaarheidsbehandelingen.* Retrieved 1 March 2015 from www.nvog. nl.

_____ 2011. Gameetdonatie in een systeem van faire wederkerigheid. Retrieved 14 March 2016 from www.nvog.nl.

_____ 2013. Kwaliteitsnorm geassisteerde voortplanting met chirurgisch verkregen zaadcellen. Retrieved 20 August 2015 from www.nvog.nl.

Pennings, G. 2005. 'Gamete donation in a system of need-adjusted reciprocity', *Human Reproduction* 20(11): 2990–93.

Pennings, G., C. Autin, W. Decleer, A. Delbaere, L. Delbeke, A. Delvigne, D. De Neubourg, P. Devroey, M. Dhont, T. D'Hooghe, S. Gordts, B.

Lejeune, M. Nijs, P. Pauwels, B. Perrad, C. Pirard and F. Vandekerckhove. 2009. 'Cross-border reproductive care in Belgium', *Human Reproduction* 24(12): 3108–18.

Pennings, G. and W. Ombelet. 2007. 'Coming soon to your clinic: Patient-friendly ART', *Human Reproduction* 22(8): 2075–79.

Raad voor de Volksgezondheid en Zorg. 2005. *Prijsverschillen voor IVF behandelingen. Grote verschillen in prijzen IVF behandelingen.* Nieuwsberichten, 21 June 2005. Retrieved 15 March 2015 www.rvz.net.

Rapp, R. 1999. *Testing Women, Testing the Fetus: The social impact of Amniocentesis in America.* New York: Routledge.

Stern, J.E., C.P. Cramer, A. Garrod, and R.M. Green. 2002. 'Attitudes on access to services at assisted reproductive technology clinics: comparisons with clinic policy', *Fertility and Sterility* 77(3): 537–41.

Stern, J.E., C.P. Cramer, R.M. Green, A. Garrod, and K.O. DeVriesl. 2003. 'Determining access to assisted reproductive technology: Reactions of clinic directors at ethically complex cases', *Human Reproduction* 18(6): 1343–52.

Ten Have, H. 1995. 'Letters to Dr. Frankenstein? Ethics and the new reproductive technologies', *Social Science and Medicine* 40(2): 141–46.

Thompson C. 2005. *Making Parents: The ontological choreography of reproductive technologies.* Cambridge, MA: The MIT Press.

Van Balen, F. and M. Inhorn. 2002. 'Introduction: Interpreting infertility: A view from the social sciences', in M.C. Inhorn and F. Van Balen (eds), *Infertility around the Globe: New thinking on childlessness, gender and reproductive technology.* Berkeley: University of California Press, pp. 3–32.

Van Balen, F., E. Ketting and J. Verdurmen. 1995. *Zorgen rond onvruchtbaarheid: Voornaamste bevindingen van het Nationaal Onderzoek naar Gedrag bij Onvruchtbaarheid.* Delft: Eburon.

Van der Burg, D. 2010. *Eiceldonatie, een overtreffende trap.* Nijkerk: Van Brug.

Veerman, G. J. M. 2000. 'Uitsluiting alleenstaande vrouwen en lesbische paren, Commissie gelijke behandeling 7 februari 2000, Oordeel 2000-4', *NJCM-Bulletin*, 1082–1094.

Chapter 3

THE COUPLES AND THEIR QUEST
FOR A CHILD

Iris (born 1974) and Johan (born 1976) are one of the couples participating in this study who visited the Radboud Clinic for medically
assisted conception. They got to know each other in 2001, when they
were both in their mid twenties. Almost immediately after initiating their relationship, they started to live together in the house that
Johan had bought when he still lived with his former girlfriend. One
and a half years later they married. Iris and Johan live in the village
where Johan grew up, close to the city of Nijmegen, surrounded by
relatives and friends from his youth. Iris was born in Nijmegen, and
she also maintains intensive contact with her parents and friends.
Both Iris and Johan have a low level of education and work full-time.
They were content with their jobs, their life, their house and their
dog; the only thing they felt they missed was a child.

Before getting married they had already decided that they wanted
to have children. They preferred to be young parents, and let their
children grow up with the children of their siblings and friends. Iris
stopped taking the contraceptive pill even before the wedding ceremony took place – though she avoided being pregnant on her wedding day as she wanted to fit into her wedding dress. After being
married for half a year without becoming pregnant, they went to
see their general practitioner, who took their concern seriously and
referred them immediately to the CWZ hospital (a general, non-aca-
demic hospital in the city of Nijmegen). Though Iris was pleased with
this quick referral, she had in fact expected that he would tell her 'to
take things a bit easy' and that they simply had to continue trying
for some more time. As she explained it herself: 'I think he immediately referred us to the hospital because I was rather emotional when

I consulted him. Normally I do not visit the general practitioner that often. He knows me very well. So, he might have grasped how bad I felt about it.'

At the CWZ some initial examinations were performed. With Iris, everything seemed to be okay, but quickly they came to realise that the quality of Johan's semen was 'extremely bad'. They were told that they would definitely need some form of advanced reproductive technology – IVF or ICSI – in order to be able to conceive. As the CWZ hospital does not perform IVF, they were referred to the fertility clinic of the Radboud Clinic. At that moment Iris was twenty-eight and Johan twenty-six years old. Examinations were repeated, and the diagnosis of 'bad quality sperm' confirmed. When the doctors proposed doing an IVF-ICSI treatment, they immediately decided that they wanted to give it a try; they felt that they did not have any other choice if they wanted to have a child of their own. After being on the waiting list for about four months – a period they perceived as terribly lengthy – they were able to start the first treatment. It was successful, and in 2005 – about two years after their first visit to the general practitioner – Iris gave birth to twins.

Liset (born 1963) and Alexander (born 1970) also visited the fertility clinic of the Radboud Clinic during the same period of time, but they came with a completely different story. They had known each other for almost two years and at the time when they met she was thirty-eight and he was thirty-one years old. They came to know each other through chatting on the Internet, and had many intensive conversations about all sorts of topics, including children and adoption, before actually meeting each other in person. Once they had met, they quickly decided to live together. Alexander, a highly educated professional, found a new job and moved to the village where Liset already lived with her children, two sons from a former relationship.

Two years after the birth of her youngest son, Liset had undergone a sterilisation. She was still upset when she talked about it, for although she had explicitly asked for a 'repairable sterilization', the gynaecologist had simply removed her fallopian tubes. Thus she knew from the onset of this new relationship that she would not be able to become pregnant in 'a normal way'. As they both wanted to have a child together – though initially Alexander had had his doubts about it – they realized they should not wait too long before visiting a doctor as she was already nearing her forties. They would have loved to spend some more time together before trying to get pregnant, but felt that her biological clock was ticking. They first consulted the general practitioner, who did an FSH (follicle stimulating hormone) test which showed that her FSH level was still low enough to allow for conception. The general practitioner then referred them to the fertility clinic of the Radboud Clinic, where the FSH test was repeated and Alexander's semen was tested as well. As all relevant values proved to be good, they were immediately placed on the IVF waiting list. At that moment Liset was exactly forty years old. They did one IVF, which was not successful. They – and in particular Liset – experienced the treatment as extremely burdensome, they were disappointed about the minimal results (few ova were fertilized), and not pleased with the follow-up services provided by the clinic. This made them decide against starting another treatment, and their quest for a child 'of the two of them' ended without achieving the desired result.[1]

The couples participating in this study all shared the same concern: they wanted a child but could not manage to conceive on their own. All of them chose to medicalize their fertility problem, a pathway that is chosen by many – though certainly not all – Dutch women and men who are confronted with fertility problems (Van Balen et al. 1995). The couples also shared the fact that they ended up at the Radboud Clinic. Despite these similarities, the couples participating in this study differed in many aspects; all of them brought their unique story to the clinic. Their stories differed from a medical point of view, but also their 'life stories' differed in terms of the circumstances they were in at the moment they realized that conceiving was not going to be that easy (as the above two cases demonstrate). Some of the couples, for example, had been in a relationship for a long time when they first visited the fertility clinic, while others had met only recently, sometimes late into their thirties. Some couples postponed childbearing for a long time, while others – once they had met each other – were in a hurry to conceive, as they felt their biological clocks ticking. Some of the study participants already had one or more children (with their current or a previous partner), though most were childless. For many of them, the fertility problem came as a surprise, while others knew from the start that having children would or might be problematic for them.

The diverse stories the couples brought to the clinic – their backgrounds and life circumstances – affected the way they (initially) perceived their fertility problem and the process that followed. In this book I do not aim to analyse and explain the couples' views, experiences and choices along the lines of these background variables and circumstances. Rather, my aim in this chapter is to give insight into the diversity of the couples visiting the fertility clinic, in terms of background features and the processes they went through.

In this chapter I first present socio-demographic background data
and draw attention to some couples' characteristics and circumstances that were shown to make a difference in the way they initially perceived, considered and acted upon their fertility problem.
Throughout the chapter I present case descriptions of some of
the participating couples, to further illustrate the diversity among
them. In the second part of this chapter I describe the processes the
couples passed through in their quest for offspring, in the biomedical health system and alternative health circles, and discuss their
considerations and actions taken regarding adoption.

Social and Demographic Characteristics

All women and men participating in the study were of Dutch nationality.[2] Four couples lived in the city of Nijmegen; all others lived in
small villages or towns within a circle of about seventy kilometres
around Nijmegen.[3] The participants' age at the moment of their
inclusion in the study (March 2004) ranged from twenty-six to fifty-
six years; with the exception of one man, they were all born between
1960 and 1980 (see Appendix 2). The largest age group consisted of
men and women born between 1965 and 1969, meaning that at the
onset of the study they were between thirty-four and thirty-eight
years old; six men and three women were older. On the whole, most
men were slightly older than their partners, though the opposite
was found as well. In two couples the man was much older than the
woman (one by sixteen and the other by twenty years). On average
the respondents in my study were slightly older than the Dutch IVF
population as found in two large Dutch studies providing average
age of IVF users.[4]

Most couples were childless when they started treatment. In seven
couples one or both of the partners had one or more child(ren): two
couples already had a child together, while three men and two
women had one or more child(ren) with former partners.

Eleven study participants had a low level of education (24 per
cent), nineteen a mid level (41 per cent) and sixteen a high level of
education (35 per cent). The level of education in this study group
is fairly comparable to the level of education of the Dutch population in general: in 2004, 30 per cent of the Dutch population of
25- to 65-year-olds held a low level of education, 40 per cent a
mid level and 29 per cent a high level of education (RIVM 2006).
The low-educated are only slightly underrepresented in the current

study group, while the highly educated are slightly overrepresented. Within the group of participants, the level of education is roughly similar for men and women. Generally, partners in a couple had more or less the same level of education, and only in one couple was the woman much more highly educated than her husband (university degree and lower vocational training respectively).

All the men and almost all of the women participating in the study were employed at the time the study started. More than half of the women had a part-time job, and seven men were working part-time; almost all of the men who worked part-time were highly educated. This reflects the common pattern of working part-time in the Netherlands (as discussed in Chapter 1). Study participants' occupations covered a huge variety of professions. All lower-educated men were employed as manual labourers, which included a mechanic, a painter, a truck driver, an agricultural worker and a road worker; the lower-educated women included two cleaners and a book-keeper. Almost all mid-level-educated men and women had administrative, secretarial or commercial functions, and one of the women owned a tattoo and piercing studio. The highly educated men included IT specialists, consultants/advisors, a social worker, a pilot and a biologist; the highly educated women were employed as a trainer, a consultant and a manager, while others worked in the field of psycho-social assistance.

Income levels ranged from no income at all to over 3,000 Euros (net income per month). More than half of the study participants (and more women than men) earned less or equal to the Dutch net modal income (which was 1,492 Euros in 2004).[5] Overall, women earned substantially less than the men (with seven having an income of less than 1,000 Euros), which is partly related to the fact that they worked on a part-time basis. Almost all couples owned the house they were living in.

The variation in levels of income is also reflected in the type of health insurance people had. More than half of the participants – and about three quarters of the women – were insured through the public health insurance (Ziekenfonds) at the start of the study, while about one quarter had private health insurance.[6] The diversity in educational level, income categories and health insurance policies of study participants reflect the situation that infertility treatments – including ARTs – in the Netherlands are widely accessible to people of various socioeconomic classes, including the lower-income classes. This is in strong contrast to what is the case in some other Western countries. In particular in the USA only 36 per cent of infertile women sought any form of medical assistance and only 1 per cent resorted to some form of ARTs, due to financial reasons (Inhorn and Birenbaum-Carmeli 2008).

Finally, about half of the women and men in the study formally belonged to the Roman Catholic Church (though most of them said they were not practicing or were hardly practising), and a small minority were Protestant. Nine persons – most of them higher-educated – did not claim any religious affiliation. This reflects a common pattern in Dutch society (as discussed in Chapter 1), where since the 1960s a process of secularization has taken place.

Facing Fertility Problems: Diverse Points of Departure

When listening to the study participants' stories, some of their cir-cumstances stood out as having made a substantial difference in the way they initially perceived, considered and acted upon their fer-tility problem.[7] About a quarter of the study participants were still relatively young – in their twenties or early thirties – when they first visited the clinic with their unfulfilled wish for a child. The majority of the study participants, however, were in their mid to late thirties or older when they first visited the clinic. The age of the women and men when first confronted with their fertility problem (in combina-tion with the duration of their relationship at that same moment) strongly affected the way they initially considered their problem, which will be discussed below.

Younger Couples

The couples in this study who were still young when visiting the clinic generally had followed the more or less traditional life course as described in the introductory case of Iris and Johan: they met in their teens or early twenties (in some cases the male partner was slightly older), started to live together and married at a young age. None of them had children from former relationships. They planned to have children soon after marrying in the hope of becoming young parents, but after a while they realized – completely unexpectedly in most cases – that becoming pregnant was not going to be as easy as they always thought it would be. They had simply thought preg-nancy would occur within a short period of time; their big concern had always been about preventing pregnancy. Therefore not con-ceiving within a few months, when they wanted it so much, came as an enormous surprise. Jeanet and Karel belonged to this group of young couples.

> Jeanet (born 1974) and Karel (born 1973) were in their teens when they got to know each other in 1991. They courted for nine years before they married in 2000. They bought a house in a small village, next to the farmhouse where Karel grew up and where his parents were still living. Karel's childhood friends and their partners became their communal circle of friends, whom they regularly saw at birthday parties, in the village pub, on the soccer field, at carnival, at the yearly village fair and so on. When I visited Jeanet and Karel at home for the interviews, they showed me the birth cards they were receiving on an almost weekly basis. By then almost all their friends had one or more children; they found themselves to be the exception, and experienced this as very problematic. They were eager to have children of the same age as their friends to let them grow up together.
>
> About one year after their wedding day they had decided that they wanted to start a family. Jeanet stopped taking the contraceptive pill, and they waited – carefully following the instructions on the leaflet – a couple of months before actually trying to get pregnant. When in 2002 Jeanet was still not pregnant, they started to worry. For a long time they did not share their concern with anybody, but at a certain moment they spoke about it with Karel's sister, a health professional, who became an important source of information.
>
> In January 2004 – after having tried to conceive in vain for two and a half years – they visited their general practitioner. They felt insecure as to whether this was the proper moment to visit the general practitioner, as they did not know anybody else with similar problems and did not have a clue about what was considered a 'normal period for trying on your own'. The doctor initiated some examinations, including a semen test at a peripheral hospital. This semen test showed that Karel's sperm was of 'bad quality' and they were immediately transferred to the fertility clinic at the Radboud Clinic.

Several of these young couples spoke about their fertility problem as the first thing in their life that did not work out the way they wanted, that they could not plan and were unable to control. Their friends and siblings, who were more or less of the same age, had mostly started to have children in the same period. Most of them had not yet encountered fertility problems within their own circle of friends and relatives, and though some of them had heard or read about IVF, the issue of not being able to conceive was one that thus far had hardly crossed their minds. Only at the moment that they found themselves not conceiving did it become an issue that they started to think, read and talk about. Most of them shared with me how uncertain they had felt about the proper moment for consulting a doctor. They had – as Jeanet and Karel stated – no clue about 'what is normal to do in such a situation', and particularly in the beginning they hardly talked about it with other people.

With the exception of one couple, all these young couples had low or mid-level education. This reflects the tendency that in Dutch society – on average – lower-educated women have their first child at a younger age than higher-educated women (Beets 2004). Moreover, I observed that almost all the couples with lower and mid-level education (thus not only the young starters) lived in the same village or neighbourhood where one or both of them grew up, and this seemed to affect the way people perceived their fertility problem. In general, these couples were still friends with, and surrounded by, the relatives and friends from their youth. Many of them – in particular the younger couples – felt confronted with lots of babies being born within this circle of friends and relatives in the same period as they themselves were struggling to have their wish for a child fulfilled. They thus felt that their 'anticipated course of life', fitting with that of the community to which they belonged, was suddenly, unexpectedly and unpleasantly disrupted (cf. Becker 2000: 30–31).[8] Almost all of them, therefore, expressed a sense of urgency to act upon their fertility problem, as they wished to keep up with the same 'pace of life' as their close friends, and with whom they wished to raise their children.[9] Contrarily, hardly any of the higher-educated couples lived in the same area that one or either of them grew up in, and though they also saw themselves confronted with other people – friends, relatives and colleagues – having babies, this was less emphasized as a factor that urged them to rush into pursuing treatments.

Older Couples

The majority of the study participants were, as with Liset and Alexander in the second introductory case, older than thirty-five years when they visited the clinic for medically assisted conception. These older couples can be divided into two types: couples who were young when they started their relationship, but postponed childbearing until a later age; and couples who got to know each other at a later stage, when in their (late) thirties or older. The couples who postponed having children did so because they wanted to 'enjoy their life together', travel, and/or build up a good life before starting a family. Marion and Kees were among them:

Marion (born 1968) and Kees (born 1968) had a longstanding relationship. They met each other when they were both twenty years
old. Though they had always liked children, for several years they
had not thought of having a child themselves. They reconstructed an
old farmhouse, kept a number of dogs and other pets, travelled a bit
and were quite happy together. Marion explained that in that period
she felt rather pessimistic about the world in general, and doubted
whether she wanted to bring a child into this harsh world. Besides,
she had serious doubts about her own capacities as a child educa-
tor. But at a certain moment things started to change. They enjoyed
taking care of their friends' baby. Marion also felt fed up with her own
negativity and decided to actually try to change her life and way of
looking at the world, something she worked hard on. She learned a
new profession, and started her own studio. She came to feel better,
and started to think about having a child. Finally, in 2001 – when
they were both thirty-three years old – she expressed her wish for a
child to Kees. Initially he was somewhat surprised, but after a short
while he agreed. Marion stopped taking the contraceptive pill.

Since Marion had had some problems with polyps in her uterus,
for which she had visited a gynaecologist in a general hospital near
the village where she lived, she did not hesitate to visit him again
when she had not managed to conceive after trying for a couple of
months. The gynaecologist reassured her that the remaining 'fleshy
growth', as he had called it, would not prevent her from conceiving,
so they continued trying. About half a year later – about ten months
after first starting to attempt to conceive – Marion and Kees visited
the gynaecologist again. Examinations were initiated on both of them,
and they discovered that Kees' sperm was of extremely 'bad quality';
in fact, they were informed that the sperm was of such 'bad quality'
that the doctor doubted whether it would be good enough even for
IVF-ICSI. In any case, they had to be referred to an academic hospital
to find out more, as the peripheral hospital did not offer IVF. That is
how Kees and Marion ended up at the Radboud Clinic in September
2003. At that moment they were both thirty-five years old.

About half of the study participants (eleven couples) did not postpone childbearing, as Marion and Kees did, but simply got to know
each other at a later stage, when in their (late) thirties or older.
Some of them spent a few years together to get to know each other
better and to 'enjoy life without kids' before they actually decided
to have children. Half of them, especially those that were around
thirty-five years or older when they got to know each other, made
this decision within a year. They felt they did not have the choice to
postpone childbearing, as the woman's biological clock was ticking.
While they had not known each other for very long, they saw

themselves suddenly confronted with fertility problems and having to decide on what to do about it. This was the case for Richard and Ria.

Ria (born 1967) and Richard (born 1964) – both with higher education – had known each other since November 2002. Ria immediately asked him if he was interested in having children. This was a crucial issue for her, because her former relationship – which had lasted ten years – had foundered on that issue. Richard was initially surprised to hear of her urgent wish for a child, but pretty soon got used to the idea and then felt confident that he shared her desire. When I visited them for the first time they had recently moved to a new house in a village near to Nijmegen. Previously Ria had lived in an alternative 'living community', where she had come across all kinds of non-traditional forms of having and rearing children (such as co-parenting, conscious single motherhood, lesbian parenthood, and so on), and she also knew quite a few women who had used IVF or other fertility treatments. Thus she was well aware that conceiving at her age might be problematic. As her former partner had not wanted to assume fatherhood for a child, she had been considering all kinds of different models for conceiving and parenting, and she also knew the critical debate regarding the medicalization of fertility problems. Richard, in his turn, had not been in a relationship for years, had been living on his own, and fatherhood had not been an issue in his life at all.

Ria had already stopped taking contraceptives before she got to know Richard; and almost immediately after initiating their relationship they started trying to become pregnant. After trying for half a year in vain she was in a panic and visited her general practitioner. She felt bad because for the last ten years she had wanted to become pregnant in her former relationship, and had not been allowed to do so; now she was allowed to but could not succeed. The doctor reassured her, saying that it could easily take between half a year up to one and a half years before becoming pregnant. He instructed her on how to make a temperature curve and invited her to return after a couple of months; given her advanced age he proposed a shorter period for trying than he would have done had she been younger. In addition, on her request, she was referred to a social worker to get some support 'to sort out some things from the past'. Ria ordered an ovulation test and they used it for some months. However, they quickly became fed up with making love at set hours and dumped the test. After one and a half years of attempting to conceive – at a later moment than the general practitioner had suggested – they returned to see him, and he immediately referred them to the Radboud Clinic.

As with Ria in the above case, some of the couples who got to know each other at an older age had, in the past, had a longstanding relationship (formal marriage or cohabitation) with another partner in which – for different reasons – no children had been born. Others, though, had one or more children with their former partner (for example Liset), which lead to a completely different situation (see below).

Strikingly, many of the older starters – and probably the women even more than the men – were (as was Ria) much more aware of potential fertility problems than the young starters were, for a number of reasons. First of all, there was their advanced age. All of them also knew other couples (friends, relatives, colleagues) that had experienced difficulties in conceiving and needed medical assistance. In addition, this group included women who had seen a gynaecologist for gynaecological complaints such as cysts, endometriosis, strong or irregular bleedings, irregular cycle, for being a DES-daughter or because they had had a miscarriage.[10][11] Though these couples were certainly disappointed when pregnancy did not happen immediately, in contrast to the young starters most of them were not fully taken by surprise. Moreover, several of these men and women expressed the sentiment that you simply cannot always get what you want; the world is not as 'makeable' (*maakbaar*) as you would sometimes like it to be. For most of them, this view clearly resulted from former confrontations with the less bright sides of life, like personal or relational struggles, or serious diseases and loss of beloved friends or relatives. They had already learnt that the course of life is not always a 'predictable, continuous flow' (cf. Becker 2000: 62). This position contrasted with the earlier described predominant reaction of the young starters, for whom fertility problems came as an absolute surprise and who felt very unsettled, as this was the first event in their lives that they could not control.

A noteworthy observation, and the opposite of what is sometimes suggested in the mass media and literature, is that the older couples in this study did not only consist of higher-educated career women who had postponed childbearing and rearing for the sake of their career (Te Velde 1991; Braat 2000).[12] While indeed the majority of the study participants – both women and men – were over thirty when they first entered the clinic, many of them were not so highly educated, and most had not consciously chosen to postpone childbearing.[13] With the ones for whom it was a conscious choice, this was motivated by matters other than the woman's career, such as the wish to travel or to enjoy life together. Different individuals' and couples' backgrounds resulted in them starting a family – or a second family – at a later age. For most of the couples involved in this study, the reason they gave for being rather late in fulfilling their wish for a child (and thus also visiting the fertility clinic at a later age) had more to do with unplanned circumstances of life, like divorce and remarriage, or because they had not met the 'right partner' earlier, than the conscious decision by higher-educated women to postpone childbearing (see also Beets 2004).[14]

Having or Not Having a Child

Being childless or already having a family – in one or another form – was another circumstance that affected the way people perceived their fertility problem. As said before, most couples were childless at the moment they visited the fertility clinic; however, two couples already had a child together, while with five couples one or both of the partners had one or more child(ren) from a previous relationship.

The two couples that had a child together had known each for a long time (between fifteen and twenty years) when they visited the clinic, and they were all past their mid thirties at the onset of the study. One of these couples, Geert and Marijke, had conceived their first child about five years ago without any medical assistance.

Marijke (born 1967) and Geert (born 1965) had known each other since 1986. In 1999 – when they were in their early thirties – they had their first child, and then after a couple of years they wanted one more. When Marijke did not succeed in becoming pregnant after one year, they first visited an alternative healer. They disliked the idea that the general practitioner would refer them immediately to the hospital, and hoped that they could find alternative means to solve their problem. When these visits to the alternative healer proved unsatisfactory, they went to the general practitioner, who did a semen test. The test showed that Geert's semen was of 'bad quality', so the doctor referred them to a peripheral hospital. As they wanted to be seen by a particular female gynaecologist – about whom they had heard good stories – they had to wait some months before being seen. They did not mind too much; they did not feel in any hurry. They ended up doing six IUIs in the peripheral hospital without achieving any result. Though initially they disliked the idea of undergoing IVF treatment for ethical reasons – they questioned whether they wanted to force a pregnancy that did not come in a natural way – at a certain moment they felt that they should give it a try. Thus the gynaecologist referred them to the Radboud Clinic, where they immediately entered the waiting list for IVF. When the semen test proved that Geert's semen was of very 'bad quality' – and that they would have to consider ICSI – they once more went through a period of reconsidering their decision on ethical grounds, as they felt that ICSI was forcing nature even more than 'ordinary' IVF. Finally, thinking about the child they already had together ('she would be worth doing it for') convinced them that they should do it.

The other couple that already had a child together had conceived through an IVF-ICSI treatment at the fertility clinic. They had gone through an extended period of treatments, including nine IUIs and four IVF treatments, before having their first child. Therefore – and also because the woman was now nearing her forties – they felt they should not wait too long before attempting to become pregnant again, as it might again take a long time. Though they felt an aversion to starting 'the hustle of treatment procedures', at the same time they felt they had no other choice if they wanted to have one more child.

Both couples were eager to have one more child ('a little brother or sister for our first child', as they often put it), but emphasized from the beginning that the fact that they already had one child together would make it easier for them to accept the potential failure of the treatment. At least, they claimed, they already had a child, and they thought the treatment process would therefore be less stressful than for couples that did not yet have a child.

This was a somewhat different scenario than for the couples where one of the partners had a child (or children) from a former relationship. Though all of them also said that at least they already had 'some sort of family life',[15] they emphasized that they would like to have 'a child of the two of us', as a kind of confirmation of their love and/or because they wanted to see their partner in their child (cf. Becker 2000: 72).[16] In the situations where the man already had a child but the woman did not, all the women added that they were eager to experience a pregnancy and delivery themselves. Thus, despite the fact that alternative family arrangements are possible and rather common and well accepted in most segments of current day Dutch society (Van Praag and Niphuis-Nell 1997), these – and in fact all – couples in this study wished to adhere to the culturally dominant family model, consisting of a heterosexual couple with their own biological children, as Becker (2000: 64) also found among the women in her middle class study group in the USA.

Knowing in Advance: No Conception without Medical Assistance

Three of the study participants who already had children – two women and one man – had undergone sterilization in a former relationship and thus they knew that having sexual intercourse would not help them to become pregnant. This created a different situation in which they knew from the beginning of their relationship that they would need some form of medical assistance in order to conceive. For the couples where one of the partners was sterilized, the need for medical assistance did not come as a surprise. These couples, soon after deciding that they wanted a child together, went to see a doctor. For them, their quest for conception started with trying to reverse the sterilization. Theoretically, men and women who have been sterilized can have the operation reversed, and if this reversal is successful, they might be able to conceive in a 'normal' way by having sexual intercourse. However, this reversal procedure is not always successful, and this was what had happened to these three couples.[17]

Knowing in advance that medical assistance would be needed affected the process people went through. First of all, they did not need to go through a period of trying on their own. Though they were therefore completely dependent on reproductive technology in order to conceive, this 'short' trajectory was also considered an advantage. Christine, for example, who knew from the beginning of her relationship that she would not be able to become pregnant with her sterilized partner, was very outspoken on this point:

> We knew from the beginning that it was a complicated story. It was not simply 'not taking the pill' . . . Maybe that is also a kind of relief, as you do not have that disappointment again and again. Others do have that. Each month they think: 'Oh shit. Again I am not pregnant'.

For these couples, once they entered the clinic for fertility treatment, the waiting period before starting actual treatment was generally shorter, because they did not need to go through a full series of examinations to find out the cause of the fertility problem (though their partners were examined as well).

Couples with a history of sterilization were not the only ones to know in advance that becoming pregnant would not be possible without medical assistance. In this study two other couples knew from the onset of their relationship that given the particular medical history of one of the partners, they would not be able to conceive on their own. One of the men, André, had undergone chemotherapy about ten years prior to participating in the study, and had his semen frozen at the time to enable him to have children in the future.[18] Therefore he and his current partner knew from the start that she could only become pregnant through medically assisted conception, using his frozen semen.

Kim (born 1978) and André (born 1962) had been in a relationship since 2001. André had a child of about twenty years old, with whom he did not have any contact. From the beginning of their relationship – which started when she was temporarily living in his house, due to personal problems – Kim and André knew that they would not be able to have children in a 'normal' way, for in 1994 André underwent chemotherapy to treat cancer. Before starting this therapy his sperm was frozen to enable him to have children later on, if he so desired. At that time he was living with his former partner, and together they had used some of the frozen sperm for three artificial inseminations (IUIs). Given the bad results, he and his then partner decided to go for ICSI treatment; this treatment was, however, never carried out because their relationship came to an end.

Six years later, André and his new partner Kim decided that they wanted a child together. André felt that he was getting older (he was forty-two at that moment) and should not wait too long to use the remaining frozen sperm, as he did not want to be older than forty-six or forty-seven years old when he would 'become a dad'. They first visited their general practitioner for a referral to the Radboud Clinic, where – to his great pleasure – they met the same gynaecologist who had treated André and his former partner in 1997. Kim, who was new to the clinic, had to go through a series of examinations before the gynaecologist could make a decision on treatment. At the same time, the quality of the frozen sperm was checked. These examinations started in March 2004, and not long after that they entered the waiting list for IVF-ICSI treatment, though she was instructed to reduce her weight and try to stop smoking before she could actually undergo an IVF treatment. Some time later, she withdrew from the waiting list, because she felt that her partner was too unsupportive (more about this in Chapter 7).

There was one more couple participating in the study that knew from the onset that they would need medical assistance to conceive. In their case the woman had had an extra-uterine pregnancy, and she had been warned against the risk of attempting to become pregnant 'normally' as this might lead to dangerous complications. Their story is as follows.

Kitty (born 1967) and Theo (born 1966) met each other in 1997, when they were both around thirty years old. In a former relationship Kitty had had an extra-uterine pregnancy and miscarried. Her situation had been critical: she had lost a lot of blood and one of her fallopian tubes had been removed. Some years before this she had been raped and she suggested that her fertility problem (blocked tubes) was due to the Chlamydia infection that she had contracted through the rape.

A couple of years after the miscarriage Kitty underwent a laparoscopy; at that time she was told that if she ever wanted to become pregnant, she would definitely have to make use of IVF. The chances of becoming pregnant naturally were still there, but she would have to prevent it due to the elevated chance of suffering another extra-uterine pregnancy. As Kitty associated sexual intercourse with having children, they hardly had sex anymore, though she and her husband both stressed that they had a satisfactory intimate relationship.

For a long period of time Kitty had not felt the desire to become pregnant. For a couple of years she had been rather depressed – for various reasons – and had undergone psycho-therapeutic treatment. She dreaded the idea of having to undergo IVF in order to conceive, but at the same time both she and her husband would have loved to become parents. In 2001 they consulted a gynaecologist in a peripheral hospital, who immediately offered to start fertility treatment. At that time they had felt that things had gone too fast, that they were not yet ready for it, and they themselves interrupted the process.

In 2003 – when both were in their mid thirties – they decided once more to start the treatment process. As they disliked the way they were treated on former occasions in the general hospital, they asked their general practitioner to refer them directly to the Radboud Clinic. Once they visited the clinic, they quickly found out that Theo's semen was of very 'bad quality', thus not permitting IVF-ICSI; some time later they also discovered that not enough semen could be found to have a PESA performed. Thus, they could not be treated at the Radboud Clinic. After some deliberation they decided to go for a TESE treatment, something that is not yet permitted in the Netherlands. For Kitty and Theo, their quest for offspring ended abroad at a fertility clinic in Germany (which was geographically speaking not far away, as they lived not far from the German border). They were one of the two cases who had to make use of cross-border reproductive care, resulting from treatment restrictions as stipulated by the Dutch ARTs policy. In 2006 – after having undergone two TESE treatments and one cryo with assisted hatching, Kitty gave birth to a baby.

Couples whose medical history inhibited them from becoming pregnant in a natural way knew from the start that sexual intercourse would not help them to conceive. Once they decided to visit the clinic with their request for medically assisted conception, they started almost directly on their treatment trajectory. Their partners' condition, however, had to be examined as well, and, as both of the above examples show, could change their situation drastically. While initially the partner with the medical history was considered the reason behind them searching for medical assistance, the other partner was also found to contribute equally to the fertility problem. This changed the dynamics among the couples and added substantial complications to the process they went through in their quest for a child, an issue to which we turn in the next section.

Couples' Quest for a Child: The Process

Thus far we have seen the diversity of circumstances that the couples participating in this study were faced with when they realized that becoming pregnant was not going to be easy. What do people do once they realize that becoming pregnant is not as easy as they had hoped for or expected? We will see that for most couples, disciplining sexual intercourse was the first step, followed (or sometimes preceded) by a visit to the general practitioner and/or a gynaecologist in a peripheral hospital. All of the couples in this study finally ended up at the fertility clinic at the Radboud Clinic (which is of course due to the way study participants were selected). Some of the couples also made use of alternative medicine, and some considered and/or actually turned to adoption.

Disciplining Sexual Intercourse

Having sex (more frequently) is what most people normally do once they have decided that they want to have a child. When couples find out after some time that becoming pregnant is not going to be as easy as they thought it would be, they often turn to planning sex: they 'discipline' their sex life. This is what Nienke and Jos did, for a while.

> Nienke (born 1968) and Jos (born 1965) had, at the time of the study in 2004, known each other for about ten years. They belong to the group who had postponed having children: they enjoyed their life together: they liked travelling, they were both highly educated and were dedicated to their jobs. For a long period they postponed making the decision about having or not having a child; they could imagine a good life for themselves with or without children. But at a certain moment things changed: Nienke started to feel like 'I do want to have a child'; and the death of her mother contributed to the feeling that she wanted to create her own family. After a while they decided

she would stop taking the pill. They were not overly worried when she did not conceive immediately, as they knew from several (older) couples in their circle of friends and colleagues that it could take some time. At a certain point she did become pregnant, but miscarried after twelve weeks. They felt deeply affected by this miscarriage, and it precipitated a visit to the general practitioner. Because she had been pregnant once, the general practitioner advised them to just continue trying for a while to conceive, and to return to him if they could not manage on their own. So they did, though at that time Nienke did not feel too happy with just advice alone, and no planned action. They bought an ovulation test – on the advice of one of her friends – and started to have sex when the test indicated that they should do so. But they soon became fed up with this, and visited the general practitioner again. At that point he did some tests, which showed that the quality of Jos' semen was not good, so they were referred to the Radboud Clinic. Additional examinations were carried out at the hospital, but nothing was found to be seriously wrong: the sperm quality was not as bad as initially observed. The doctor therefore sent them home with the message that they could not find an explanation for the fact that they had not conceived thus far; he advised them to continue trying by themselves for another year or so, and that they might enhance their chances of conception by having sex at the moment of ovulation.

To better plan their sex life, some women started (as did Nienke) to keep a record of their ovulation, because they had heard about this from others or read about it on the Internet.[19] Generally, most women started measuring their ovulation on the instruction of their general practitioner or gynaecologist. Some bought sophisticated ovulation tests – with appealing names like 'Maybe Baby' – to help with the measuring, in order to have sex at the right moment. Some couples were very strict about having sex at the right moment, but in general couples were far from enthusiastic about the whole process. The interview excerpt below, part of the second interview with Nienke and Jos, shows just how much they disliked having planned sex:

> Nienke: It puts your relationship pretty much under stress – having sex on command. At a certain moment I really had had enough of the sex. I really felt like 'do we have to do it again?'
> Jos: Yes, that is also what we said to each other: 'It is getting clinical'. Yes, sex becomes clinical. You have to do it then and then . . .
> Nienke: Now, we are doing it less [both laugh]. Are we not? Yes, last Monday evening I intended to go to sleep, but my ova were almost collapsing so we had to!

Jos: Or the other way around: 'We have to . . . but we have already done it'. [Laughter]
Nienke: Yes, I'm really curious to know how others do that. [She changes her voice] 'Come on, do not whine! Just go on.' [Normal voice] Do other couples always feel like having sex? Or are they just doing it because they have to?
Jos: To have to . . . it gets clinical.
Nienke: I don't think it is positive for the experience of sexuality.
Jos: The romance . . .
Nienke: Yes. We do have two kinds of sex: one because we must, and one for fun. And sometimes we do have periods that we say: 'But not now.'

With some laughter – but also with frustration – other couples told me stories about tests that did not function well, thermometers that broke, and the problems they had with having sex at the right moment. Some of them expressed, like Nienke and Jos, their concern that the obligation to have sex at set times was spoiling the quality of their sex life. The negative effects of infertility and infertility treatments on couples' sex lives have been discussed in other studies as well (e.g., Greil et al. 1990; Becker 2000). They found that couples' sex lives were adversely affected due to having to have scheduled intercourse, because sexual intercourse became a means to an end, the act of intercourse became a reminder of the couples' infertility and couples felt their privacy invaded as health staff required information about their lovemaking. A few couples in the current study were absolutely reluctant to have planned sex, as they felt this would not only spoil their sex life, but their entire relationship. Annelies, for example, was very clear about this:

Annelies: I said, 'I'm not going to keep a record of my temperature'. Because then you have to do it on command.
Bart: We did it for a short while.
Annelies: Yes, only two months to know about the ovulation . . . Normally people do that for one year! So, I said, 'no, we are not going to do that' . . . We never had planned sex. We have said to ourselves, 'what happens, happens', but we are very happy now, and we have gone through a lot! It is not going to happen to us – and I know several of these examples – that our relationship is going to collapse because of this. That is not going to happen. Absolutely not!

For Annelies, as well as for some other couples, good sex thus symbolized a good and intimate relationship (cf. Greil 1991: 120). As Greil claimed for the USA, in Dutch society sex also has a 'culturally

assigned meaning' of creating (or reflecting) intimacy between partners and is considered pivotal for a successful relationship.[20] While
some couples felt fed up with having sex on command and therefore stopped doing so after a while, others seemed to be much more
resigned to having planned sex and spoke about it as an unavoidable
part of the process they were in.

Medicalizing the Wish for a Child

Once the couples participating in this study found that disciplining
sexual intercourse would not bring the expected results, they opted
to (further) medicalize their wish for a child. In this section I sketch
in broad strokes the medical trajectories that they went through
from the moment they took their first steps in the medical field. For
most couples the first step was a visit to their general practitioner,
while some couples went directly to the gynaecologist that they
had already been referred to for another reason. [21] Some of these
latter couples wanted to find out whether they, with their particular gynaecological problem, could expect to become pregnant at all
(and they did thus not immediately expect to be treated); for some
others, a miscarriage was the immediate reason for consulting a
doctor.

For the study participants, the period of 'trying by themselves'
before visiting a doctor varied from two months up to two and a half
years; most of them, however, went for a consultation after about
one year of trying to conceive on their own. A similar pattern of
help-seeking was found by the national study on behaviour in case
of fertility problems (NOGO) in the Netherlands.[22] Typically, almost
all the young couples in the current study waited more than a year
before they consulted the doctor, while most of the older couples
waited less than one year before they did so.

Some of the older couples initially felt reluctant to enter the
medical field, as they said they were aware of the pitfalls of the
medical treadmill. These couples also expressed how difficult it was
not to use the medical options, as they were so readily available.
They felt that the mere existence of medical options obliged or
pressurized them to make a choice, and it was hard to say no to
starting treatment. It is noteworthy that this type of pressure –
resulting from the mere existence of medical options – was referred
to more than pressure coming from people surrounding the couple.
All couples stressed – when I asked during the interviews – that it
had been their own decision to seek medical help for their fertility
problem. They all said they did not feel at all pressurized by elders,

other relatives or friends to do so (some of them had not even told others about their fertility problems). Some explicitly emphasized that this was their own choice, and that they would have been upset and reluctant if they had felt such a pressure from parents or others. At the same time, several of the couples – and certainly most of the young couples as we saw above – found it difficult to be confronted with the birth of children of close friends and relatives, as they were eager to let their children grow up with their friends' children. Though these couples did not refer to explicit external pressure to seek medical assistance for their fertility problem, it might be that – on a less conscious level – they were affected by the dominant societal norm to have children. Dutch couples that voluntarily choose to remain childless have reported some form of pressure from their environment (Van Balen and Gerrits 2001a; Nobis 2007). It might be assumed that such a pressure – however subtle – is also exercised on couples who have problems conceiving, and that this affects their decision to seek medical assistance.

Consulting the General Practitioner

In the Netherlands women cannot directly – on their own initiative – visit a gynaecologist. They first have to visit their general practitioner, who can – but not necessarily has to – refer a woman (or couple) to a gynaecologist. In 1998 the Dutch association for general practitioners (NHG) and NVOG agreed on a division of tasks among general practitioners and gynaecologists with regard to sub-fertility problems (NVOG 1998). These guidelines leave space for personal interpretation. When seeing the couples participating in this study that had not managed to conceive, the general practitioners – according to the couples – responded in various ways. In general, they performed some basic medical examinations (including a sperm test) and often they also instructed the women on how to keep track of their ovulation by means of a temperature curve and thus how to plan their sexual intercourse. When the couple had been trying to conceive for less than a year, often – though not always – the general practitioner attempted to reassure them that getting pregnant might take some more time. When the woman had had a miscarriage, which was interpreted as a sign that the couple in principal had the capacity to conceive, couples were also encouraged to continue trying on their own.

Some of the couples who were sent home to continue trying were not at all satisfied with this advice. At that time they were strongly convinced that they would not be able to conceive on their own, and felt that their concerns were not taken seriously. When looking back during the first interview (which took place after they had been given an indication for IVF) some couples felt that history had proved them right in thinking that there would be problems, and they had therefore wasted precious time in 'only trying by themselves'. Generally, these couples returned to the general practitioner earlier than they were advised to. One woman, Margriet, who wanted to avoid 'being sent home without any action being taken', found a way to speed up the initial process. As she knew from friends that her general practitioner requested a temperature curve before taking any action, she had kept record of her ovulation before visiting him. While some women and men perceived the period of trying for themselves (and the advice to do so by their general practitioner) as a waste of time, others were completely satisfied with receiving reassurance only, and were pleased to not immediately enter the 'medical treadmill'. Sooner or later, however, all couples participating in the study were transferred to the clinic, either directly to the Radboud Clinic or first to a peripheral clinic.

Referral to a Peripheral Hospital

Two-thirds of the couples visited a peripheral hospital before they came to visit the Radboud Clinic. Some only went to a peripheral hospital to have their semen tested (with the test results being explained to them by their own general practitioner), while others actually consulted the gynaecologist in the peripheral hospital. When the test results showed the sperm quality to be very bad – which was quite often the case in this study group – and IVF or ICSI treatment was expected to be immediately needed, the couples were directly referred to the Radboud Clinic, as the peripheral hospitals were neither licensed to offer IVF treatments, nor did they have the required laboratory infrastructure to do so. Other couples – whose semen test results showed to be of a fair quality and/or the woman's cycle was found to be irregular – underwent low-tech treatments in the peripheral hospital. These low-tech interventions included hormonal treatments to regulate the cycle or the moment of ovulation and artificial inseminations. The number of low-tech treatment cycles the couples underwent in the peripheral hospitals varied from two to nine. As none of these low-tech treatments lead to an ongoing pregnancy and the birth of a child, at a certain moment the couples were referred to the Radboud Clinic.[23] After having tried a number of unsuccessful low-tech treatments in peripheral hospitals, several couples almost felt relieved that they could finally go to the Radboud Clinic for more advanced treatment. They no longer expected that low-tech treatments would bring them a solution. Only one couple – Anne and Joost – had undergone a series of IVF treatments in another academic hospital nine years before they came for an IVF treatment in the Radboud Clinic.

> Anne (born 1971) was twenty-five years old when she and her partner Joost (born 1968) decided that they wanted to have a child. At that moment they had known each other for about five years. After about one year of unsuccessfully trying to conceive, they visited the general practitioner who referred them to a peripheral hospital. Initial examinations showed serious adhesions in Anne's fallopian tubes, most probably resulting from a Chlamydia infection which Anne perceived as an unpleasant souvenir from a former relationship. At that moment she was given the choice between operations on her fallopian tubes or undergoing an IVF treatment. As the peripheral hospital, which she had visited at that time, could not do the operation, but offered IVF treatments in collaboration with another academic hospital, they opted for IVF. The first IVF treatment was initially successful but ended in a miscarriage after about twelve weeks. They followed this with a second and third IVF; in their last IVF treatment many ova were fertilized and were of good quality, and eight of these embryos could be frozen for use in a later cycle (cryopreservation or cryo). She underwent one cryo, which again was unsuccessful. At that point they decided to obtain a second opinion from gynaecologists at two different academic hospitals, one of which was the fertility clinic at the Radboud Clinic. Both gynaecologists advised her to do the operation. As Anne was pleased with her experience with the gynaecologist at the Radboud Clinic, she and her husband decided to stick with this hospital for further treatment. Together with this gynaecologist they decided that they would first use their frozen embryos before doing the operation, so they contacted the hospital where the embryos were preserved only to find out that they had been discarded without Anne and Joost having given their permission. That was an enormous shock for them, and they did not understand how this could have happened; but at the same time they did not want to sue the hospital as they felt that 'this won't help us to get the embryos back'. Subsequently, they decided to first do the operation before opting for another IVF treatment. Both fallopian tubes were removed, and after a while, when she had recovered from the operation, they decided to go for one more IVF treatment. As she had been pregnant once for twelve weeks, the health insurance was willing to pay for one more IVF treatment, so this was done in the spring of 2004 and proved to be successful. Nine

months later Anne and Joost – who had by this time reached the age
of thirty-four and thirty-seven – became parents. It had taken them
four IVF treatments in two different clinics and nine years of their life
to finally achieve their goal – a child of their own.

Ending up at the Radboud Clinic

At the moment the couples participating in the study visited the
Radboud Clinic for the first time, they had thus gone through quite
different trajectories. Some of them had yet to undergo any medical
examinations at all; some had been tested but still did not know
what impeded them from conceiving; others had been tested and
had a fairly good idea of why they could not become pregnant; and
still others had already undergone a series of treatments at another
hospital. Once entering the Radboud Clinic, an initial or additional
diagnosis was performed and – in most cases – treatments were
initiated.

The clinical practices at the fertility clinic of the Radboud Clinic,
and the way couples responded to these practices, are central
issues in the following chapters; in this section I merely sum up
the couples' diagnoses, treatments and outcomes. In ten out of the
twenty-three couples, a factor affecting the male partner was diagnosed as the single cause of the fertility problem (this is higher than
the average contribution of male factors to infertility, which is normally estimated at around one third [NVOG 1996, 1999]).[24] In only
four cases was a female factor found to be the single cause of the
fertility problem; in four couples both partners contributed to the
fertility problem; while for five couples the fertility problem was
unexplained.[25]

Most couples participating in the study (nineteen) underwent
IVF or related treatments (it should be noted that sixteen of them
were specifically selected for that reason – see inclusion criteria
in Chapter 1). Two couples were still undergoing low-tech fertility treatments at the moment I contacted them for the last time to
collect data (August 2006), and two couples did not undergo any
fertility treatment at all (one couple split up just before starting their
first IUI treatment, and the other withdrew from the IVF waiting
list).[26]

Finally, eleven of the twenty-three couples (about fifty per cent)
ended their quest for conception with the birth of one or two
child(ren) (two women gave birth to twins). Eight of the eleven
pregnancies leading to the birth of these children resulted from

IVF/ICSI treatments at the Radboud Clinic; two children were conceived through TESE treatment abroad; and one couple spontaneously became pregnant after two IVF treatment failures. In addition, one of the couples adopted a child before the study was finalized.

Complementary and Alternative Medicine

The medicalization of fertility problems did not stop at the boundaries of the formal health care system. In pursuit of their goal to have a child of their own, several couples demonstrated pragmatism in the use of Complementary and Alternative Medicine (CAM).[27] Half of the couples (twelve) visited one or more alternative healers, generally in the same period as they visited the fertility clinic. The percentage of couples that sought help from alternative medicine in the current study is substantially higher than the 17 per cent, which Verdurmen (1997) found in her study of couples with fertility problems in the Netherlands.[28]

In the present study, couples with higher education were more inclined to seek help from alternative medicine than people with lower education: in six out of the twelve couples visiting an alternative healer, one or both partner(s) were highly educated, while only two men with lower education visited an alternative healer. Some of the couples explained that they did not opt for alternative types of medicine because they knew that this could not provide a solution for their type of fertility problem (e.g., removed ovaries or sterilization of the man). CAM used by the couples included acupuncture, Chinese herbal medicine, homeopathy and extra-sensory perception (*paragnost*). In addition, beds were removed to prevent the negative working of radiation (*aardstralen*), candles were burnt and medallions worn in the hope that clinic treatments would be more effective (see Coulson and Jenkins (2005) for a long list of CAM options for infertility).

Ambivalence about the use of alternative medicine was sometimes expressed, in particular by those couples that were not used to visiting alternative health care providers. However, they used two types of arguments to justify its use for their problem: first, they felt that they should try anything that might possibly help them to become pregnant, including alternative medicine; and second, many of them were of the opinion that 'if it does not do any good, it does not do any harm either'.

Couples made use of CAM for two interconnected reasons: either to actually – physically – improve the conditions for getting pregnant, and/or to feel more relaxed when undergoing IVF treatment in the clinic in the hope that this would increase their chances of success. The perceived effectiveness of the alternative medicine was judged accordingly. One woman, for example, was satisfied with the alternative medicine used because her irregular menstrual bleeding stopped as a result of the homeopathic medicines she had taken (which she had actually started taking to treat haemorrhoids); and another said that her mucus became thicker due to the acupuncturist treatment. While most couples saw some form of positive effect from the alternative medicine – even if only that it calmed them down – others were sceptical or disappointed by it, and set their own limits. One couple, for example, perceived the use of dried human placenta as an ingredient for a Chinese medicine as one step too far; they were relieved when they found out that this medicine was not available in the Netherlands. Others were disappointed about the way they were treated – long waiting times, paying lots of money and being given false hope, receiving vague diagnoses or advice – and decided not to return to that particular healer. Though none of the participants claimed that they actually became pregnant through the use of CAM, some felt that the good results of an IVF cycle, which had been undertaken concurrently with alternative medicine, were partly due to the alternative treatment.[29]

Few couples spoke about their visits to alternative healers with clinic staff. Some thought that doctors and nurses would not like them to visit alternative healers and therefore purposely avoided talking about it; others just did not mention it, and said they did not mind whether the hospital staff would approve of it or not. Twice I was present when couples spoke with the attending doctor about the use of CAM (a visit to an acupuncturist and the use of homeopathic medicines respectively). In the first case the doctor reacted positively, responding that she was an acupuncturist herself (though she did not do fertility patients), and she added that couples should do what they felt good about. In the second case the doctor was sceptical; she could not imagine how the homeopathic medicines could have resolved the woman's irregular bleeding. The woman was upset about the doctor's negative reaction (though she did not show this in the presence of the doctor), but she herself felt that she had prevented an operation by taking these medicines.

Health professionals at the Radboud Clinic certainly did not encourage 'shopping around' in alternative health systems, and a number of times I heard doctors express their concerns about the use of alternative medicine; besides being sceptical about its effectiveness, they were worried that it would raise false hopes and that couples would spend too much money on it. Despite these concerns on the part of health professionals, some of the couples were fairly pragmatic about its use, and even when they did not really understand or share the basic principles of these alternative health systems, they merely hoped that it would bring them closer to their desired goal.

Adoption as a Last Resort

In theory, adoption and fostering are non-medical ways to resolve the problem of childlessness. In practice, however, few couples participating in this study were in favour of these solutions. All couples preferred to have 'a child of their own'. At its best, adoption was seen as a last resort.[30] Van Balen et al. (1995: 20) also found that only 5 per cent of Dutch couples with fertility problems opted for adoption. Several of the men and women in the current study had strong objections to adoption; most of them did not seriously want to consider adoption before having exhausted all medical means to conceive a child of their own (cf. Becker 2000). Three couples, and in particular the women (all highly educated), were positive about adoption right from the beginning of the medical trajectory, though they also preferred first to attempt to have a child of their own by using available medical technologies.[31] During the course of the study six couples (one quarter of the study group) signed up for adoption, including the three couples who were positive about adoption right from the beginning. The other three couples drastically changed their views about adoption as a possible solution for childlessness along the treatment process, as was the case for Chris and Mireille.

> Chris (born 1967) and Mireille (born 1974) met each other in 1997, and their wish for a child dated from 2002. When they did not manage to conceive they consulted their general practitioner, who referred them immediately to the Radboud Clinic. It became clear straight away that Chris' sperm was of extremely 'bad quality', and so they were directly entered onto the waiting list for IVF-ICSI. In that time they had spoken about adoption, but did not really want to consider it. As Chris expressed it: 'I want to think positively about the ICSI treatments'. They did four IVF treatments, which Mireille experienced as incredibly burdensome, both physically and emotionally.

In the last interview I spoke again with them about the possibilities
of adoption and the use of donor semen.

> Chris: Yes, we spoke about adoption, possibly . . .
> Mireille: And a year ago, you should not have asked me, because then
> I would immediately have said 'no' . . . Yes, things are just changing
> a lot. You are going to think differently about it, because when treat-
> ment fails, you choose to stay as just the two of us, or – possibly – for
> adoption.
> TG: . . . And did you ever speak about the possibility of using donor
> semen?
> Chris: Yes, but with donor semen you have the risk that at the end
> you [I] say, 'It is yours, it's not mine'. That is not what I want. That is
> the most difficult thing. Therefore, I say that I do not want that. And
> therefore I rather prefer adoption, because then it is for both of us . . .
> You start together, and – let me say it like this – it is equally for both
> of us.

In the course of the interviews couples expressed different types
of feelings and arguments for and against adoption. With regard
to arguments against adoption, the feeling that an adoptive child
would never really be your own child was paramount, reflecting the
value in Dutch contemporary culture that is attached to the 'primacy
of biology' when defining parenthood (cf. Becker 2000: 238). As
most adopted children in the Netherlands come from abroad (from
China, or African or Latin American countries) it is likely that the
child would not look like its adoptive parents and therefore couples
felt it would be difficult for the child to identify with them.[32] In addition, the role of genetics in a child's constitution also played a role in
some people's arguments; they thus 'chased the blood tie' (Ragoné
1996). One man, for example, stressed that it has been proved that
some behaviour, like criminality for example, is genetically defined,
and that made him hesitate about going for adoption and the use
of donor semen alike, because 'you never know what you will get
in your house'. Linked to these ideas about genetics is the couples'
preference for having a child of 'the two of them together', as an
expression or confirmation of their love for each other, and in the
hope that they recognize each other's and their own features in their
child.[33] This argument was emphasized by couples where one of the
partners already had a child of his or her own. Adopting a child was
then considered rather a step backwards (because the child would
not have any genetic links with either of them) instead of a step
forwards: it would not bring them closer to the realization of their

desire to have a child of the two of them together. Consequently, none of the couples who already had a child (from one or both partners) opted for adoption.

Another major argument against adoption was based on the assumption that adoptive children are likely to be more problematic to educate than a child of your own. First, because they are not well attached, and this was in particular thought to be problematic when the child would be older (no longer a baby) during the adoption process. Secondly, adopted children may want to eventually search for their roots, which could cause tension and uncertainty in the future. When talking about this, women and men often referred to *Spoorloos* (meaning literally 'without a trace'), a Dutch television programme that supports adoptive children in their search for their biological parents. If such a search is successful, the reunion between an adopted child and his/her biological parent takes place in the presence of the camera, and is observed by many people on TV (see also Kaptein and Van Berkel 2002: 59). These kinds of programmes – and similar stories in popular magazines and on the Internet – shape and confirm people's ideas about the importance of biological bonds between parents and children, and about the risks involved in adoption. Aside from the influence of this public representation of adoption, it should be noted that several couples were also influenced by their own nearby – predominantly negative – experiences with adoptive children. While these couples readily admitted that their own negative experiences did not automatically imply that adoption never works, it was obvious that the dominant discourse surrounding adoption was more negative than positive.

Bureaucratic and financial obstacles were also referred to as major arguments against adoption. For couples in the Netherlands an adoption trajectory may take three to five years from the first moment couples sign up to adopt; they have to be screened – both medically and by a branch of the Ministry of Justice (Raad voor de Kinderbescherming) – and they have to attend a preparatory course of six sessions. In addition, Dutch adoption law has defined that the age difference between the child to be adopted and the oldest parent should not be more than forty years; and in principle, the adoptive elders should not be older than forty-one; however, for people older than this exemptions can sometimes be made (Heida 2001: 120). The age criteria, the extended selection and approval procedures and the long waiting time were perceived as major obstacles. Peter summarized his practical arguments against adoption thus:

We have thought about it. And when you think about it, no, I do not
want it, because it entails many disadvantages. You have to wait for
five or six years, and I am thirty-five now, and then I will be forty-
two. And I also think the costs are ridiculous – very high ... The
waiting time is the worst. I understand that they have to investigate
everything well, that they want to place the children well, but that it
has to take this long, I think it is a shame! There the story ends for me.
I will just be too old then.

Some couples argued that they would not be able to stand any
more waiting: they felt that because of the extended period of trying
to become pregnant, their life had already been in a waiting room
for too long. They felt that, once having finished the treatment, they
would finally want to go on with setting up their life, without again
having to wait for something to happen. The costs involved in adoption formed another major obstacle. These costs include expenses
for the information sessions and the residence permit for the child
(around 1,200 Euros), mediation costs, which may differ from 7,500
to 22,700 Euros, plus travel costs to pick up the child (Van Duin
2005). Some couples explicitly compared the costs of adoption with
the costs of one more IVF treatment (at that moment around 2,200
to 3,200 Euros per treatment), which did not contribute to a positive
consideration of adoption: one can pay for quite a number of IVF
treatments with the costs of one adoption.

Finally, an argument against adoption at a more ideological or
political level that was mentioned by only a few couples is that
adoption does not really solve the problem for the children involved.
Abandoned or orphaned children should be taken care of in their
own country, in their own environment, instead of being transported to the Netherlands to solve the problem of childless couples.
If people really wanted to do something for these children, they
argued, they should financially support them over there.

Contrarily, helping those children who are in poor conditions
and 'sharing our affluence', was in fact the motivation most often
mentioned by those women (and one man) who were in favour of
adoption from the onset. Ria, who was one of them, said the following, before undergoing any form of treatment:

I certainly would consider adoption. I think it must be wonderful to
be pregnant, but if we will not be able to achieve that, I see space
in our life for an adopted child – or children – who are in need of
care. There are so many children who do not have a pleasant life,
and we could offer them a nice life. Such a child, of course, is not

your biological child, and that makes a difference . . . But that does not mean that it will not be your child in other ways, emotionally, in everything. Yes, I am rather positive about it.

Like Ria, other women (and one man) also mentioned emotional reasons for being pro-adoption: they felt they could easily love a child that was not biologically their own and thought this was a good alternative to help create a family. Two of the couples who were initially negative about adoption also used the latter argument for adoption – though less enthusiastically – after a number of failed IVF treatments: as they could not create a family by giving birth to their own child, they decided to opt for adoption as a last resort to resolve their childlessness. That this was not an easy step to take is clearly illustrated by the following excerpt from Louise's diary, which she wrote before starting the third IVF treatment:

> We made a difficult decision: we have signed up for adoption. Cry-ing, I completed the forms for the Ministry of Justice. For a long time we could not believe that it would come this far for us, but now I am more than ever convinced that we will not have children ourselves. It is a very big step to sign up for adoption. It is as if you have already given up and accepted that no children will come. Terrible. But the desire to educate children – even when they are not our own – is too big.

Yet, even when this initial step to adoption was set, the couples often continued hoping for a child of their own.

At the end of the data collection period three of the six couples who had signed up for adoption managed to conceive on their own, and stopped adoption procedures; three other couples continued the adoption procedures. One of these couples, who from the beginning had been in favour of adoption, had – against the rules – already started the adoption procedures in the period that they were still doing IVF treatments. On the day that they were confronted with a miscarriage after their third IVF treatment, they also received an invitation letter from the adoption organization to attend the 'adop-tion course'. They perceived this as a positive coincidence; it helped them to say goodbye to the IVF treatments, even though they still considered doing another IVF treatment at a later moment. About two and a half years later they finally went to pick up their child in China. Some years later – long after the study had ended – they sent me a card, announcing the arrival of their second adopted child, again from China.

Conclusion

This chapter shows the diversity of the couples with fertility problems participating in this study and of the processes they have gone through in their quest for a child. In addition, I have drawn attention to a number of trends and patterns affecting their views, experiences and choices.

First, I contrasted younger and older couples. Most of the younger couples had less education, which reflects a similar trend in Dutch society with regard to age and child bearing (Beets 2004). The older couples, however, were not only highly educated career women who postponed childbearing for the sake of their career (as they are often depicted in the mass media and literature), but included women and men of different levels of education who, for several reasons or life circumstances, did not start having children at an earlier phase. Typically, the older couples were in a hurry to visit the clinic and initiate fertility treatments as they felt their – and in particular the woman's – biological clocks were ticking. Most of the younger couples in this study, however, were also found not to want to lose precious time, though they had a different reason: they wished to keep up with the same 'pace of life' as their siblings and friends from their youth. Clearly, they hoped to avoid 'a disruption of their [culturally] expected life course' (Becker 2000: 62). Further, the fact that all these couples – low-, middle- and high-income groups – had equal access to infertility treatment, including high-tech ARTs, reflects the Dutch ART and health insurance policy, which aims to make all treatments affordable to all.

With regard to the help-seeking behaviour of the couples – their quest for conception (Inhorn 1996) or for a child – we have seen that, for almost all couples in this study, seeking medical advice in the formal health care system was their first choice, rather than seeking alternative solutions such as alternative medicine, adoption or doing nothing. A similar pattern of help-seeking was found in the nationwide study on people's choices when confronted with fertility problems (Van Balen et al. 1995; Verdurmen 1997). Some older couples initially felt reluctant to enter the medical field, as they expressed an awareness of the pitfalls of the medical treadmill, while others stated that the mere existence of the medical options obliged or pressured them to make a choice, making it difficult not to enter the medical system. This type of pressure – the mandate from technology (Sandelowski 1993: 49) – was referred to more often than any form of social pressure (and will be further addressed in Chapter 6). Couples stressed that it was their own choice to go for medical treatment, though it might be that, on an unconscious level, they have been affected by the dominant norm in Dutch society that having children is still seen as a basic and integral part of growing up, even when voluntary childlessness is accepted to a certain extent (Nobis 2007).

Couples' strong preference for having a child of 'the two of us' points to the 'imperative of genetics' and their wish to adhere to ideals of the traditional family. The couples where only one of the partners had a child (or more than one) from a former relationship were keen to also have a biological child with their current partner, but did not consider adoption (as none of them would have a genetic tie with an adopted child). Dominant (cultural) discourses, which were negative about adoption and emphasized the role of genetics in people's personality, and the existing bureaucratic and administrative adoption regulations in the Netherlands, were for most couples seen as being prohibitive against adoption. The couples that seriously considered adoption did so only after all medical treatments had been explored.

Couples' quests for children did not stop at the boundaries of the formal health care system. Half of the couples participating in this study consulted CAM at one moment or another. They did so either to actually, physically improve the conditions for becoming pregnant, and/or to feel more relaxed when undergoing IVF treatment in the clinic. Hardly anything is known about the use of CAM in the case of infertility. My findings suggest that on the one hand CAM has the potential to exploit desperate infertile people and its use may lead to disappointment and scepticism; on the other hand CAM seems to provide some sort of support, care or attention that the couples did not (expect to) find at the Radboud Clinic.[34] In the chapter that follows I move from the trajectories of the couples to the patient-centred care as offered and experienced at the Radboud Clinic.

Notes

1. Their dissatisfaction about the treatment will be discussed in more depth in Chapter 5.
2. Only one female participant did not have Dutch nationality; she was born in a neighbouring country, but had lived in the Netherlands for about twenty years and spoke fluent Dutch.

3. These characteristics were part of the set criteria defined for participation in this study, namely that couples should reside within the IVF Region Nijmegen, that at least one of the couple had to be 'autochthon' Dutch, and both had to speak fluent Dutch (see Chapter 1).

4. De Boer et al. (2004) reported an average age of women using IVF for the first time of 32.3 in 1985 and 32.9 in 1994; Lintsen et al. (2007) report an average age of 33.6 among women using IVF for the first time in the period from 2002–4. These study groups are not fully comparable with my study group as in the current study not all participants used IVF and some of them were not first time IVF users.

5. See www.gemiddeld-inkomen.nl (Retrieved 21 March 2015). The net modal income refers to the income that most people have.

6. This refers to the couples' insurance status in 2004. In 2004 people earning less than 32,600 Euros Gross Income were mandatorily insured by the public health insurance (Ziekenfonds). In 2006 the Dutch health insurance system changed, and subsequently the distinction between private and public health insurance no longer exists (see also Chapter 2).

7. Most of the information presented in this section was collected by the 'Timeline' method: I asked the couples to compose their reproductive life history, using a long piece of paper and post-it notes (see Appendix 1 for more information on this method).

8. In addition, Becker (2000: 30–31) observed that women participating in her study referred to the 'metaphor of life as a journey', which enabled them to see the hardship they had to go through as part of a 'process of integrating disruption and restoring a sense of order, and thus continuity of life'. Becker (ibid.: 62) further argues that the tendency in the USA 'to focus on continuity in life rather than on disruption can be seen as a cultural ideology that informs people's efforts to ameliorate infertility'. A similar tendency can definitely be observed in the Netherlands as well.

9. Strikingly, the only highly educated couple among the young starters commented that most of their friends had not yet started having children, and they often received the comment that they should not worry too much as they 'were still young' and 'had plenty of time'.

10. DES daughters are women who were exposed to DES (Diethylstilbestrol®) before birth (in the womb). Research has confirmed that DES daughters are at an increased risk for – among others – infertility. Retrieved 23 March 2016 from www.cdc.gov/des/consumers/about/index.html.

11. Miscarriage had also occurred to women among the younger starters, though less frequent.

12. Both authors argue that Dutch (highly educated) women postpone child bearing because they find it difficult to combine parenthood and a professional career, partly as a result of failing government support to facilitate this. Without intending to deny the importance of structural

measurements enabling women and men to better combine work and child rearing, my study findings do not support the idea that postponing childbearing and the subsequent use of IVF at a later age result from the lack of structural measures.

13. When I shared this observation with some of the clinic staff, they thought that this applied to their patient population in general, though they also met women (couples) who consciously postponed childbearing for career motives.

14. In a study among women on the waiting list for oocyte freezing in a Dutch clinic a similar pattern was found: while all women participating in that study were higher educated, none of them referred to their career as a reason to postpone childbearing. Rather, they referred to not having a partner with whom they could plan a family as the major reason for postponement. They all preferred to create a 'traditional' family, having children of their own partner (De Groot et al. 2013).

15. With the exception of one man who did not have any contact with his child.

16. Becker (2000: 72) observed that women much more than men underlined the importance of recognizing their partner in their child. This was less outspoken among the Dutch participants in this study; I heard both men and women make similar comments.

17. In the case of the sterilized man, the attempt to reverse the sterilization failed; for one of the women the sterilization was successfully reversed, but subsequently it was found that one of her fallopian tubes was obstructed; for the other woman, undoing the sterilization was not an option at all as her fallopian tubes had been removed during the sterilization procedure without her being aware of it (see the case of Liset and Alexander, presented at the beginning of this chapter).

18. Since the end of 1980s men at the Radboud Clinic have been offered the option of freezing their semen before undergoing chemotherapy.

19. A number of menstrual cycle monitors have been developed to detect the fertile window of the menstrual cycle, mainly for contraceptive purposes. Reliable data on most of these systems are still missing. Braat et al. (1998) did a small-scale test of a saliva test in the Radboud Clinic, and found that the test was unreliable for predicting the fertile period and therefore should be discouraged. Thus, in contrast to its widespread use, medical staff at the Radboud Clinic did not consider keeping a temperature curve to be an effective means of measuring the hormonal cycle.

20. In a study among Dutch couples 'sexual problems' were reported by 24 per cent of the men and 28 per cent of the women as a reason for divorce; it was the third most mentioned reason, after 'communicational problems' and 'incompatible characters' (Van den Troost 2005: 18). Gender dynamics in Dutch conjugal relationships are discussed further in Chapter 7.

21. Only one couple visited an alternative healer before going to their general practitioner, as they thought the general practitioner would immediately refer them to the hospital, a step they had hoped to avoid.

22. In the NOGO it was found that 72 per cent of the couples who visited the general practitioner for their fertility problem did so after one year of trying to conceive in vain (Van Balen et al. 1995: 20). For more information on this study see Chapter 1.

23. For two couples these treatments at one point resulted in a pregnancy, though both ended in a miscarriage.

24. It is acknowledged that the estimation of male factor fertility is a rule of thumb rather than based on scientific evidence (see also NVOG 1999).

25. These are the couples' diagnoses as registered in the computerized data files of the Radboud Clinic.

26. For the latter couple, the reason for withdrawing was due to the expected burden of the treatment in combination with a non-supportive husband (see an extensive discussion of Kim and Andre's case, Chapter 7). With regard to the other couple, the reason they split up was – as they both said – not related to their fertility problem.

27. The use of Complementary and Alternative Medicine for infertility in Western countries has been observed, but thus far few studies have examined this issue (as exceptions, see Verdurmen 1997; Coulson and Jenkins 2005).

28. This might either be due to a selection bias or to the way data was collected. Regarding the latter, it might be that in this study – as I spoke intensively and frequently about all phases of the couples' trajectories – couples remembered or mentioned more visits to alternative healers, even when these were occasional events, than what they would mention in a one-time interview contact. In one case a woman explicitly told me in the third interview that she had initially hidden her visit to an alternative healer from me as she thought I might disapprove of it.

29. Coulson and Jenkins (2005: 2) mentioned that patients described encounters with a CAM provider in terms of a person who was 'really interested', 'who listened really carefully to what I was saying' or 'who seemed to understand how I feel'. From this, the authors contend, doctors in the biomedical system could learn to refine their listening and counselling skills.

30. The issue of fostering was hardly mentioned by the couples, and therefore will not be included in this section.

31. Two of these women had been thinking of adoption anyhow, even when they thought they would be able to conceive 'normally'. One of these woman said she did not necessarily need to exploit all medical options before deciding about adoption, and the other (together with her husband) had been thinking of creating a family of both their own *and* adopted children.

32. On a yearly basis around 1,100 children are adopted in the Netherlands (Van Hoksbergen 2002).
33. The genetics argument – as we will see in Chapter 7 – was also used by some of the couples for whom the use of donor semen could have been a solution. Some of the men dreaded that if their wife conceived with donor semen they would feel that the child was more connected to their wife than to them, and that they would not consider it to be their own child (cf. Ngemera 2001: 52–54).
34. More studies are needed to better understand the role (and potential) of CAM in infertility care.

References

Becker, G. 2000. *The Elusive Embryo: How women and men approach new reproductive technologies.* Berkeley: University of California Press.

Beets, G.C.N. 2004. 'De timing van het eerste kind: Een overzicht.', *Bevolking en Gezin* 33(1): 115–42.

Braat, D.D.M. 2000. 'Donor-eicellen: Wanneer en bij wie?', in W.C.M. Weijmar-Schultz (ed.), *Fertiliteit en ethiek, een kind tot (w)elke prijs?* Symposium WPOG, 10 November 2000. Groningen: Instituut Wenckebach.

Braat, D.D., Smeenk, J.M., Manger, A.P., Thomas, C.M., Veersema, S., and Merkus, J.M. 1998. 'Saliva test as ovulation predictor', *The Lancet,* 352(9136): 1283–1284.

Coulson, C. and J. Jenkins, 2005. 'Complementary and alternative medicine utilisation in NHS and private clinic settings: A United Kingdom survey of 400 infertility patients', *Journal of Experimental and Clinical Assisted Reproduction* 2(1): 5.

De Boer, E.J., Van Leeuwen, F.E., Den Tonkelaar I., Jansen, C.A.M., Braat, D.D.M., and Burger, C.W. (2004). 'Methoden en resultaten van in-vitrofertilisatie in Nederland in de jaren 1983–1994', *Nederlands Tijdschrift voor Geneeskunde,* 148(29), 1448–1455.

De Groot, M., Dancet, E.A.F., Repping, S., Stoop, D., Goddijn, M., Van der Veen, F., and Gerrits, T. (2013, June). 'The voice of Dutch women with anticipated gamete exhaustion who consider oocyte freezing to increase their chances on shared parenthood', *Human Reproduction,* 28: 66.

Greil, A.L., K.L. Porter and T.A. Leitko. 1990. 'Sex and intimacy among infertile couples', *Journal of Psychology and Human Sexuality* 2(2): 117–37.

Heida, A. 2001. 'Juridische aspecten van reproductieve technieken', in S. de Joode (ed.), *Zwanger van de kinderwens: Visies, feiten en vragen over voortplantingstechnologie.* Den Haag: Rathenau Instituut, pp. 108–21.

Inhorn, M.C. 1994. *Quest for conception: Gender, infertility, and Egyptian medical traditions.* Philadelphia: University of Pennsylvania Press.

Inhorn, M.C. and D. Birenbaum-Carmeli. 2008. 'Assisted reproductive technologies and culture change', *Annual Review of Anthropology* 37: 177–96.

Kaptein, M. and D. Van Berkel. 2002. 'Is bloed dikker dan water? Over zoekacties en het belang van de bloedband', in F. Van Balen, D. Van Berkel, H.Bos, Y. de Roode, J. Verdurmen (eds), *Van adoptie tot eiceldonatie. Op zoek naar oplossingen voor onvruchtbaarheid.* Nijkerk: Uitgeverij van Brug, pp. 47–73.

Lintsen, A.M.E., Eijkemans, M.J.C., Hunault, C.C., Bouwmans, C.A.M., Hakkaart, L., Habbema, J.D.F., and Braat, D.D.M. 2007. 'Predicting ongoing pregnancy chances after IVF and ICSI: a national prospective study', *Human Reproduction* 22(9), 2455–2462.

Ngemera, D.B. 2001. 'Dutch men experiencing infertility, infertility treatment and involuntary childlessness'. Amsterdam: University of Amsterdam (Unpublished MA thesis). Retrieved 23 March 2016 from dare.uva.nl.

NVOG. 1996. *Richtlijn. Oriënterend fertiliteitsonderzoek (OFO).* Retrieved 1 March 2015 from www.nvog.nl.

———— 1998. *Landelijke Transmurale Afspraak. Subfertiliteit.* Retrieved 1 March 2015 from www.nvog.nl.

———— 1999. *Richtlijn. Onderzoek en behandeling mannelijke subfertiliteit.* Retrieved 1 March 2015 from www.nvog.nl.

Nobis, E. 2007. *Geen kinderen geen bezwaar. Waarom niet alle vrouwen moeder willen zijn.* Amsterdam/Antwerpen: Uitgeverij Contact.

Ragoné, H. 1996. 'Chasing the blood tie: surrogate mothers, adoptive mothers and fathers', *American Ethnologist* 23(2): 352–65.

RIVM (Rijksinstituut voor Volksgezondheid en Milieu). 2006. *Nationaal Kompas Volksgezondheid, versie 3.7.* Bilthoven: RIVM.

Sandelowski, M. 1993. *With child in mind. Studies of the personal encounter with infertility.* Philadelphia: University of Pennsylvania Press.

Te Velde, E.R. 1991. *Zwanger worden in de 21ste eeuw: Steeds later, steeds kunstmatiger.* Utrecht: Oratie, Rijksuniversiteit Utrecht.

Van Balen, F. and T. Gerrits. 2001a. 'Kinderwens in context', in S. de Joode, (ed). *Zwanger van de kinderwens: Visies, feiten en vragen over voortplantingstechnologie.* Den Haag: Rathenau Instituut, pp. 28–37.

Van Balen, F., E. Ketting and J. Verdurmen. 1995. *Zorgen rond onvruchtbaarheid: Voornaamste bevindingen van het Nationaal Onderzoek naar Gedrag bij Onvruchtbaarheid.* Delft: Eburon.

Van Duin, J. 2005. *Toename adoptie vraagt extra zorg.* Retrieved 1 September 2008 from www.pedagogiek.net.

Van den Troost, A. 2005. *Marriage in Motion: A study on the social context and processes of marital satisfaction.* Leuven: Leuven University Press.

Van Hoksbergen, R. 2002. 'Vijftig jaar adoptie in Nederland. Een historisch-statistische beschouwing'. Utrecht: University of Utrecht, Afdeling Adoptie. Retrieved 1 September 2008 from www.pedagogiek-online.nl.

Van Praag, C.S. and M. Niphuis-Nell (eds). 1997. *Het gezinsrapport; een verkennende studie naar het gezin in een veranderende samenleving*. Rijswijk: Sociaal en Cultureel Planbureau.

Verdurmen, J. 1997. 'Keuzes bij onvruchtbaarheid. Besluitvorming bij onvruchtbare paren'. Ph.D. dissertation. Amsterdam: University of Amsterdam.

Chapter 4

DAILY PRACTICES IN THE
PATIENT-CENTRED CLINIC

Together with Dr J. Kremer, head of the IVF department, I walk for
the first time through the corridors of the fertility clinic. This morning I received permission to do my study. So, when Dr Kremer suggested taking a tour through the clinic, of course I eagerly agreed.
We enter the clinic from a back door and the first stop we make is at
the waiting room for IVF patients. The waiting room is a small niche
of about three metres in breadth, with chairs on both sides, a small
table with some magazines, a tea and coffee thermos, cups, sugar
and milk. Most of the wall on one side is covered by a notice board,
on which is displayed all kind of information sheets. I take a quick
look and comment to Dr Kremer: 'So, this is where my study starts'.
He looks a bit puzzled and as I am fully aware that having a medical
anthropologist around is a new phenomenon for him, I quickly add,
'The things that you put on the wall give me an indication of what
you, staff members, think is important for your patients to take notice
of'. I point to some of the things I noticed, including a summary of
the results of the yearly users' satisfaction study, an overview of the
'complaints and suggestions' and how they were dealt with by staff
members and a small notice book where people can jot down their
experiences with the treatment in the clinic. There is also a sheet of
paper, stating in big letters: 'This is an academic hospital, therefore
student staff are often present during treatment and consultation
hours. Please, let us know if you do not appreciate this'. In addition,
I see that next to the notice board, in a nice frame, is displayed the
clinic's DIA certificate – the Dutch Infertility Award. This prize was
awarded to the fertility clinic for being the most patient friendly IVF
clinic in the Netherlands and they received the prize for a second year

from Freya. Dr Kremer smiles a bit at my observations and then we continue our tour. (Diary TG)

From the first moment I entered the Radboud Clinic I was struck by the amount of attention given to the voices and views of the women and men who visit. Clinic staff showed themselves to be strongly aware of the fact that the people visiting their clinic had needs and preferences that were not purely medical-technical, but had to do with the way they would like to be treated and informed. It is part of the Radboud Clinic's patient-centred policy to attempt to address these needs and preferences. In this chapter I describe how this patient-centred policy is employed in daily practice – thus focusing on the actual dynamics and interactions between the health staff and women and men visiting the clinic – and the study participants' experiences and views thereof. The chapter is divided along the lines of four themes that stood out as major issues in the interviews and observations, which are: interpersonal aspects of care, privacy, the provision of information, and psycho-social support. Subsequently I address the question of how this particular context – the patient-centred clinic – affects decision-making about (further) use of reproductive technologies.

Interpersonal Aspects of Care

Not Being Treated as a Number

I am sitting in the corridor. Close to me a couple is waiting for their embryo transfer. One of the nurses passes the couple, when suddenly she recognizes them. She stops, turns back to them and greets them in a friendly way. Then she asks, 'And how have things gone after the ova pick-up?' A short conversation develops and at the end the nurse wishes them good luck. (Diary TG)

The above observation is an example of just one of the many occasions in which I noticed the friendliness and personal involvement of clinic staff members regarding the women and men visiting their clinic. They often seemed to remember people's faces, their names and one or another relevant medical or personal detail, which they demonstrated to the women and men visiting the clinic. Friendly greetings, handshakes and the question, 'How are you?' were part of the daily routine when encountering patients in the consultation rooms and sometimes in the corridor as well. Staff members often showed genuine interest in how couples' treatments developed. They followed treatment processes by means of information provided in formal staff meetings, but also through less formal collegial encounters in staff rooms or in the corridors. In particular, the couples who were doing IVF or a related treatment and who visited the clinic regularly during a short period of time often became quite familiar with the IVF staff. While preparing for the ova pick-up or for the embryo transfer, which takes some time, all kinds of conversations would develop. Often they were about the treatment procedure or the stress involved, but they could also be about a shared interest in dogs or music. Despite the seriousness, the stress and sometimes pain of the medical proceedings, it was not rare to hear an animated conversation or laughter coming out of a treatment room or in the corridor.

When I asked the couples to reflect on the way they felt treated at the fertility clinic, the first comment almost all of them made was one or another positive statement about the friendliness of the people working at the clinic. Often they referred to nurses or doctors, but some of them also added positive remarks about a helpful lady at the reception desk or about the gentle laboratory technician who phoned them at home to explain the outcome of a laboratory procedure. Apparently, being treated nicely and respectfully by staff members was important to the couples (cf. Halman et al. 1993; Inhorn 2003). They were pleased at 'not being treated as a number' – as several of them commented – and obviously appreciated that. Many added that they had not expected to find this kind of human attitude or personal touch in an academic hospital. As Ria explained:

> It is much more personal than I expected it to be. They do, I don't know how many treatments a year! In fact it is a factory which is doing this and still you have the feeling that you are treated very personally.

Most emphasized that they felt well listened to and that there was often plenty of time to ask questions. This made them feel that they were being taken seriously and were in good hands. Marijke and Geert, who had strong doubts about initiating high-tech treatments for ethical reasons, felt relieved by being cared for in such an attentive way:

> It felt that much okay, that we said to each other, 'Yes, here we dare to do it'. It gave us a safe feeling.

Some of the couples said that in fact they liked all the staff members they met. As one of the women said, 'It is as if they select their staff based on their friendliness'. However, personal sympathies and antipathies existed as well and both were sometimes strongly expressed. As Mireille, who was quite irritated about the impersonal way she felt she was dealt with by one of the doctors, cynically said:

> That doctor would be better not handling patients . . . She is not really caring or concerned about people.

When making these types of remarks about individual staff members, couples often added that personal preferences are normal in human relationships and that staff members may have bad days as they themselves can have bad days. In addition, they recognized that people and their styles are different, so they could not and did not expect to have a good rapport with each and every staff member. This meant that a doctor that was almost glorified by one woman ('She is absolutely *my* doctor') was depicted as distant and impersonal by another. Sometimes couples were positive about a doctor or nurse in particular because they felt they got special attention or treatment, or an extra chance because of his or her personal involvement and concern: 'If it were not for her, I would not have got the chance to do this treatment'. Some people felt disappointed about a less positive encounter or the distant attitude of a medical doctor at a certain moment, as this contrasted so much with what they were used to. As Annelies, who compared the two ova pick-ups that were done by different medical doctors, said:

> That first doctor was very impersonal with us . . . If you compare her with the last one! She was much nicer. She was really joking with us. But the other one only spoke with the nurse, not with me!

In general, though, couples felt positive about the committed and friendly way in which they were dealt with most of the time; and some of them had even experienced the friendliness as slightly overdone at a particular moment. For example, one couple described one of the staff members as 'too familiar – that did not fit us' and another as 'too servile – she doesn't need to cringe for me'.

Fertility treatment trajectories often take years, and over the course of these years couples and clinic staff may come to know each other quite well. The extended trajectories lend themselves to building good and close relationships, which most couples appreciated. It struck me, for example, how pleased one of the men participating in the study was when the gynaecologist recognized him, even though he had not been in the clinic for several years (many years ago he had undergone fertility treatments at the Radboud Clinic with his former partner). Some of the couples addressed the doctors (and nurses) by their first names, which was probably also due to the fact that staff generally introduced themselves using their first name, they signed with their first names when they chatted on the Digitale Poli and because some of them were rather young (often younger than the couples).

Couples who stopped treatment without having reached the desired result sometimes came to the clinic to say goodbye and to thank the clinic staff for the care and support provided to them over time; some then indicated that they found it difficult to definitively say farewell. For them, not returning to the clinic implied that they had put an end to their attempts to have a child of their own (which was both painful and a relief at the same time); but it also implied, as some of them explicitly said, that they would no longer be in contact with the clinic staff to whom they had become personally attached. Couples whose treatment had ended successfully sent birth cards to the clinic in which they expressed their gratitude and occasionally couples visited the clinic – proudly and happily – to show off their baby. Clearly, for many of the couples, the clinic staff, the persons with whom they came to share their emotions, concerns and hopes and whose judgements they (often) came to trust, played a pivotal role in their quest for a child.

Plenty of Time

This afternoon I have been sitting in the corridor for a long time. I had planned to attend the consultation hour of one of 'my' couples, but I have been looking at a closed door for a long time. Finally – half an hour later than expected – the doctor opens her door and takes leave of the couple with whom she had been consulting. Then she comes to me and says, 'Whew! That was a difficult one. The outcome of their examinations was bad. I had to explain a lot and they reacted emotionally. So I really had to give them some extra attention'. Then she rushes away to pick up 'my' couple in the waiting room. When she returns she is apologizing for letting them wait so long. (Diary TG)

A good patient–doctor relationship can only develop if people get sufficient time to talk with their attending doctor. The time scheduled for different types of consultation and treatment sessions at the fertility clinic varied substantially and depended to a large extent on the amount of information that had to be exchanged. Generally, the medical interventions themselves did not take that long.[1] The pre-IVF consultations, in which lots of information was provided and couples received injection instructions, were exceptionally lengthy. Other consultations – for example when a control ultrasound was performed or an IUI done – were scheduled to take only ten minutes and in practice they rarely took longer. For ova pick-up and embryo transfer, thirty and fifteen minutes were planned respectively and only in exceptional cases was more time needed for these treatments.

Overall, clinic staff could and often did spend a large amount of time with the women and men visiting the clinic. In particular, they spent a lot of time on the anamnesis (a complete case history, as recalled and recounted by a patient), explaining treatment options and procedures, talking through treatment results and discussing and deciding upon the way to proceed. The couples were pleased with – and surprised about – the time staff in general could spend with them and this contributed to their overall positive feelings of being taken seriously, being well-informed and well-treated (cf. Franklin and Roberts 2006). Marijke, for example, told me about their intake at the clinic:

> She [the doctor] asked us a number of times if we had any questions. We thought, 'Do they have time for this?' We were absolutely amazed by that.

The importance of couples getting enough time and attention was clearly underlined by a few negative remarks couples made about doctors who were occasionally in a hurry: running away quickly after having done an embryo transfer or not taking enough time to talk about disappointing results. These kinds of situations immediately led to irritation. Birgit commented on such a situation:

> That was really tough. I think she could have done it differently . . . More carefully . . . It was during a control ultrasound and the doctor – a female one – found it difficult to tell me that there were only two follicles. Of course, I understand this is routine work. One leaves the room and the other comes in. But at that moment, I think she should have talked with me separately.

Too Many Different Faces

> Yes, we have seen different medical doctors. I see that as a disadvantage. But of course, that is difficult to schedule.

Couples visiting the Radboud Clinic have a high chance of seeing several doctors and being attended by a (partly) different group of staff members, during the different phases of their examination and treatment trajectory. Most study participants disliked this.

In the examination phase and when undergoing low-tech treatments, couples were mostly seen by trainee gynaecologists, who stayed at the department for only half a year. In that period they tried to follow up on their own patients, but they did not always manage to do so. Moreover, as these phases of treatment often took longer than half a year, there was a big chance that couples would see trainees from more than one rotation. One couple commented that in that part of their trajectory alone they might have seen fifteen different doctors. Though this is probably an extreme case, it is still part of the reality. While couples may have seen many different faces, all trainee gynaecologists working at the fertility clinic were informed about their situation. On a weekly basis they met to discuss all 'cases': the trainees gave a presentation about the examinations and treatment results thus far and suggested a treatment plan. Questions were asked, comments were made, alternative options discussed and finally a decision was reached on how to proceed. In principle, this meeting enabled all trainee gynaecologists to take over each other's patients. I noticed several trainees explaining this system to the couples when they apologized in advance that they might not see the same doctor at their next visit. As one of them told a couple with whom she was planning their next appointment:

> It might be that by then I will no longer be here. But that is not a problem. We discuss everything in a group. The doctor in fact knows you, even if you have not seen him [or her] before. There is a big chance that you won't see me then, because I am leaving on the first of May. (Doctor, Observation of consultation)

That the attending doctor was well-informed about their situation, however, only partially solved the problem from most of the couples' perspective, as we will see later.

When couples went through one or more IVF cycles it was also most likely that they would see several different IVF doctors and nurses and sometimes a gynaecologist as well. The IVF team also had their meetings to decide upon and keep updated on couples' treatment trajectories. On a daily basis, the IVF staff met to plan the work for the coming day(s). These meetings were attended by all IVF doctors and IVF nurses on duty, one or more of the laboratory technicians and at least one gynaecologist. They looked at and discussed the progress of the follicle growth and the results of ova pickups. Some cases were looked at in more detail, for example when there was uncertainty about the amount of hormones to administer, about the interpretation of women's complaints or whether or not to continue hormonal stimulation for another day.

Notwithstanding these systems of collegial consultation and information, several of the couples I followed in the study made critical comments about the multitude of doctors they had seen. Though most of them said that they in a way understood that 'things cannot be organized otherwise', they clearly expressed their preference for seeing only one or at least fewer doctors. They had various reasons for this. Some of them saw the fact of seeing several different doctors as problematic because they had – despite the systems of collegial interaction – experienced miscommunication between doctors. They felt that they constantly had to be alert and to update the doctor attending them. This concern was more often expressed with regard to the examination stage and low-tech trajectory than with the IVF trajectory.

Others indicated that they disliked seeing several different faces, as they preferred to undergo such an intimate treatment trajectory in a more personal ambience (cf. Inhorn 2003; Blonk et al. 2006). They felt that the treatment process (and the IVF treatment in particular) would be much more personal if you could go through it with only one doctor, or at least with fewer doctors. José, for example, was explicit about this:

> If I could say how I would prefer to have the treatment, then I would like to have the same medical doctor during each ultrasound control . . . At least, I would like to have the same doctor for the ova pick-up and the embryo transfer and also the same nurse . . . But preferably I would have one person . . . Seeing different faces again and again makes it very impersonal.

José and her husband felt that this medically assisted way of conceiving – under the close surveillance of various onlookers – contrasted sharply with how they had always thought conception would occur: in the intimacy of a relationship. Some couples, who by chance had seen the same doctor or nurse (practitioner) in all or most sessions of one treatment cycle, expressed satisfaction with that.[2]

Finally, a reason couples gave explaining their wish to see fewer doctors was the differences in doctors' personal styles. This was, for example, very notable in the way they performed the ultrasound control sessions during IVF treatment: women and men perceived a big difference in the way the doctors communicated what they saw when doing the ultrasound controls.[3] Several referred to one doctor (and I observed this as well), as she hardly explained what she saw on the screen and only rarely provided couples with information about the number of follicles that were growing, while the others generally shared this information with them.

Another concern – related to the desire for intimacy mentioned above – was the total number of people that were present during consultation hours and treatment sessions. The Radboud Clinic is situated in an academic hospital and consequently medical and nursing students doing their internships are present at all times. Thus, the chance of having an extra person joining a consultation or treatment session was high. This implied that at the ova pick-up or embryo transfer, three or four persons (a doctor, a nurse, a laboratory technician and a trainee) could be present in the treatment room. Patients were always explicitly asked whether they agreed to the presence of an extra onlooker and in general most people did accept, whether they are particularly happy about it or not. A few times I heard people object to an extra onlooker and that wish was always respected. One of the female study participants was absolutely against the presence of any extra person, as she felt it was an enormous disturbance to her privacy. She had refused the presence of a male medical student who wanted to attend her ova pick-up and she was also the only one among the study participants who did not want me to observe her clinical encounters.

The sex of the attending doctor was another issue of concern for some women, who had a preference for seeing a female doctor. None of them, however, expressed this preference when making an appointment. Clinic staff, though they are aware that some women have a preference, normally did not honour such requests, as the staff felt this was not practical from a logistical point of view. Moreover, as the head of the department told me when I asked, they maintained the position that in principle everybody – male and female doctors – should be able to deliver good quality care to everybody. Only in exceptional cases, for example if a woman had had a traumatic experience, were they inclined to honour a woman's request to only be seen by a female doctor.

Privacy (or Not)

Uncomfortable in the Waiting Room

Roos: No, that is not really a pleasure when you see all those women wandering around with their big bellies . . . Practically it might not be possible to do it differently at this moment [she knows that the Radboud Clinic is constructing a new building].[4] But it is not that I like it . . . On the other hand, it is not that I cannot see pregnant women with big bellies. In a way it is also funny. You think, maybe, who knows, it will be me in a while.

Henk: Oh, these big bellies. In general, I don't mind. Hopefully, at some point it will be us . . . But it [the waiting room] is a kind of passage to other departments. So, people for all kinds of different departments pass by. And then you are sitting there in a kind of monkey cage.

Privacy was highly valued by women and men visiting the fertility clinic (cf. Inhorn 2003; Blonk et al. 2006). They did not like to be exposed like 'in a monkey cage', as Henk eloquently put it. From my conversations with the couples, I learned that this urge for privacy first of all has to do with the intimate nature of the reason for their visit: the need for medical assistance for procreation. Instead of having others involved in such an intimate aspect of their life and relationship, understandably they would have preferred to conceive a child 'on their own'. In addition, assisted conception involves talking about, examinations of and treatments upon the sexual organs, which are intimate parts of the body. And finally, intimate and personal body materials – sperm and ova – are spoken about in detail, taken out of the body, re-worked in the laboratory and replaced in the woman's body. In the clinic, all these intimate subjects – their wish for a child, their sexual organs and their body materials – have to be shared with professional others. As long as this was restricted to professionals others, most study participants seemed to accept as unavoidable this sharing of intimacy, but beyond that, they preferred to be in charge of what they shared and with whom. This urge for privacy forms a major reason why women and men felt embarrassed if one of these private issues became public, as they felt happened at times in the clinic, in particular when sitting in the central waiting room or in the queue for the 'seed room', as it was called.

The fertility clinic had two waiting rooms: one for patients coming for initial examinations and low-tech treatments and one for couples undergoing IVF treatment. The first waiting room was also used for gynaecology patients in general; thus fertility patients were mixed up with other gynaecology patients, including those who came for pregnancy control, which several of the study participants did not like. Moreover, as Henk referred to above, the waiting room, which was surrounded by glass, was next to the entrance that led to other departments; thus it was almost unavoidable that those passing would turn to look at the people waiting. One couple recalled with some sense of humour how they had found out that they had been seen in the clinic by the man's pregnant niece: one day, when he had encountered his niece in a market, she had remarked, 'You don't manage [to get pregnant], eh!' Initially, they thought that his mother had been talking about them visiting the Radboud Clinic, but then they found out that the niece had seen them in the hospital when they had walked from the waiting room to the corridor for 'fertility problems'. Though the couple was not hiding their fertility problems and medically assisted quest for conception, they felt embarrassed that other people could simply find out without them being aware or in charge providing this information.

Contrary to the waiting room as described above, the waiting room for the IVF department was at the end of a corridor, where hardly any other patients passed. Though it allowed more privacy, several people spoke critically about this waiting room as well. They felt it was too small a space and was therefore hardly possible to avoid contact with others (some couples did, however, see this as positive as it enabled them to exchange experiences). In addition, people coming out of the ova pick-up room – occasionally in a wheelchair or on a stretcher – had to be transported through the waiting room to the recovery room, which was also felt to be a disturbance of one's privacy.

Lining up for the 'Seed Room'

Marijke: My husband hated that little room. But okay, that is generally known and that hopefully will be different when the new building is ready ... At a certain moment it was really a queue. It also made me laugh! I had to hide behind the *Libelle* [Dutch women's magazine]. I was sitting in the waiting room and there was a row of chairs, say, for the men. And at a certain moment Geert [her husband] asked me, 'Do I have to queue over there as well? More and more men are coming' ... He felt that was really embarrassing. But for the rest, things are very discrete.

With the clinic layout as it was during the time of the study, in the period when couples underwent fertility examinations and treatments, men had to hand in their semen to the laboratory. In case a thorough examination of the semen was needed (during the examination phase) they had to hand it in at a laboratory located some distance from the fertility clinic. When it was intended for direct use – either for artificial insemination or IVF – they had to hand it to the laboratory near the IVF treatment and waiting rooms. The 'seed room' was located next to both. Men were instructed to deliver semen not longer than one hour after it had been 'produced'; if they were able to come to the clinic from home within an hour, they could produce it at home and simply hand it in at the laboratory, but for those who did not live nearby they had to produce semen at the clinic. Men generally felt relieved if they were able to produce it at home (though this could also give rise to stress when travel time took longer than expected because of traffic jams or road diversions). Clearly, those who had no choice other than to produce sperm at the hospital were not at all pleased with the location of the 'seed room', which was next to the IVF waiting and treatment rooms and adjacent to the toilet. Once having entered the room, the men locked the door and switched on a button;[5] with the button switched on, a red light above the door indicated that the room was occupied, which was meant to avoid disturbances. However, when visitors went to the toilet and found the first door closed, they often tried the second door, unaware that this was the door to the 'seed room'. Almost all men participating in the study that had to make use of this room commented negatively about it, because of its location and because everybody knew what you were or had been doing when you entered or left it. Producing semen by means of masturbation was felt to be an intimate act, and the fact that others knew what they were doing made them feel their privacy was being intruded upon.

In addition some people also commented on the lack of privacy at the reception counter, as other people could easily overhear what was talked about. Staff members were aware of these criticisms about the clinic (see also Blonk et al. 2006) and they were taken into account when the new building for 'Mother and Child' was constructed. The construction of this building was announced on a huge billboard, so most study participants were aware of this and referred to it when commenting on the limitations of the clinic accommodation. My fieldwork ended the same month the clinic moved to the new building, so I was unable to do any observations there. In the new building the fertility clinic, including its waiting room, is separated from the rest of the gynaecology department and is not a thoroughfare to other departments; this allows for more privacy, and women and men coming for fertility problems are no longer confronted with pregnant women while waiting for their treatments. In addition, the new clinic has two 'seed rooms', which are located in a discrete place, removed from the eyes of onlookers.

Abundant Information

Plenty of Information

Eight o'clock in the morning. The phone rings for the first time. I am sitting in the IVF staff room next to one of the nurses, who today is in charge of answering patients' questions during the daily phone information hour. I have headphones in order to be able to hear the full conversation. The nurse picks up the phone and we hear the voice of a woman. After some friendly greetings back and forward, the nurse asks what she can do for her. The woman answers, 'This coming Friday I have to do a pregnancy test. What pregnancy test do you recommend?' The nurse answers that there are several good pregnancy tests, but that it is important to choose one that is easy to read. She gives the name of a test that is easy to read and mentions some other good ones as well. The woman then tells a story about her friend who had had a vague test result that led to confused feelings, which she herself would rather avoid. After the nurse has acknowledged this concern, the woman comes with another question: 'Can I do the test one day earlier than I was told at the clinic?' The nurse tells her that she may do so, but in that case she still has to do another test on the fifteenth or sixteenth day, to be sure. The nurse wishes her all the best in the coming week and they end the phone call. After this first phone call, five other calls follow with all kinds of questions, varying from doubts about the colour of vaginal secretion to the interpretation of examination results. Some of the questions the nurse can answer herself. For other queries she refers the women (only one man phoned that day) to a phone appointment with one of the doctors. (Diary TG)

Each weekday the fertility clinic started as described above: answering questions and concerns from women and occasionally men. Clinic staff spent a large part of their time informing the women and men visiting the clinic about the treatment and answering their questions. Many issues were covered, including explanations about the outcome of examinations and potential steps in treatment, risks and possible side-effects of examinations and treatments, expected results in terms of success percentages and the meaning and implications of actual results. Often, this entailed translating complex scientific information into language and images understandable to lay people. Another large part consisted of explaining procedures: how and what had to be done and when and where, in order to allow examination and treatment procedures to run smoothly. This included instructions about where and when to give blood or to hand in sperm, about taking medications at set moments and about when to do a pregnancy test. Some of the information exchanged was similar for all couples; other parts had to be adapted to the specific situation of a couple. The fertility clinic had set up a series of guidelines about what information had to be given at what moment, by whom and how.[6] Case-specific information was given during individual consultations in the clinic or by phone. In individual sessions, women and men were encouraged to ask questions, to phone the clinic if they had any remaining questions or doubts and to read and consult other available information materials. Among all the consultations I attended – with the exception of the encounters for ultrasound control as part of the IVF treatment – there was not one session in which I did not hear the nurse or doctor asking 'Do you have any questions?'

It is generally known that patients find it difficult to remember what a doctor has told them during a consultation (Hammarberg et al. 2001). The ability to retain information varies greatly and it has been shown that as much as 50 per cent is forgotten as soon as five minutes after a consultation. This is particularly the case and might even be worse when the processing of information is inhibited by anxiety, for example when the information is given in the same session as bad news is delivered. Moreover, people have different preferences for how information is transferred to them – verbal, written or audio-visual – and differ in the amount and level of information that they can absorb at one time. Therefore, a general rule in patient education is that information needs to be given repeatedly, in a variety of forms, and should be adapted to the individual knowledge and capacities of the receiver. In infertility care in particular, it has been stressed that information needs to be given throughout the course of treatment and not only at the start (Hammarberg et al. 2001; Kremer et al. 2007). Moreover, communication experts have emphasized that when transmitting information about health, one should not only appeal to the rational part of a human being, but also touch their emotional side, as this may strengthen the impact of the message transferred (Chetley et al. 2007).

The Radboud Clinic had, apparently, taken seriously the advice and lessons learned from communication science and health education and they informed their patients through several means and on many occasions. Over the course of the years the clinic had developed several written and audio-visual materials to support the explanations given verbally in consultations. The clinic's website gave practical and logistical information about the clinic; presented all staff members, including their photographs; outlined studies in progress, and so on. A number of brochures provided detailed information about specific examinations and treatments, such as the OFO (initial fertility examinations), laparoscopy, IVF, ICSI and PESA. Couples starting IVF treatment could also borrow a video or CD-ROM containing information about the IVF procedure and providing an example of how a couple experienced their treatment. The clinic had also made use of materials developed by others. Clinic staff frequently encouraged couples to peruse further information on the websites of Freya or NVOG; and a CD-ROM designed by a pharmaceutical company to explain the application of the pen that is used to inject the follicle growth-stimulating hormones was handed out to couples before starting the IVF treatment.

In addition, three times a year the clinic organized a plenary education evening for couples who were on the waiting list for IVF treatments. During this evening one of the gynaecologists gave a brief plenary talk about the IVF treatment (procedures, success rates, risks, etc.). Following this talk, people could watch the IVF video on a big screen and visit an information market. In a lounge several stands were set up to provide the future IVF users with information. These stands were partly occupied by the clinic's own staff: secretaries, nurses, laboratory staff, IVF doctors, the clinical psychologist and social worker and the man in charge of the Digitale Poli (see below). The patient organization Freya; an adoption organization; Fiom (an organization providing psycho-social support to people confronted with fertility problems and childlessness);[7] and a bookshop (carrying books about childlessness, fertility problems and adoption) were also represented at the information market. Visitors had about three-quarters of an hour to roam around the market. After, they were invited to return to the plenary room, in which a couple who had undergone IVF treatments shared their experiences with the audience. A couple whose treatment had not been successful was sought for this endeavour (the IVF video already shows a successful couple) as they wanted to avoid creating the picture that IVF treatments were always successful, though it was not always possible to find a couple that wanted to share the emotions of such an experience. The evening ended with a question-and-answer session and one of the gynaecologists responded to the questions that women and men had written on pieces of paper.

When couples were about to start IVF treatment, the pre-IVF consultation was held. In this lengthy consultation an IVF nurse went through all the steps of the IVF trajectory and gave instructions on how to administer the injections. At the end she gave a small tour through the department to show the couple the different spaces in which the IVF treatment was going to take place (the ultrasound control room, 'seed room', laboratory, room for ova pick-up and embryo transfer and recovery room). After this session with the nurse, one of the IVF doctors informed the couple – once more – about success rates, risks and possible side-effects of the treatment. Repeatedly, in this and at other sessions, I heard nurses and doctors tell the couples that they did not need to worry that they would not be able to remember all the information given.[8] They referred them to other places – brochures, video, DVD – where they could find the same information. Besides, I often heard them say, 'The information will be repeated again and again in little pieces throughout the treatment', and 'If you feel unsure, just phone us!' And indeed, over the course of the IVF trajectory, couples did get several written 'short time reminders' explaining the next step to be taken.

On top of all these informative means and events, in 2004 the clinic started the Digitale Poli for couples undergoing IVF treatments. The Digitale Poli allows couples to have access to their medical files through the Internet and to communicate with fellow couples in treatment and health professionals about their experiences and concerns. The Digitale Poli began from the principle of patient empowerment, i.e., from the idea that better-informed patients are more actively involved in the treatment process and decision-making and therefore would be better prepared to accept negative treatment outcomes.

Feeling Well Informed

Due to the many efforts made by staff to adequately inform the women and men visiting the clinic, most of the couples I spoke with, and certainly those who were undergoing IVF treatments, said they were satisfied with the amount of information they received. When I asked them in the first interview if they felt they knew enough to make an informed decision about the next step of examinations or treatments, all of the couples – with one exception – answered affirmatively. They felt that a lot of time and effort was invested in informing them properly. Some of those following the IVF trajectory described what they had to digest as 'an overwhelming amount of information'. Women and men who had read, seen and attended everything possible – more often women and higher-educated people than men and lower-educated people – felt that there was some repetition in the information provided and therefore they had even become a bit bored when watching the video or attending the information evening, as they 'already knew everything'. Others spoke about their personal preferences for oral or audio-visual information over written information and were therefore glad that they could choose the means that fitted them best. Some said that as they were not 'big readers', they were pleased they could watch the video at home or attend the information evening. In particular, some of the lower-educated men and women said they found it difficult to immediately and fully follow all the information given. Still, they appreciated the efforts undertaken, as Joost, for example, described:

> They take time for you. You can ask how and what. You get all your questions answered in understandable language. Not in Latin or Greek – short and clearly.

Though most people used and appreciated the different sources of information, for many the information they received directly from the doctor – and sometimes from the nurse – was most highly valued, as 'this concerns our own situation'. Several explained how they built up their body of knowledge, switching from one source to another, and emphasised the crucial role the doctor played in this:

> Then I hear something in the clinic and when I do not fully understand it, I go to the Internet and get some more information. But that is general information. When I am back in the hospital I will ask the doctor again, 'What does that mean for me, in my case?'

Here, we see the importance of a good personal relationship with the doctor, who knows everything about you and whom you can trust. The medical doctor is also supposed to take the individual's level of education and understanding into account, as Vince, a male participant and biologist by training, said:

> In the beginning I felt he started at a very low level with his explanations. I understand that, as of course he does not know at first who is sitting in front of him. He does not immediately know that we are highly educated.

The Digitale Poli seems to fit perfectly with this need for personalized information and contact. The eight couples in my study who participated in it were all satisfied with this innovative project, in particular because it gave them access to their personal records.[9] In addition, some liked the idea that they could put forward any questions or concerns to the clinic staff on the Digitale Poli, who would reply as soon as one of them came online. As Roos recalled:

The day before I had the ova pick-up I was online and she [referring to one of the IVF doctors] was online as well. So I could ask her some questions directly and she answered them immediately. That was really luxurious. Where else would you find that?

The importance of being well informed about one's personal situation is maybe best illustrated by the complaints of some couples who were not satisfied with some of the information they had received. Some of them complained that different doctors gave different information about something important, for example, the interpretation of the semen results, the amount of hormonal medicines to be taken or the next step in treatment. Most of these complaints referred to the phase of initial examinations or low-tech treatments. One man, a highly educated professional, who had been irritated by different interpretations of test results and subsequently different treatment options offered, became upset when he recalled the situation:

In my own job I am used to working with checklists. So, why don't they use checklists, which clearly indicate what to do in each situation?

Although there was overall satisfaction with the information received by the couples participating in this study and undergoing IVF treatment, still some felt there was a lack of information at certain instances. This concerned pieces of standardized information that according to the IVF department should have been routinely provided, but according to the couples they never received.

Psycho-Social Support and Empathy

Available Support

Annelies is telling me how stressed she was when she had the second IVF treatment: 'That tenth day is just awfully stressful. And then it goes wrong [she started her menstruation] and you completely collapse. Then you have to phone the hospital . . . In a way it is a pity that they do it like this. I would rather go there. I find it a bit crude, the way things end then [she refers to the fact that after a failed treatment couples do not immediately see a doctor at the clinic]. Though they [the nurses] talk with you on the phone; they really do!'

Subsequently, she tells me a lengthy story of how she had cried and shouted on the phone ('I'll never do a treatment again!') and how the nurse had consoled and encouraged her. As she had some preserved embryos, the nurse had encouraged her to at least do a cryopreservation treatment, as that would be far less burdensome than a full IVF treatment ('You don't need to inject yourself when doing a cryo'). While at that very moment she had not been able to listen well to what the nurse said, she appreciated enormously that the nurse had spoken with her at length. The nurse had promised to phone her back after a couple of days and she did indeed do so. The nurse had asked how she felt and Annelies had told her that she had not yet changed her mind about doing another treatment and that she and Bart, her husband, would go for a holiday. The nurse had remarked that that was a good idea and had promised to phone again after their holiday. And again she did so. In the meantime, Annelies and Bart had decided that they wanted to go for another treatment. When I asked Annelies how she had felt about the fact that the nurse was pressuring her like that, she answered, 'At that very moment it did not interest me at all. But later on, I was and still am very glad that she did it that way. For me, she did it very well. She knows me very well by now. I need this kind of approach . . . For me it is okay. I don't know if this is good for others, but I assume that she is experienced enough to know whom she has to handle like this and whom not'.

Fertility treatments and in particular repetitive IVF treatments are generally considered to be emotionally demanding and stressful (Greil 1997; Verhaak et al. 2002; Verhaak 2003; Greil et al 2010). Empathic behaviour by staff and adequate psycho-social support are considered key to making treatments more bearable, minimizing stress and improving the well-being of women and men undergoing treatments, and even limiting drop-out rates (Alper et al. 2002; Smeenk et al. 2004). The Radboud Clinic has recognized this and over the course of the years has established a system to support couples in treatment. Preparing couples for the potential emotional and physical demands of the treatment started in an early phase. Before entering the IVF waiting list, they were warned about the intensity of the trajectory and that they had to think hard before deciding to start a treatment. During the IVF treatment, at various moments, doctors and nurses showed couples that they were aware that this was not an easy thing to go through. In particular, when performing the ova pick-up, which many women experience as a painful event, nurses and doctors showed understanding and compassion; they encouraged the women and tried to support them as much as possible. Another moment when most people needed extra attention was when they received bad results, either from examinations or from a treatment, as we saw in the case discussed above

(Observation consultation). The potential burden of treatment was also addressed in the different preparatory educational efforts, including the video, at the information evening and the pre-IVF consultation. In the video and at the information evening couples who had been in treatment told their 'experience stories', in which they emphasized the emotional burden of going through IVF treatment. In the pre-IVF session the nurses also paid attention to the possible psychological burdens of the treatment. They posed questions to try to find out in 'what mood people are initiating the treatment' in order to inform the IVF doctors about possible stress factors which they should take into account.[10] Couples were informed that they could make an appointment with the social worker or be transferred to the psychologist if they felt the need to do so and this offer was repeated during the treatment trajectory, when couples – or actually most of the time women – demonstrated that they experienced the treatment or outcome as stressful. Clinic staff in their monthly meetings discussed the situations of the women and men who were visiting the social worker or the psychologist, and strategies to maximize support for the couples/women were developed. Clinic staff also referred the couples to external support groups: they advised couples to contact Freya for information and support, and Freya's brochures were available in the waiting room; the clinic also collaborated with Fiom in the organization of discussion groups for people with fertility problems. These discussion groups took place three times a year and focused on the emotional dimensions of coping with fertility problems and undergoing fertility treatments.

Empathy Rather than Psycho-Social Support

Of course, they do not have ages to dwell long on everything, but . . .
Yes, it was okay. I have not once left [the clinic] with an after-effect.
They do not ask you at each visit 'How do you feel?' but I also do not
expect them to always ask that. That is just impossible.

In the interviews couples frequently commented on how they perceived the way in which clinic staff supported them throughout their treatment trajectory. In general, they appreciated it when clinic staff showed them some form of empathy – demonstrating that they were aware that it was not an easy trajectory to go through – though they did not always expect, nor were they constantly given, intensive emotional support. Differences among staff members' styles were referred to as well. Several couples recounted small gestures – some of them I observed myself – which were highly appreciated. For example, some couples told me that their doctor had said, when phoning them, 'I know that you are eagerly waiting for this result. So, you are the first I am calling today'. Other couples recalled that their attending doctor or nurse had also shown their disappointment about a negative outcome, something they perceived as a sign of their personal involvement and understanding of their situation.

While couples did not always expect explicit emotional support, at some moments some of them said that they appreciated more attention to the psycho-social burden of treatment, for example when they were confronted with bad news. After a failed IVF treatment couples were offered an appointment for an evaluative talk with one of the IVF doctors. Some of them eagerly accepted this offer as an extra chance to talk about their experiences with a medical doctor, sometimes to get emotional support, but more often in the hope of getting more insight into the reason for the treatment failure. Others did not see the added value of such a conversation and therefore felt they should not bother the IVF staff, as they 'would not be able to change the outcome' and 'you have to get over it yourself anyway'.

From conversations with the couples participating in the study, it also became clear that for most of them, visiting the clinic's social worker or psychologist was not their preferred way to receive emotional support while in treatment. They appreciated the possibility being offered and saw it as recognition of the burden of treatment, but they were not generally disposed to make use of it themselves. Of the twenty-three couples I followed, only one visited the hospital social worker. A few of the other couples considered or were advised to visit the clinic's social worker, but chose not to do so, 'as long as we can handle it ourselves'. They postponed it, saying, 'Maybe, if the next treatment will not be successful, we will go there'. Couples seemed to show a kind of resistance to letting their quest for a child become too dominant in their lives. They were aware of other people being 'completely obsessed' and 'putting their relationship under pressure' by their wish for a child, and they seemed to want to avoid letting things go that far. In a way, it was as if visiting the clinic's social worker was like admitting that you were reaching that stage of becoming obsessed with treatment. Boivin et al. (1999) also noted a relatively low uptake of professional counselling by people attending a fertility clinic. The authors suggested that this low uptake might be related to the level of distress the women and men experienced, and that they had been able to receive good support from informal sources (i.e., spouses, relatives and friends), while some did not take up these services due to practical constraints (such as not knowing who to contact or potential costs). The latter was certainly not the case for the couples visiting the Radboud Clinic – they all knew that they could visit the clinic's social worker or psychologist – but most of them found other ways of addressing their need for psycho-social support. Some did visit other professionals to address these needs.[11]

Next to seeking professional psycho-social support, most couples emphasized the importance of talking intensively with each other as a major form of emotional support. Sharing with each other how they felt about going through this trajectory, crying with each other if they felt the need to do so and supporting each other – including doing fun things together for distraction – was what they highly valued. For one woman, the fact that she could not share her feelings and fears about the up-coming IVF treatment with her partner was her reason for cancelling it. The different ways in which they felt about and dealt with the coming treatment caused serious relational problems between this couple (see also Chapter 7). Men and women developing relational problems, because of differences in the way they perceived and dealt with their fertility issues and the infertility treatment and/or not being able to share their feelings or support each other, were regularly spoken about in the social work meetings.

Most couples (women more than men) also shared their experiences with and received support from others such as good friends, colleagues, or relatives; and many of them said they often felt best understood by people 'who have experienced this themselves'. The need to share experiences was also given as a reason for some of the users of the Digitale Poli to chat with others, though this need was not equally shared among all of them. Among the eight couples that had access to the Digitale Poli, half of them – again mostly the women – were active users of the chat room, while the others only read what people wrote or incidentally posed a question or remark. Likewise, Freya's chat boxes were only actively used by a small minority of the couples I followed. Most of them told me that they read what others wrote, but they themselves did not feel inclined to add their own experiences, because they felt these issues were too private to share with people you do not know, even when using a nickname. Thus overall, couples appreciated the empathy clinic staff expressed, but were not dependent only on them to help them bear the emotional demands of treatment.

Decision-Making: Multiple Dynamics

The patient-centred practices in the Radboud Clinic thus shape an ambience in which patients generally feel at ease, well listened to, well-informed and well-supported. Overall, couples participating in the study appreciated the way fertility services were provided at this clinic, reflecting fertility patients' needs and wishes in general (cf. Schmidt et al. 2003; Blonk et al. 2006). How then, in such a context, were plans made for (further) use of ARTs? How did these patient-centred practices affect couples' decision-making?

Enabling Informed Decision-Making

Jeanet and Karel are listening attentively to the doctor's explanation of the outcome of the initial examinations. They come to know that on Jeanet's side no irregularities have been found and it is once more confirmed that – as expected, given the outcome of previous semen analysis – Karel's semen is of extremely bad quality: the amount of motile sperms was around half a million. The doctor further explains about the large amount of sperm needed for fertilization ('The normal amount of sperms is supposed to be around twenty million') and informs the couple that the reason for the low sperm-count cannot be explained. She adds that the chance of becoming pregnant with Karel's amount of semen is very small, though 'We won't say that it will never happen'. After some remarks back and forth about the bad news, the doctor mentions that there are, however, some ways to handle this problem. Using a large book with colour pictures she explains the differences between artificial insemination, IVF and ICSI. She proposes that given the extremely low sperm-count, ICSI treatment is most appropriate as it 'brings the sperm even closer to the ova'. The doctor speaks quite fast, but in between she stops to check whether the couple is still following her. They both nod their heads affirmatively and say they can follow her explanations. Every now and then Karel raises a question, while Jeanet keeps silent. The doctor repeats a number of times that they do not need to remember everything that she is telling them now; they will get written information to read at home. She also emphasizes that they have to think hard about it before making a decision. At a certain moment she says, 'You have to realize that it is not an easy thing, such a treatment. You have to think hard about it, before making a decision. The woman has to take medicines and emotionally it is quite burdensome. You will get additional information about this. But it is important to recall that you *really* have to think about whether you *really* want this. Once you get started, you easily forget this'. Then the conversation continues about blood tests that have to be done in case they decide to start the treatment. Here the doctor gives them the option to first think about their decision or to go ahead and do the tests before making a decision, as they can always decide later on not to start the treatment. 'If you don't want it, you don't have to do it'. Karel says that he would prefer to do the blood tests now, as they can always decide later on what to do. Jeanet agrees with him. The doctor says she would have done the same if she were in their position. After some more explanations about procedural issues they leave the room.

This observation concerns the consultation following initial fertility examinations, which was an intensive communication event. The doctor not only had to deliver and explain the outcome of the examinations and pay attention to the emotional response of the couples (which I did not elaborate on in the above example), but also had to provide insight into possible steps for the future. These possible steps included: doing nothing, starting low-tech treatments, starting IVF and related treatments or doing further examinations. If the initial examinations did not suggest any serious or clear obstacle to conception, doctors at the Radboud Clinic were not supposed to propose any form of treatment – this was called the expectative policy – as long as the couple had not been trying to become pregnant for a period of at least two and a half years (though this also depended on the age of the woman). If a minor problem (according to NVOG standards) had been diagnosed, low-tech treatments were always offered before starting the more intrusive IVF treatment. When obstacles were diagnosed that clearly impeded conception and for which IVF was an indication, IVF and related treatments (ICSI or PESA) could immediately be offered. Sometimes additional examinations had to be performed, for example, to obtain more insight into the cause of semen problems, before any treatment could be initiated.

Similar intensive consultations were also held after a series of failed treatments (either low-tech or high-tech) in order to evaluate the results of these treatments and discuss possible next steps in treatment. The content and type of communication in these consultations were of course never the same; yet some overall features can be distinguished which clearly reflect the clinic's patient-centred policy and may affect decision-making.

First, doctors made sincere attempts to clarify and interpret the results of examinations and/or failed treatments thus far and explain further possible steps and their estimated prospective. They hoped this information was understandable and in response to the couples' questions. They realized that patients were not able to capture everything immediately and encouraged them to read things over at home and contact them if things were not clear.

Second, doctors often explicitly pointed to the clinic's expectative policy and their position on not offering more intensive treatment than needed. For example, as one of the doctors told a couple:

> We here [in this clinic] are very much in favour of taking a good look at what is the problem. We do not want to over-treat or offer a treatment that we know will not help you to get pregnant. (Observation, consultation)

This was a remark I also overheard many times in staff meetings, when clinic staff were preparing for these consultations. The clinic definitely seeks to present itself as an institution that does not promote the unnecessary medicalization of fertility problems.

Third, and this is particularly relevant with regard to IVF and related treatments, doctors emphasized and warned people that these treatments could be demanding, emotionally and physically, and that they entailed some risks while success was not guaranteed (more details about how risks and rates were dealt with follows in Chapter 5). In the above case we saw that the doctor explicitly advised the couple to think twice before starting IVF and thus to make a conscious decision rather than automatically stepping into a treatment trajectory (it should be noted that this was not always as explicitly emphasized in other consultations I attended). As mentioned previously in this chapter, aside from the consultations, couples had ample opportunities to receive additional information and talk through their questions and concerns with clinic staff; they were definitely not supposed to make decisions overnight. All couples (except one) told me that they felt well enough informed to make a decision about the next step in the treatment process. The patient-centred practices in the Radboud Clinic thus certainly enabled conscious deliberation and decision-making about treatments, though this does not mean that women and men made decisions based on a purely rational assessment of information.

Missed Opportunities

While the patient-centred practices at the Radboud Clinic definitely enhanced informed decision-making, I also observed a contradictory tendency taking place. Clinic staff did not always 'practice what they preached': I observed that couples were not always explicitly asked if they indeed wanted to start treatment and/or to switch to another treatment type or cycle. For example, though the doctor in the case of Jeanet and Karel, above, provided information about the treatment, explicitly warning the couple about the demanding features of IVF treatment and advising them to think twice before deciding to pursue it, she still acted with the unspoken assumption that the couple – once provided with the examination results – would want to be informed immediately about treatment options and indeed consider starting treatment. She did not question *if* the couple wanted to be informed about treatment options or *if* they had considered starting any form of treatment at all. When reading my fieldwork notes it struck me that at this stage I rarely heard doctors explicitly asking whether the couple indeed wanted to initiate fertility treatments, or whether they would prefer to leave it as it was and not start any medical interventions.[12] Here we come across a dynamic that may somehow direct couples into starting treatment automatically – a mechanism Pasveer and Heesterbeek (2001: 92–97) also noticed and referred to as a 'false start' – and may draw them into the 'medical treadmill'. I see this as a 'missed opportunity' in the practice of patient-centred medicine.

'Doctors are Doers'

Doctors – in their commitment to resolve their patients' problems – seemed to assume that when people came to the clinic with a fertility problem, they want to be medically treated. Some of the doctors did, however, criticize their own inclination to act – to offer treatment – as the following remark by one of the trainee gynaecologists nicely illustrates:

> You know what it is, Trudie? If we here [she points to the consultation room] have found the reason for the fertility problem, we immediately offer treatment. We should not do that. It would be better if we first ask them *if* they want to be informed about possible treatments. For some it may be fine once they know what the problem is. Maybe they do not want to be treated; maybe they would rather do nothing, or go for adoption. We should talk about adoption as well.

The head of the IVF department also showed his awareness of doctors' inclination to act – to treat – as he commented more than once, when discussing this issue: 'Doctors are doers. Doctors are trained to act, to help people, to cure patients, not to do nothing'. He thought that this rendered it difficult for doctors not to offer treatment in the first place.

Doctors, however, were not the only ones who thought it was obvious to go for treatment; I also noticed the same inclination with the nurses. For example, when responding to the phone calls in which couples informed the clinic staff about a treatment failure, they made encouraging remarks such as, 'Don't give up hope – a further try might be successful'. While such expressions were unquestionably meant to be consoling and encouraging, they also demonstrate the assumption that there would be a next try. In the case described in the introduction of the section on psycho-social support – where we saw that the nurse followed up a couple (Annelies and Bart) for some weeks after the IVF failure, to encourage her (them) to do at least one more treatment with the frozen embryos – the double sidedness of such reactions is well illustrated. While the nurse's follow-up action was undoubtedly meant to support the woman and reflected her dedication to her work and to the couple involved, such an action could also be viewed as putting pressure on the woman (couple) to undergo further treatment. Apparently, the woman involved took the nurse's approach as a well-meant action to support her, as became clear from her answer to my question of how she felt about the nurse 'pressing' her in that way:

> With hindsight I am glad that she [the nurse] did so. She knows me very well by now. She knows I need this kind of approach.

Even when in this case the woman did not personally mind the nurse's support (or insistence) and even when the nurse's intention was not meant to steer the patient in the direction of further treatment, the nurse's action may definitely have had that effect. In addition, most women and men participating in this study also seemed inclined to go for treatment (and not only for diagnosis) once they had decided to visit the clinic; most apparently came to the clinic to have their problem 'fixed'.

'Avoiding Getting Caught up in the Medical Treadmill'
However, not all couples were equally keen to immediately set in motion the first or next step of treatment, as considered appropriate or logical from a medical point of view. This was the case, for example, for Nienke and Jos, who were very explicit about this. From the very first moment they entered the clinic they were scared of the potential perils of the medical treadmill. When the initial fertility examinations did not indicate a clear cause for their fertility problem, they did not mind being sent home to try for themselves

for a while (thus following the clinic's expectative policy). After that period they returned to the clinic and were indicated for artificial inseminations, which they started, though with some ambivalence. They tried three artificial inseminations with hormonal stimulation, none of which were successful: Nienke only produced one egg per cycle (instead of the two or three that were hoped for) and she reacted strongly to the hormonal treatment and experienced the insemination as painful. Nienke and Jos lost all confidence in the treatment ever being successful. In the consultation following these three failed treatments the doctor suggested not continuing with inseminations (even though the normal series of six IUIs had not been completed) and – in the same sentence – announced that she would put them on the IVF waiting list. Nienke told me that she had immediately reacted to the doctor's assumption that 'we automatically wanted to go for IVF', a treatment that she dreaded would be even more demanding and invasive than the inseminations. She clearly recalled her reaction at that moment:

> I thought, 'Why so?' I had the feeling that this is not my body anymore; this is not my life anymore. I felt different. My upper legs were still swollen. I asked her what an IVF treatment would entail, as artificial insemination was already so burdensome.

At that moment Nienke had immediately told the doctor that she felt she (the doctor) was going too fast. The doctor had – according to Nienke – immediately picked up on the meaning of her words and changed her position: she then responded adequately to the queries and concerns Nienke and Jos expressed and she also immediately supported the couple's suggestion to 'taking some months to think about it'. While she was pleased with the doctor's second reaction, Nienke said that she had felt once more that you have to be assertive when entering the medical field 'to avoid getting caught up in the medical treadmill'. After that session, when at home, she and her partner decided not to continue further treatment and when I later spoke with them on the phone, they felt relieved about their decision. As Nienke proudly said:

> I do not want my life to be defined by my wish for a child. I define the trajectory of my life and not medical science.

'The Imperative of Three Treatments'

The way in which fertility treatments were presented also played a role in the observed tendency to continue treatment once couples had begun the process: they were generally presented as trajectories and not as if they were supposed to be immediately effective the first time (cf. Sandelowski 1991). Couples at the Radboud Clinic were advised to start with a series of six low-tech treatments and if these low-tech treatments failed – or in some cases immediately after the initial diagnosis (thus depending on the diagnosis) – a series of three IVF treatments was proposed. In addition, the clinic's average success rates were not only indicated per treatment but per three treatments (see Chapter 5), thus also suggesting that doing more than one treatment was normal. Moreover, at the educational evenings I heard a gynaecologist say that most couples undergo up to three IVF treatments (if previous treatments fail) and only a limited number surpass this. It is noteworthy that the number of three treatments was not based on clinical insights, but on the fact that Dutch health insurance only paid for up to three IVF treatments.[13] In one of our conversations the head of the IVF department used the expression 'the imperative of three treatments' to indicate that – according to his impression – couples saw it as normal, almost as a right, to do three treatments.[14] In this study, this limit of three treatments – which is thus set by health insurance regulations – was indeed found to be an important point of reference for the couples participating in the study, as the interview excerpt below illustrates:

> TG: You are starting now with the first treatment. Do you have any idea – if needed – how many treatments you will do? Did you already talk about that?
> Iris: We now think . . .
> Johan: Certainly three times.
> Iris: Yes, we want to go to the limit. Then you can definitely say, 'Here it finishes and now it stops'.
> TG: Yes.
> Iris: And we should not go further than that, because then you are making yourself mad. Yes, that is what we think.

Couples entering the trajectory seemed to consider the IVF treatment – as Iris and John did – as a 'package deal': once having made an informed decision in the beginning, in principle they considered that decision 'valid' for up to three treatments, as long as pregnancy did not occur, the experienced treatment burden (emotional or physical) was not too high and their prognosis was not too bad. The 'imperative of three treatments' was thus found to be crucial and had two implications. On the one hand, couples came to see it as normal to think in terms of doing three treatments; on the other hand it also indicated a kind of final limit, that helped them define when 'enough was enough' without later on regretting that they had not done enough.[15] Though not all couples in the study perceived three treatments as an absolute end point, at least it formed a kind of temporary end point, a moment at which they had to consciously reconsider whether they wanted to pursue further IVF treatments and pay for them themselves or not. This does not mean that couples did not reflect on their decision to go from the first to the second IVF treatment or from the second to the third, nor that they never consciously considered this decision with clinic staff; yet these steps were far more obvious (compared to the step to surpass the line of three treatments) as long as there was no good reason *not* to do so. There is thus a commitment of, 'Yes we will go for three treatments, unless . . .', rather than an agreement in which a whole new decision must be made at each new step. The fact that after the first and the second failed IVF treatment an *optional* evaluation was offered (though couples did not always use that opportunity), while after three failed IVF treatments an evaluation session was part of standard procedures, once more underlines that, if needed, three treatments were considered the norm, both from the perspective of the clinic and from the couples involved.[16]

In sum, doctors' professional inclination to act, the unspoken assumption both on the part of doctors and (most) couples to start treatment once couples had entered the clinic, in combination with the 'imperative of three IVF treatments', meant that doctors did not always explicitly ask *if* couples wanted to start and/or continue treatment. This was, as I have noted, a missed opportunity within a framework of patient-centred medicine. Doctors' *and* couples' inclination to act thus (may) have drawn people into the medical treadmill, despite the clinic's policy and doctors' firm stance against such a situation. This inclination to act, however, was neither infinite nor compulsory. Couples could and did escape from this unspoken assumption, but this required assertiveness and agency. In the current study three out of the nineteen participating couples who were indicated for IVF set their own boundaries and withdrew from (further) treatment even though they were allowed to start or do further IVF treatments according to the clinic's medical regime *and* according to health insurance regulations.[17] For these three couples their particular circumstances and views meant that they did not consider starting or continuing treatment up to three IVF cycles. One of these couples was Jos and Nienke, whose situation was considered above: they had several reasons for not moving from low- to high-tech treatments. The circumstances and views of the other two couples whom this concerned will be presented elsewhere in this book (see Chapter 5 and 7).

Conclusion

In this chapter I have shown how the Radboud Clinic put its patient-centred policy into practice and that, overall, couples visiting the clinic appreciated the care – the information and personal attention – they received from the clinic staff. However, some specific aspects of care were disliked and criticised. These criticisms reflected in particular the need women and men felt for privacy and intimacy when dealing with such personal and sensitive subjects as infertility and medically assisted conception.

Regarding decision-making, I distinguished two dynamics. First, the patient-centred practices are described – are *intended* – as empowering and enabling informed and deliberate decision-making. Second, certain practices and dynamics were observed which (may) have had the opposite effect, which I referred to as the missed opportunities in the practice of patient-centred medicine. In particular, the maximum of three IVF treatments, as covered by health insurance, was found to be crucial. This maximum had two implications: on the one hand couples came to see it as normal to think of doing at least three treatments (the imperative of three) and on the other hand it indicated a kind of final limit, which made them less inclined to go – automatically – beyond these three treatments. In addition, as I have shown, the inclination to start and continue treatment, from the side of clinic staff as well as from most couples, implied that couples were not always explicitly asked if they indeed wanted to start treatment and/or switch to another treatment type or cycle. In many cases couples would not even notice this, or they were not troubled by it, as they indeed wanted – and might even be more eager than the doctor – to start or continue treatment. In other cases, however, as illustrated in this chapter, this automatism may have upset people and required them to be assertive and exert their agency to avoid starting treatment against their will. Not consistently and repetitively raising the question of whether people indeed want to start or continue treatments may draw people into the medical treadmill (cf. Pasveer and Heesterbeek 2001).

Yet, on the other hand, one may question whether, given the 'Yes, we will go for three treatments, unless . . .' type of agreement, not repeatedly asking couples if they indeed want to go on, but rather routinizing the treatment, might be more preferable from the point of view of the couples, as they do not then have to re-think their basic decision. This might give them peace of mind; the more so as they have put their trust in the doctor. After all, the chance of success with the first treatment is small and it is prob-ably more realistic to think you will not belong to the few lucky ones, than to expect that you will. Giving patients more choice and a voice, which has become an increasingly central feature of contemporary Dutch (Western) medicine – as it fits with the idea of patients as critical consumers of health care, who are making informed choices and can be held responsible for their choices – is not necessarily always better, as it may also add to the burden and responsibility of patients (see Mol 2006; Trappenburg 2008). Thus, in first instance not repeatedly asking couples if they want to do one more treatment may be seen as a missed opportunity in patient-centred practice. Yet, at the same time, for some couples this may – once they have made their first well-considered step into the IVF trajectory – be the preferred approach. How best to talk about pursuing further treatment is situational and may be dif-ferent with different couples; therefore, explicitly soliciting couples' views on how they would prefer to go about it might be the most patient-centred approach.

Finally, I want to draw attention to the unintended conse-quences of patient-centred practices. What do all these practices – the information provided, the Digitale Poli, staff's expressions of concern, empathy and commitment – do to the women and men in treatment, when we consider them through a Foucauldian lens as disciplining and normalizing practices (Sawicki 1991; Cussins 1998; Pasveer and Heesterbeek 2001). From this perspective, the amount of information and support provided and the bonds created between doctors and couples can be regarded as practices which may strengthen people's 'medical gaze' (Foucault 1977), in terms of how they come to look at their body, bodily processes and solu-tions for their fertility problem. Strengthening the medical gaze may make couples more inclined to think only in medical terms and solutions. Their increased understanding of bodily processes and treatment procedures, for example, may enable couples to better follow and understand the treatment outcomes at all stages of an IVF treatment cycle. In Chapter 6 I will further elaborate on how this also affects the way couples come to think in terms of success and failure at each treatment stage, which in turn may make them more eager to do one more treatment. Moreover, the commitment, concern and empathy as shown and expressed by clinic staff may increase the couples' trust in and their dependency on staff and the clinic, which may interfere with the way they assess the risks and rates of fertility treatments, as will be elaborated in Chapter 5. Further, while couples are and feel well prepared, supported and monitored to avoid risks and bear the heavy toll of treatment, this also results in them becoming used to the idea that a substantial portion of burden – both physical pain and psychic stress – is normal with IVF. This, in turn, may make them more inclined and prepared to bear this burden and thus more persistent in continuing fertility treatments, as will be further argued in Chapter 7.

In sum, all these patient-centred practices may render couples more inclined to continue with treatment, even in the face of uncertain prognoses and/or the significant physical and emotional toll of continued treatment. Patient-centred practices – which aim to, and succeed in, fostering informed decision-making – may thus also interfere with processes of conscious and deliberate decision-making, and bias decision-making towards (further) medical treatment. This analysis points to the paradox of patient-centred practices. In the chapters that follow, these practices and their effects will be further described and scrutinized.

Notes

1. The first intake and the consultation where the results of the examinations were discussed were supposed to take between half and three-quarters of an hour. For gynecologists half an hour is planned, and for the less experienced trainee gynaecologists – who do most of the initial examination consultations – three-quarters of an hour is planned. According to my observations, however, these consultations took much longer (implying that others had to wait), as unexpected situations and results needed more time for explanations, discussions and support, as illustrated above.
2. One of them recalled that the IVF doctor herself had also been pleased to have followed them through all of their treatment. Occasionally, I heard IVF doctors make similar remarks. Apparently, clinic staff also seemed to appreciate being able to follow up on couples during the course of their trajectory.
3. It has been observed that the different styles of clinic staff makes it difficult to measure patients' satisfaction with infertility care (Sandelowski 1993; Greil 1997; Malin et al. 2001).

4. At the time I was carrying out the study, a new building for 'Mother and Child' was being constructed at the Radboud hospital. This building was opened the month I ended my fieldwork.

5. The room was small, containing a bed, a water basin, towels, and a small table with some magazines such as *Playboy*.

6. In this chapter I only mention the type of information dissemination activities that are undertaken. In other chapters I go deeper into the content of the information that is given, and how couples handle this information.

7. Fiom was initially created to provide support to young women who had an unwanted pregnancy.

8. Clearly, the importance placed on patient information and communication requires staff that are able and willing to do so (cf. Franklin and Roberts 2006).

9. The Digitale Poli started as a pilot project in the period I was conducting fieldwork and only some of the couples undergoing IVF treatment could join. Currently, all IVF couples are offered the opportunity to participate in the Digitale Poli.

10. These questions included, among others, one about what they feared most about the IVF treatment and another about any negative experience they might have had in hospitals in general. The idea behind these questions was that the IVF staff would then be sensitized to possible stress factors. However, during the period in which the fieldwork took place, IVF staff members concluded that in fact nothing was being done with this information, as it was kept separate from the IVF treatment form. Therefore, they started to develop another system to alert attending medical doctors about couples that might need some extra attention in one or another form. This system was still in development when the fieldwork ended.

11. A few women visited a social worker or psychologist outside the hospital just before or during their treatment trajectory (though in all these cases the women said that their fertility problem or treatment trajectory were not the only or primary motive for these visits). In addition, about half of the couples visited an alternative healer over the course of their treatment trajectory to decrease stress (see Chapter 3).

12. Likewise, while adoption was at times referred to as an option in the consultation room, it was hardly ever given serious attention, and certainly not in the initial phase immediately after the initial diagnosis. The limited attention placed on adoption at this stage seems to affirm the notion (prevalent among couples, see Chapter 3) that adoption is only an option after all medical means to have a child of one's own are exhausted.

13. This was the case except for the period of January 2004 to January 2007, during which time the first IVF treatment was temporarily not covered by health insurance.

14. This, he added, made it sometimes complicated for them (the doctors) to convince couples that had had bad results in the first or second IVF that it was not useful to do another treatment, given their bad prognosis.

15. Some of the couples in the study, when indicated for a third treatment, were inclined to postpone it. They did so because they wanted a break – to be free from the injections and clinic visits – between the second and third treatment; but they also dreaded that once they had done the third and thus final treatment (as most of them saw it) then treatment options would be over and, if not successful, they would definitely know that they would never have a child of their own. They felt that they wanted to postpone that final moment and some also hoped that the quality of the man's semen would improve in the meantime.

16. Clinic figures confirm the picture that most couples restrict themselves to three (or maximally four) treatments. Of the total of 467 couples who started their first IVF cycle at the Radboud Clinic in 2004 (the year that the couples participating in this study also started), 45 couples (9.6 per cent) underwent four IVF cycles and 15 couples (3.2 per cent) did five or more IVF (as of September 2008). These numbers do not include the couples who did more than four IVF treatments of which one or more treatments were cryo preservations (for these treatments no hormonal stimulation, nor a follicle aspiration, has to take place). If these couples were included, the total number of couples undergoing four or more treatments would increase from 60 to 97.

17. Smeenk et al. (2004) also demonstrated that not all couples continue IVF treatments up to the three insured options, even when doctors allowed them to do so: they found that about one-tenth of couples undergoing IVF treatments decided to refrain from further treatments after a failed first IVF treatment and about one-fifth did so after a second failed treatment. Part of the sample of this study came from the same clinic where the present study was carried out.

References

Alper, M., Brinsden, P.R., Fischer, R., and Wikland, M. 2002. 'Is your IVF programme good?', *Human Reproduction* 17(1): 8-10.

Blonk, L., J.A.M. Kremer and T. ten Haaf. 2006. 'Het ontwikkelen van een patiënttevredenheid vragenlijst.', *Tijdschrift voor Verpleegkundigen* (7–8): 54–57.

Boivin, J., L.C. Scanlan and S.M. Walker. 1999. 'Why are infertile patients not using psychosocial counselling?', *Human Reproduction* 14(5): 1384–1391.

Chetley, A., Hardon, A., Hodgkin, C., Haaland, A., and Fresle, D. 2007. *How to Improve the Use of Medicines by Consumers*. Geneva, Switzerland: WHO.

Cussins, C.M. 1998. 'Ontological choreography: Agency for women patients in an infertility clinic', in M. Berg, and A. Mol (eds), *Differences in Medicine: Unraveling practices, techniques, and bodies*. Durham, NC: Duke University Press, pp. 166–200.

Foucault, M. 1977. *Discipline and Punish: The birth of the prison*. New York: Vintage.

Franklin, S. and C. Roberts. 2006. *Born and Made: An ethnography of preimplantation genetic diagnosis*. Princeton: Princeton University Press.

Greil A.L. 1997. 'Infertility and psychological distress: A critical review of the literature', *Social Science and Medicine* 45(11): 1679–704.

Greil, A.L., K. Slauson-Blevins and J. McQuillan. 2010. 'The experience of infertility: A review of recent literature', *Sociology of Health and Illness* 32(1): 140–62.

Halman L.J., A. Abbey and F.M. Andrews. 1993. 'Why are couples satisfied with infertility treatment?', *Fertility and Sterility* 59(5): 1046–54.

Hammarberg, K., J. Astbury and H.W.G. Baker. 2001. 'Women's experience of IVF: A follow-up study', *Human Reproduction* 16: 374–83.

Inhorn M.C. 2003. *Local Babies, Global Science: Gender, religion and in vitro fertilization in Egypt*. New York: Routledge.

Kremer, J., M.J.A. van Eijndhoven, J. van der Avoort, B. Cohlen, D. Braat. 2007. 'Zorg over de grens. Geen grip op kwaliteit van buitenlandse fertiliteitsbehandelingen', *Medisch Contact* 62(33/34): 1342–46.

Malin, M., Hemminki, E., Räikkönen, O., Sihvo, S., and Perälä, M. L. 2001. 'What do women want? Women's experiences of infertility treatment', *Social Science and Medicine* 53(1): 123–33.

Mol, A. 2006. *De logica van het zorgen. Actieve patiënten en de grenzen van het kiezen*. Amsterdam: Van Gennep.

Pasveer, B. and S. Heesterbeek. 2001. *De voortplanting verdeeld. De praktijk van de voortplantingsgeneeskunde doorgelicht vanuit het perspectief van patiënten*. The Hague: Rathenau Instituut.

Sandelowski, M. 1991. 'Compelled to try: The never enough quality of conceptive technology', *Medical Anthropological Quarterly* 5: 29–47.

——— 1993. *With Child in Mind: Studies of the personal encounter with infertility*. Philadelphia: University of Pennsylvania Press.

Sawicki, J. 1991. *Disciplining Foucault: Feminism, power and the body*. New York: Routledge.

Schmidt, L., Holstein, B. E., Boivin, J., Tjørnhøj-Thomsen, T., Blaabjerg, J., Hald, F. and Andersen, A. N. 2003. 'High ratings of satisfaction with fertility treatment are common: Findings from the Copenhagen Multi-centre Psychosocial Infertility (COMPI) Research Programme', *Human Reproduction* 18(12): 2638–46.

Smeenk, J.M.J., C.M. Verhaak, A.M. Stolwijk, J.A. Kremer, and D.D. Braat, 2004. 'Reasons for dropout in an in vitro fertilization/intracytoplasmic sperm injection program', *Fertility and Sterility* 81(2): 262–68.

Trappenburg, M. 2008. *Genoeg is genoeg. Over gezondheidszorg en democratie.* Amsterdam: Amsterdam University Press.

Verhaak, C. 2003. 'Emotional Impact of Unsuccessful Fertility Treatment in Women'. Ph.D. dissertation. Nijmegen: Radboud University Nijmegen.

Verhaak, C.M., Smeenk, J.M.J., Kremer, J.A.M., Braat, D.D.M., and Kraaimaat, F.W. 2002. 'De emotionele belasting van kunstmatige voortplanting: Meer angst en depressie na mislukte eerste behandeling' *Nederlands Tijdschrift voor Geneeskunde* 146(49): 2363–66.

Chapter 5

INFORMATION AND INTERPRETATION
RISKS AND RATES

Today, Birgit and Harry, one of the couples participating in my study, are attending the pre-IVF consultation to prepare for their first IVF treatment, which they will start next month. When I enter the consultation room, the doctor is in the middle of her explanation about potential treatment risks. After exchanging greetings, she carries on. 'When doing the follicle puncture, there is the risk of infection. An infection may happen', she tells them. Birgit and Harry are both listening attentively and the doctor continues. 'There is also a chance that a small vessel in the vagina will bleed. That is not a real problem. If it is bleeding too much, we simply squeeze it. Bleeding in the belly is more serious. Generally, such a bleed stops automatically. Very rarely is an urgent operation needed to resolve it. That chance is very small, but it may happen'. 'But it may happen', Birgit repeats the last words of the doctor. Both Birgit and Harry nod their heads, indicating that they have understood what the doctor is telling them. The doctor continues, 'And then the stressful waiting time starts . . . Not all ova will be fertilized: generally around sixty per cent. Rarely, no fertilization at all takes place. But it may happen'. 'But it may happen', Birgit again repeats. 'Next, there is the risk of having an extra-uterine pregnancy', the doctor goes on. 'But my fallopian tubes are obstructed', is Birgit's immediate reaction, 'is that still possible then?' The doctor confirms that even then an extra-uterine pregnancy may occur. Then she tells them that there is a chance that she could become pregnant with twins. Birgit immediately reacts, 'Yes, we would very much like that'. Birgit explains that they had had some doubts about starting the treatment, as she is getting older [she is thirty-seven]. She thinks that having twins – 'two children in one go', as she puts it – would

be ideal, as she would probably be too old to do another treatment.
The doctor listens attentively to the woman's story, but reacts plainly,
'Here we see twin pregnancies as a risk. Twin pregnancies are often
more complicated and there is also more chance of having complications at delivery'. Birgit nods, indicating that she has heard what the
doctor told her, but says firmly, 'If there are two [children], they will
be most welcome'. She looks at her husband and he confirms this.
Before moving onto the next topic, the doctor makes a final remark
about twins: 'If you have two embryos replaced and you become
pregnant, then you have a twenty-five per cent chance of becoming
pregnant with twins'. (Observation Pre-IVF consultation)

Nowadays, it is widely acknowledged that IVF treatments are
not without medical risks and that success cannot be guaranteed. Since the advent of IVF in the 1980s, these potential risks and
the relatively low success rates have become highly debated issues.
Critics have questioned why medical doctors encourage women
to take the physical and emotional risks involved in the use of
advanced reproductive technologies, as long as IVF efficacy remains
relatively low and nobody can give any guarantee that the treatment will be successful (see summary of critiques in Van Balen
and Inhorn 2002: 15). Most women (and men) undergoing fertility treatments are not really sick, so why, then, would they or do
they take these risks? In particular, such medical risk-taking has
been questioned in cases where an otherwise healthy woman is
being treated – and thus undergoes risks – for her husband's infertility, as is the case when couples opt for IVF-ICSI. While initially
these critiques and concerns were predominantly heard beyond
medical circles, since the 1990s representatives of the medical field
have also expressed their concerns more and more about the risks
involved in IVF treatments and the efficacy of treatments. They
have been actively seeking ways to improve the situation, and
nowadays (potential) users – certainly in Western clinics – are often
informed about the drawbacks of IVF (see, e.g., Ten Have 1995;
Weymar Schultz 2000; De Joode and Fauser 2001). At the Radboud
Clinic, couples doing IVF treatment, like Birgit and Harry above, are
– as an important element of patient-centred practices – abundantly
informed about IVF success rates and medical risks that are potentially involved in IVF procedures.

Social scientists and representatives of the medical field have critically examined and debated the way information about ARTs, and
in particular about their efficacy and risks, is presented in clinical
settings as well as in the public media, and how this affects the way

(potential) users consider and interpret this information or – to put it differently – how lay users construct their own perceptions of risks and rates.[12] Linking to these debates, this chapter discusses how and what information about success rates and risks the Radboud Clinic presented to the couples and how this affected couple's views of pursuing IVF treatments.

IVF Success Rates: What Do They Tell Us?

[C]ouples can be informed on the probabilities (what is likely) and possibilities (what is conceivable) of the success, failure and risk associated with a course of action. In the case of medical treatment options for infertility, these probabilities and possibilities are necessarily based on some prior accounting of outcomes in other infertile people who may be more or less similar to (in terms of such factors as diagnosis, severity of disease, duration of infertility and age) the couples receiving this information. Despite the wide variations and rapidly changing protocols in implementing any one therapy, such accountings may be based either on outcomes in categories of therapies (such as ovulation induction and in vitro fertilization) or on outcomes within specific variants of a therapy (such as specified dosages of particular drugs and a specific duration and time for their use to induce ovulation). (Sandelowski 1993: 248)

Information on success rates provided to (potential) IVF users is generally based on published national and international data and/or on a clinic's own experiences and statistics (Sandelowski 1993: 247). The reliability and relevance of these data for the women and men receiving this information, however, has been questioned and criticised for a number of reasons: for example, as Sandelowski argues in the above quotation, because the variations in therapies and changes over time complicate the applicability of aggregated data to new groups of users.

Similar critical remarks have been made about the presentation of outcome data per treatment centre, without distinguishing differences among types of patients (such as the age of the woman, the type of clinical indication for IVF and the number of previously failed treatments) (Kremer et al. 2002). IVF clinics that appear to be highly successful based on overall statistics may only be treating the easiest patients or selecting patients for whom treatments are most effective (e.g., young women with relatively mild problems such as blocked fallopian tubes) (Turiel 1998, in Inhorn 2003:

161). Single and highly generalized success rates do not give any information about individual success rates and may distort people's expectations.

Another major point in the presentation of IVF results pertains to the definition of what is considered a successful IVF. Clinics and/or national statistics may report as successful treatments their total number of 'chemical pregnancies' (apparent on pregnancy tests) or all pregnancies confirmed by ultrasound or the total number of deliveries (Inhorn 2003: 161). These results are normally given in percentages of a total number of IVF attempts, yet the definition of an IVF attempt differs as well. What moment in the IVF cycle is considered the start of an attempt? Is the success rate presented as, for example, the percentage of confirmed pregnancies out of all women who started taking hormones or out of all embryos transferred (see also Turiel 1998, in Inhorn 2003: 159-162? In the publication of results for Dutch IVF centres, a successful IVF treatment is defined as the chance for an ongoing pregnancy, confirmed by an ultrasound of fetal heart action at ten weeks after the ova pick-up, per started IVF cycle (Kremer et al. 2002; Kremer 2007). This definition has been criticised for two reasons. Firstly, couples do not undergo IVF treatment in the hope of achieving an ongoing pregnancy, but in the hope of having a healthy child, so only that should be seen as a successful outcome (Fauser 2002; Inhorn 2003). Secondly, the argument has been put forward that multiple pregnancies should no longer be seen as a positive outcome, given the manifold possible complications, thus calling for a distinction to be made between single and multiple pregnancy outcomes.[3]

Scholars also refer to confusing and even misleading presentations of outcome results, in particular in countries where IVF centres are commercial institutions, where success rates are used for marketing purposes and doctors' incomes directly depend on the number of treatments their centre performs (see, e.g., Becker and Nachtigall 1994: 515; Fauser 2002; Inhorn 2003); though it has been remarked that doctors in other settings may also be inclined to present good figures (Fauser 2002).

Finally, it has been argued that any presentation of medical facts by medical experts – and in particular to lay audiences – involves some sort of interpretation and 'fact choosing' (Sandelowski 1993: 249), while the premises guiding the interpretation and choices are not always made explicit, as this would be too complicated to understand for most lay people.

Information about Success Rates

Couples considering starting IVF treatments at the Radboud Clinic were told that the clinic's average success rate for this treatment was around 20 per cent per treatment cycle. Distinctions for different categories of treatment were made: success rates for ICSI were slightly higher (around 25 per cent), as women undergoing ICSI were generally younger, while success rates for cryo preservation treatments (in which frozen embryos are used) were much lower (10 per cent). The clinic's success rates were presented in terms of the percentage of ongoing pregnancies out of the total number of started cycles (i.e., from the moment that hormonal stimulation with medicines begins); an ongoing pregnancy was defined as an ultrasound-confirmed, intact, intra-uterine pregnancy, minimally ten weeks after the ova aspiration.

In addition to figures about the estimated success rate per single IVF treatment, couples were also given an indication about the average chance of conceiving after three consecutive treatments. In the IVF brochure this was stated as follows:

> The final success rate after a complete IVF treatment (consisting of one or more attempts) is 40–50%. (FertEndo n.d.: 3, translation TG)

Many couples also spontaneously quoted the phrase below, which was repeated at each and every plenary information evening and was often heard in the consultations as well:

> Half of you won't get pregnant and will leave the hospital without a child after three completed IVF treatments.[4] (Gynaecologists, plenary education evenings)

While the presentation of this cumulative success rate after three IVF treatments may have given a slightly more optimistic picture than the success rates per treatment – and at the same time confirmed the idea that it is normal to do more than one treatment – both percentages seemed to deeply affect couples' views on success rates.

Not Creating False Hope

> I think it is good. Because you think that if we do it in this way [using IVF], we will be successful. But they [the doctors] really show you that it does not simply happen, that it is difficult to become pregnant. It is not nice to hear, but it is really good that they point it out clearly.

Almost all couples said they definitely wanted to be informed about these limited success rates (only two women said they would rather not as it made them feel pessimistic). The vast majority, however, thought it was important to be realistic, not to have false expectations and to be prepared to bear the disillusion of treatment failure. The experiences of couples whose IVF treatments failed repetitively – to whom they were introduced at plenary information sessions – strongly impressed the couples who still had to start their treatment. They realized that a 'negative experience story' was purposefully chosen to make people aware that undergoing IVF treatment does not give you any guarantee of success. As Bob expressed:

> Yes, they do that purposefully! To make people realize that it is not always Hosanna!

The plenary information evening was often referred to as *the* event at which people came to realize the relatively low success rates. One of the couples recalled what they remembered about that evening:

> Harry: They clearly said a few times that the probability you will *not* get a child with IVF or ICSI continues to be lower than the probability you *get* a child.
> Birgit: And at a certain moment he [the doctor] said literally, 'Of all you present here, only fifty per cent will have a child after the [three] treatments and fifty per cent will not have a child'.
> Harry: It is good you realize that.
> Birgit: More than clear. You must be very simple if you do not understand that. Yes, and that is very important.

Another man, Tim, also referred to what he heard during the plenary information evening when he underlined the importance of being well informed about the limited success rates:

> In itself they bring it [he hesitates over how to express himself] . . . It is tough to hear, the way they clearly point it out there. But on the other hand, it helps you not to let your hope grow out of proportion. Your hope has to remain realistic . . . You are tempted to think at some moments: this is artificially controlled, the success rate will be higher than if you do it on your own. After all, there is a reason that you are visiting the hospital. And if nobody tempers that hope . . .

The fact that you go to the hospital, a place where you normally expect your health to be improved and your problem solved, was often referred to, for example by Theo:

> Normally, in the hospital you expect to leave the door 'cured'. In this
> case it is different . . . The chance that you fail is there and that chance
> is bigger than the chance that you succeed. Much bigger! And I think
> it is important that they tell you this.

Clearly, such expressions underline the high expectations people
have from biomedine and reproductive technologies, which – as
have been argued by several scholars – may result from the over-
reporting of successes, 'miracle babies', at the expense of the reporting of failures and flaws of these technologies (cf. Franklin 1997;
Van Dijck 1998; Layne 2003: 95).

Despite this, having once started the IVF trajectory, all couples had
fully taken in the fact that there was no guarantee of success. With
regard to success rates, it became clear that couples in the Radboud
Clinic were certainly not provided with false hope, as has been suggested by some authors (see, e.g., Becker and Nachtigall 1994). For
the couples in this study, the '50 per cent success rate' statement
underlined the fact that even after three cycles there was not any
guarantee of success, and that seemed to be a daunting message.
Still, the information provided – and the limitations thereof – lead to
multiple individual considerations and interpretations.

What Does it Say about Us?

Success rates are based on average results over a certain period of
time. As they are averages, they cannot be used to give an accurate
prediction of the exact chances of the individual couples involved.
Consequently, couples struggled to give meaning to all the different figures and percentages they were confronted with during
treatment.

In consultations hours, doctors and couples talked about the
couple's chances and sometimes doctors made rough personalized
chance estimations, taking into account various criteria such as the
age of the woman, the quality of the man's sperm and the smoking
pattern of both partners. Rarely, however, were hard figures given
in the consultation room. The clinic doctors told the couples that
they could not predict how an individual couple would do in a treatment cycle, first of all because they could not foresee how women
would react to the hormonal treatment.

Yet couples who made use of the Digitale Poli had access to information about their individualized estimated success rate at the start
of the treatment cycle; and after each step in the treatment cycle
– follicle stimulation, follicle aspiration, fertilization and embryo

transfer – this individualized rate was adapted. The more steps the couple successfully passed through, the higher their personal estimated success rate became. At the same time, people were told that the last phase, when the embryos have to nestle, was the most difficult one. This was, for example, made explicit at the plenary information evening when a woman in the audience asked at which stage an IVF treatment most often fails. The gynaecologist responded:

> Of every hundred couples, ninety reach the follicle aspiration and eighty-five reach the embryo transfer. After that – up to the pregnancy test – most failures occur. That is still a black box. That has to do with the implantation, the uterus mucus, an embryo that does not develop. (Gynaecologist, plenary education evening)

Men and women participating in the Digitale Poli might – the further they came along in the treatment trajectory – be confronted with an increase in their personalized estimated success rate, which would in turn increase their hope. Yet at the same time they were supposed to bear in mind that overall most couples did not pass the last phase successfully.

At the time the study was conducted not all couples had insight into their personalized estimated success rates via the Digitale Poli, and those who did not felt that the way percentages were presented was far too general, and lumped together all sorts of cases (cf. Sandelowski 1993). They were aware that success rates depend on several criteria, and therefore felt that these averages were not really helpful for estimating their own individual chances. Besides, some of them expressed the feeling that an IVF attempt can ultimately only result in two ways – either succeeding or not succeeding. Theo, for example, commented:

> Those percentages do not tell you anything at all. It does not say anything! You can just as easily belong to the group that succeeds or to the group that fails . . . It does not say anything. How would it help you? Whether it is ten or five, or thirty or hundred! It simply has to succeed.

Thus, for Theo, as he interprets the percentages, there are only two possible outcomes: succeeding in having a child or not. This type of reasoning relates to what Tijmstra (1987, 2003) refers to as 'binary thinking': 'A chance is a chance and for me it is yes or no' (Tijmstra 2003: 145, my translation). People do not rationally – mathematically – assess the risks figures or success rates provided, they just think 'for me it is yes or no'.

Birgit and Harry were also outspoken about the limited value of averages, and in particular about lumping together different sorts of diagnoses (cf. Sandelowski 1993):

> Birgit: One person is not like the other. If you compare me with my sister-in-law [undergoing IVF for a different reason], I can still become pregnant spontaneously, so I think I have a better chance than she has. And that is not explained [on the clinic's website]. Everything is lumped together. It is not split up into various types of problems.
> Harry: [Agreeing] They should, for example, split it up in three sorts.
> Birgit: Yes. For example, problems of the ovaries, bad quality sperm and bad quality ova.
> Harry: Now it is: either it is successful or it fails . . . They just throw it in one big pile!

Other couples also commented on the limited value of the generalized success rates and regretted that the data were not more specific. One of the couples was seriously upset that the doctor could not give them a more specific figure regarding their chances. They had known at the start of their first treatment that their chances were low (in particular because the woman, Liset, was almost forty years old) and because their first treatment had failed. During the consultation hour in which this failed treatment cycle was evaluated, the couple tried to find out exactly what their estimated success rate was at that very moment. That information, they felt, would help them to make an informed decision about whether or not to continue the treatment. They had serious doubts about doing another treatment because Liset had experienced the first one as extremely burdensome, both physically and psychically, and they did not find the negative outcome encouraging at all. When the attending IVF doctor asked them what they themselves thought about doing another treatment, the man, Alexander, questioned their chances:

> Alexander: What is our chance, based on the existing information? We know that when we started we had a chance of 10 per cent. How is that now? Lower or higher?
> Doctor: That chance has not become less. Your chances of becoming pregnant did not decrease . . . We cannot do too much. Your chances also have not increased. And your chances were already lower [than the average]. We can only say that you are allowed to do one more treatment, if *you* want it. (Observation Consultation)

The couple was obviously not satisfied with this answer and thought it far too vague. Besides that, they felt that the IVF doctor had originally depicted the situation as more optimistic than in reality it had been (according to Alexander she had mentioned a higher number of follicles and ova than were actually produced).[5] In the end, only two ova were fertilized and the quality of the embryos had not been good at all. The doctor's misrepresentation of the facts, the lack of (in the couple's view) clear standards to judge whether a treatment went well or badly, and the fact that their question about the estimated success rate in their specific case was poorly answered, irritated Alexander and Liset throughout the consultation and thereafter. The doctor, in her turn, told me afterwards that she could not give them a more precise estimated success rate, of for example 9.4 per cent, as she felt the couple wanted to hear. This case emphasizes the need of some couples to know their personal estimated success rates – and the more precise the better – in order to be able to make an informed decision. For this couple the low estimated success rate and the imprecision about it was one of the reasons they chose not to do a second IVF treatment.

Having access to personalized information about estimated success rates by means of the Digitale Poli affected the way couples perceived the treatment and their individual chances. These couples were confronted with changing percentages during the course of the treatment, which they eagerly watched, discussed and interpreted. One couple, for example, saw on the Digitale Poli that their chances were constantly 'only one percentage below the average'. This made Christine, who had not been too positive about their own chances, happily comment:

> After all, we are maybe going according to the book! We are like the average!

Another couple, Ria and Richard, felt that this personalized information strengthened their position when negotiating with the clinic staff about a next treatment attempt. They worried that they were not going to be allowed to do a second IVF attempt, because in the first treatment Ria had only produced three ova, of which only two were fertilized. They had prepared themselves well, using the information from their personal medical file on the Digitale Poli to convince the doctor to allow them to do another treatment. As Richard recalled:

> We had seen on the website [Digitale Poli] that up to the embryo transfer our chances were below the average. After the embryo transfer there was a gigantic green arrow pointing upwards, indicating that our chances had increased [compared to the average]! . . . If they had not allowed us to continue, I would have confronted her [the IVF doctor] with these facts.

In the end, this couple did not need the data to convince the doctor, as they were simply allowed to do another treatment. Nevertheless, having detailed insight into their personalized estimated success rate at each step of the treatment meant that this couple not only became much more positive about their chances, but they also felt better equipped to negotiate with clinic staff.

Thus knowledge of personalized estimated – and changing – success rates, presented in the Digitale Poli, affected people's views in various ways. It not only affected the way they saw their chances (either as more positive or more negative), but also strengthened their capacity to negotiate with the doctors about further treatments. The presentation of more personalized success estimates can be seen as an important step in moving away from the presentation of 'misleading' – or probably rather meaningless – generalized information and supports informed decision-making.

Speculating about Your own Chances

As stated above, averages were found to be too general to be really insightful when couples assessed their own situation. Still, men and women – once confronted with these averages – started to speculate about their own chances. Again, the statement that 50 per cent would ultimately go home without a child and 50 per cent with a child served as an important point of reference. Margriet recalled how that statement affected her:

> The effect is like that of a bomb! Everybody immediately looks at his neighbour and thinks, 'Who of us will become parents and who will not become parents?'

Christine also remembered exactly what she thought at that moment at the plenary information evening:

> It was special to see that we are definitely not the only ones. You look around in that room and you think: Gee, all of them! And then you look around you . . . at the end so many per cent . . .! That will be okay! I compared it with being in a lecture hall at the university.

Some of you will fail the exams, some not. 'I will belong to those who succeed', I thought.

Couples applied various criteria to estimate their personal chances. They had learned about these criteria from the doctors or on the Internet. The age of the woman was one of the criteria they frequently applied. Women nearing their forties were not too positive about their chances and that was confirmed by what they were told at the plenary education session:

> Yes, that is what was strongly emphasized. The doctor [gynaecologist] told us that if you are around forty, and you have never been pregnant before, and she mentioned one more factor, then it decreases your chances. Yes, that's what she clearly stated.

While the age factor tempered the hopes of the relatively older women, for the younger ones it was a reason to be optimistic. This was so for Louise and Erik, for example, though at the same time they realized that their optimism was probably not realistic:

> Erik: Yes, I am really having good hopes. That is the problem that all people seem to have. The figures say your chance is only 40 per cent, but everybody apparently thinks they have an 80 per cent chance or something like that. Maybe I am a bit too positive . . .
> Louise: Yes, our chances of course are [good]. We are both young, we do not smoke, we do not drink.

Smoking, excessive drinking and being overweight (for women) were frequently referred to by staff members as factors diminishing the chances of conception. These lifestyle factors were explicitly discussed and – if necessary – followed up during intake and other consultations. This was what one of the couples heard when the attending doctor at the end of the intake summarized their situation:

> We have to look at the quality of your sperm [which was frozen] and see how your [the woman's] fertility chances are. Your age is positive [twenty-six]. You have been pregnant before; that is also positive. You still are a bit overweight, though you already lost a lot. You smoke, which is negative, but you are saying that you will stop. We then also have to look at the position of the ovaries: can we reach them? (Doctor, consultation)

Men and women were encouraged to stop smoking and to drink alcohol moderately; and if the woman's body mass index was higher than thirty they first had to lose weight before they could enter the IVF programme (though not all doctors were equally strict in the application of this principle). In particular, stopping smoking and losing excess weight troubled the men and women to whom it referred, as they found it quite demanding. Some deliberately postponed a treatment to allow for the effects of stopping smoking to become visible in the quality of the sperm and see their estimated chances enhance. Marion and Kees, for example, were very pleased to hear that Kees' sperm had improved substantially after he had stopped smoking (the mobility increased from 20 to 40 per cent). The laboratory technician, however, had indicated that the improvement was not per se due to his stopping smoking, as Marion recalled, slightly indignantly:

> Yes, he told me, 'It is good enough for ICSI'. I told him that I knew that, but that we had specifically asked for this sperm test to know more than that. 'It is good enough for ICSI', the man repeated again. I told him again that I knew that. It was good enough for ICSI before. But my husband stopped smoking and we wanted to know whether it had improved. And then he said that it might be because he stopped smoking, but not necessarily so.

Women and men were informed about criteria that may increase or decrease their chances, but at the same time they were taught that these criteria – and changes therein – still did not explain the full story. Couples came to understand that there was quite some uncertainty around IVF and its efficacy. They did not therefore immediately conclude that positive factors would indeed work out positively for them, as Margriet's comment below nicely illustrates:

> I dare not say anything about chance. Only about hope! They say that if you have been pregnant once, then it will be easier. But that was two years ago! Does my body still understand how it works?

Lower than Expected

Peter: I was shocked . . . that percentage is much lower than I thought. I thought IVF is a big chance.
TG: And you had not heard that percentage before?
Peter: No. Not really . . . I thought it was something like 40 to 50 per cent. But then you hear it is in fact only 20 per cent [per cycle]. I did not know that.

Several men and women were, like Peter, disappointed when they first heard about the relatively low success rates, in particular some of the younger couples who did not know any other people who had undergone IVF treatment and therefore had not heard stories about treatment failures. Some of the couples who had previously undergone IUI treatments – which have a success rate of around 10 per cent per cycle – were pleased to finally enter the phase of IVF. They had high expectations of the IVF treatments:

> For the first time I had the feeling that we were going to do something that really gives you a chance.

However, their enthusiasm was tempered when they came to know the actual rates for IVF treatments. They had expected the success rates of IVF to be much higher. One of the couples participating in the Digitale Poli was disappointed once they saw their personal estimated success rates. They had not known before that they were this low; they only came to know it the day they opened their medical file on the Digitale Poli:

> Bob: Yes, then we were really disappointed ... We looked in our personal file [on the Digitale Poli] and there we saw that we had a chance of 10 per cent.
> Sylvia: Thirteen.
> Bob: Or thirteen, yes.
> TG: And what was that based on?
> Sylvia: On my age ... And that was really sobering. Apparently we were never told this before. We were not informed about this. Maybe in general terms, but not specifically about our case.
> Bob: That is important to know. Then you know what your chances are.
> Sylvia: What you are choosing for. Because we both thought, '13 per cent only!' [both laugh]. 'What are we doing this for?'

While the low estimated success rate made Sylvia and Bob – as some other couples – hesitant about starting treatments, they still continued. On the other hand, as discussed in the previous chapter, for Nienke and Jos, the estimated success rates in combination with some other concerns made them firmly decide not to enter the IVF trajectory after three failed IUIs. For them the estimated success rates were not worth all the possible troubles, as Jos said, feeling fairly annoyed:

> And the success rate – after all those attempts, they say it is still only 50 per cent!!! That was truly disappointing, that chance of success.

Compared to Nature

We do not have hopes of that [natural conception] anymore. If we were not doing ICSI, our chance would be only 1 per cent. So, we do not have hopes of that. . . . That is, of course, extremely small – 1 out of 100 per cent. That is what she [the doctor] said. If that is really so, I do not know.

Estimated success rates may be perceived as low, yet when couples compared their chance of conceiving through IVF with their chance of conceiving via natural conception, they found that IVF success rates were not too bad (cf. Sandelowski 1993). This was particularly so when there was a clear diagnosis of the fertility problem and couples knew that their chances of conceiving 'on their own' were extremely low or even nil, as was the case for Karel (quoted above) and his wife. As his sperm was found to be of very bad quality, he and his wife felt that their chances of conceiving increased substantially when making use of IVF and ICSI. At times doctors – in particular when there was a clear diagnosis of the fertility problem – also compared a couple's chance of conceiving with treatment with their chances in a natural cycle.

One of the couples had an interesting conversation about their procreation chances if they were living in the 'animal kingdom'. This dialogue left little doubt about how they saw their own chances:

Henk: If you think of the race to have a child, we are in the last ranks.
Roos: Yes. If we lived in the animal kingdom we would be 'the dying family'.
Henk: Yes. [Laughter]
TG: Though in the animal kingdom, the male would . . .
Roos: Yes, indeed, the male would visit another female.

It is a Like a Lottery

While many of the couples tried to – more or less rationally – apply medical criteria to estimate their chances, at the same time most of them also realized that even by applying these criteria nobody could predict the outcome of the treatment. They felt it was like participating in a lottery: at the start you never know whether you will belong to the lucky ones. Men and women used metaphors to express how they felt about their chances, by saying such things as 'it is just like a lottery' or 'it is just as clear as mud'. Doctors also took part in looking at IVF treatment in this way, in particular during the last stage of the treatment cycle, the phase where the embryo has to nestle. This is the period in which the largest proportion of treatment cycles fail, and as we saw before, the failures at this stage cannot be clearly explained. Doctors explicitly share the unpredictability of this treatment stage with the women and men in treatment. One of the doctors referred to this stage as 'the flaw of the IVF treatment'. It was also during the embryo transfer stage that I heard some of the doctors make joking remarks hinting to the lottery-like feature of this phase of the IVF treatment cycle. For example, they referred to the presence of one or another person – e.g., a particular intern, themselves or me – which 'may bring luck'. Or, when the pregnancy test or ova retrieval was planned for a special day, like Mother's Day, St Nicolas' Day (5 December) or Easter, then it was remarked that 'that must bring you good luck!' The day of the embryo transfer was also the moment that men and women most often asked me to 'keep my fingers crossed', which indicated their awareness that at that moment few other means were left to influence the treatment outcome than trying to get good luck on your side.[6]

Some men and women expressed that they had a kind of feeling about the amount of chance and luck they expected (or hoped) to have. Several preferred to position themselves as 'a positive thinker': they would be among the lucky ones. Marijke, for example, who strongly emphasized the importance of having good fortune in order to succeed, was fully confident about a positive outcome for them:

> I just think I will become pregnant. That is what I simply think. I want to think that.

Contrarily, a few of the study participants were inclined to be more pessimistic about their own chances, like for example Johan who described himself as someone who is pessimistic by nature and who had little hope of being successful:

> I have really bad thoughts. I think, 'again this will not succeed'. But I should not say that too often, because I will bring her [his wife] down as well, you know? So, I hope it will be successful, but the chances are low. Twenty-five per cent! One out of four! So, I don't think we will belong to those [lucky ones]. That is how I think.

In sum, independent of how couples attempted to – rationally – make sense of and speculate about the likelihood of success based on the provided information, three things were fairly clear for all of them. First, IVF success rates were considered to be low, for some of them far lower than expected. Second, compared to their chance of conceiving when not doing treatment, IVF increased their chance; though some felt this increase was very meagre. Finally, they knew they all had a chance to succeed, yet – given the lottery-like characteristic of treatment – it was unpredictable how big that chance was.

Risks: Facts and Perceptions

Information about Risks

Couples visiting the Radboud Clinic also received plenty of information about the risks potentially involved in IVF procedures (through brochures, at the plenary information evening and during individual consultation hours) and when couples were about to start their first IVF treatment, they were informed once more about the possible risks during the extended pre-IVF consultation, using a checklist of issues. Potential risks that were most stressed in the different educational sessions were the risk for ovarian hyperstimulation syndrome (OHSS) and the risk of twins. Regarding OHSS, it was stressed that it could be serious and may even lead to hospitalization; at the same time it was said that nowadays it rarely occurs and that to avoid OHSS women's follicle growth (when hormonally stimulated) was intensively monitored and couples themselves should be aware of the symptoms as well. The risks of multiple or twin pregnancies, for example the increased chance of miscarriages, early birth and complications for the pregnant mother and baby were also pointed out on several occasions. Infections or bleeding resulting from the ova retrieval were just briefly mentioned and the same applies for the increased chance of miscarriages and ectopic pregnancies.

With regard to possible risks for the children born from IVF or IVF-ICSI procedures, for both procedures the message provided was reassuring: couples were told that most studies thus far showed hardly any or no more innate distortions in children born from IVF-ICSI than in children that are conceived 'normally'. With regard to ICSI, however, it was added that much less was known about its effect on the children as the treatment had not been conducted for very long and thus the first children born through ICSI were – at that time – only between ten and twelve years old. On several occasions I heard doctors refer to the NVOG patient brochure on ICSI (NVOG 2001), which detailed possible risks and also pointed to contradictory research findings. These contradictory study findings were also mentioned in the brochure, in the plenary educational sessions and sometimes in the pre-IVF consultations. The importance of studies to follow up on children born from ICSI was underlined and it was mentioned that the Radboud Clinic was undertaking such a study.[7]

The increased risk of cancer – of the ovaries, breast or uterus – in women who had undergone IVF treatment was addressed in the plenary session, but was only spoken about in vague terms on other occasions, like 'no long-term effects on women are known'. The message given at the plenary educational session was predominantly reassuring: though they referred to a study (conducted some time ago) that showed an increased risk of ovarian cancer in women who had previously undergone IVF and which subsequently received much media attention and caused some anxiety among IVF users, the presenting gynaecologist explained that since then other studies (including a large study undertaken in the Netherlands, the so-called Omega study) had not shown an increased chance of any type of cancers of reproductive organs. They added that caution should still be taken (i.e., not using more hormonal medicines than needed) and emphasized the importance of follow-up studies to assess the long-term effects in women who had undergone IVF treatments.

Thus the overall way in which risks in IVF were presented at the Radboud Clinic can be summarized as one of expressing concern, raising awareness about possible risks and acknowledging knowledge gaps. At the same time couples were reassured that risks were not 'irresponsibly high', that to a large extent they were kept 'under control' (e.g., by transferring maximally two embryos) and that serious efforts were being made to gain more insight into the long-term effects. Women and men visiting the Radboud Clinic were thus confronted with a lot of insights into potential IVF risks. How then did couples participating in this study and receiving this information – as average lay people – take up and interpret all this information? Before addressing this question I briefly look into what social scientists have said about the construction of lay risk perceptions.

Lay Notions of Risks

Lay notions of risks are known not to be (purely) based on a rational assessment of risk as defined by medical or epidemiological science, namely the 'likelihood or probability of some adverse outcome' (Becker 2000: 79). Rather, lay notions of risk are shaped in context – in the 'circumstances and constraints' (Gabe 1995: 8) of people's everyday lives and experiences (Becker 2000: 80). Rapp (1999), in her study on amniocentesis, noticed a gap between statistical risk figures and phenomenological experiences. In particular women with a lower level of scientific literacy developed 'a practical sense of community epidemiology' (ibid.: 176), drawing conclusions based on factors irrelevant to testing. In a USA-based study, Becker and Nachtigall (1994) found, for example, that risk perceptions of women undergoing IVF were shaped by the women's strong desire to have children (their 'biography'); their bodily knowledge; dominant cultural values regarding the use of fertility technologies as the proper means for solving fertility problems; and by women's ongoing experiences in the health care system. For example, women who had pre-existing reproductive health conditions (such as DES or polycystic ovaries) and men whose fertility problems were attributed to previous medical treatment (such as radiation therapy for cancer) expressed more concerns about the possible risks involved in IVF treatment compared to study participants who did not have such experiences; these concerns, however, were not translated into less willingness to take risks (Becker 2000: 83).

Lay risk perceptions are thus not static, but evolve over time as a result of experiences and influences of various sorts. Researchers have found that people's favourable risk perceptions concerning prescribed medicines and medical technologies are related to their recognition of the direct benefits of these medical interventions and with trust in the medical and pharmaceutical professionals offering these interventions (Slovic 1992, quoted in Gabe 1995:4). Franklin (1997), in her turn, has pointed to the impact of representations of IVF – its procedures, its potential risks and so on – in the pamphlets of clinics and pharmaceutical companies: while they may give technically accurate descriptions, at the same time they may 'fail to convey several important aspects' (ibid.: 104) and hence affect people's expectations and views. Further, social institutions such as the mass media also play an important role in framing public perceptions of risks (Gabe 1995). Inhorn (2003: 189), for example, has referred to the role of the mass media in Western countries – so-called 'risk societies' (Beck 1992) – in promoting a dominant discourse preoccupied with health and safety risks, a discourse which profoundly moulds people's risk perceptions about IVF treatments, in particular concerning the use of hormones as part of these treatments. How then did the participants in this study assess the extended information they received on the risks of IVF, and how did this affect their risk perceptions?

You Have to Know Everything that May Happen

Margriet: Yes, I think they have to give this kind of information. Maybe some women do not want to know it . . . but people have to have the chance to make a decision based on information and you cannot do that if they only tell it to you afterwards. I really think so. I think if you begin something, then you have to know everything that may happen. [Her husband nods his head affirmatively]. Only then can you make a decision about starting or not starting. It is people's right to know this.

Almost all couples participating in the study underscored – as Margriet did – the importance of obtaining information on the risks involved in IVF treatment before starting. Only then did they feel they could make an informed decision. Some also referred to the hospital's legal obligation to fully inform patients about the pros and cons of any treatment. Overall, couples felt the clinic staff warned them extensively about possible risks. Mireille and Chris, for example, felt they were well informed about 'all potential disadvantages' of all parts of the treatment. As Mireille put it:

Yes, they tell you about everything that can go wrong. They don't only tell you the good part of it, but also what can go wrong during the treatment and possibly with the children afterwards.

Two out of the nineteen women undergoing IVF treatments in this study would have preferred not to hear all this 'negative information'.[8] It frightened them, as they immediately thought that everything that might possibly go wrong would actually happen to them. Both women said that they were the kind of people who never read medicine information leaflets out of fear of immediately feeling all possible adverse effects. One couple recalled – with a bit of amusement in hindsight – their conversation in the car when they drove back home after their pre-IVF consultation hour:

Bart: She [Annelies, his wife] was really scared, because they started to tell us all the possible side effects. This can happen! And that can happen! And then she said in the car back home, 'I am not going to do it!' [Annelies nods her head, confirming what he is saying, and laughs loudly]. Then I thought, 'better they had not told her'. They mentioned a long list of all possible side effects. Still in the car she said 'I am not going to do it. It is far too dangerous!'

Despite Annelies' initial concerns, she and her husband initiated IVF treatments, as did most of the participants in this study.[9] For two participating couples, however, the potential risks was among the reasons why they did not start or (further) pursue IVF treatment. Yet all participants had their thoughts and concerns about the potential risks.

How Frightening is It?

Some of the couples explicitly said that what they heard about the potential risks did not really scare them off. For example, Marijke, one of the women who had serious doubts about starting IVF treatment on ethical grounds, said that what she heard about the physical risks did not make too much of a negative impression on her:

> No, the risks were not such that I thought, 'Oh, I am frightened to do it'. No.

Louise, one of the higher-educated women who had read a lot about all kinds of issues surrounding IVF treatment, including scientific articles she downloaded from the Internet, shared that feeling:

> I knew it already [the risks]. I knew what could go wrong. For me it was not new at all. I think it is okay to talk it through once more: what does it [the treatment] look like and what are the risks? But I did not hear anything about which I thought, 'I have to scratch my head and think whether I still want to do it'.

Some of these women contrasted the risks of IVF with risks they were exposed to in other medical procedures or risks involved in 'normal' pregnancies or delivery and did not see the potential risks of IVF as unbearable or extremely high. Birgit, for example, recalled the lengthy operation she had undergone to undo her sterilization:

> I am not really put off [by the potential risks]. It is not that you will die from it. I have had that sterilization undone. That was a much higher risk! Then I was 'under the knife' for four-and-a-half hours.

While for Birgit her previous health care experiences meant that she was not too worried about the possible risks involved with IVF, for some others previous experiences did increase their concerns about risks. This was particularly so with regard to the hormonal medicines, for which two types of concerns can be distinguished, namely short-term and long-term. Women who had suffered from substantial side effects due to hormonal medicines taken in previous treatments (such as IUI) expressed more concerns about the immediate side effects in IVF treatment as well;[10] while women (and men) who had had a close relative – a mother, an aunt or grandmother – suffer from breast or cervical cancer expressed more long-term concerns. Some of the participants also referred in this context to a Dutch celebrity (Guusje Nederhorst) about whom it was publicly known that her recent death from breast cancer had occurred after having undergone IVF treatment. In this context some women also hinted at a kind of generally (society-wide) acknowledged and shared concern about hormones. For some of the women the fear for the long-term impact of hormonal medicines became stronger along the treatment trajectory, when they experienced the bodily impact of these medicines. Marion, for example, after two IVF treatments, feared more and more the impact of the medicines and became reluctant to continue treatment:

> Yes, if you see how those hormones are dominating and taking over your body, then you think it is all rubbish, a lot of hormonal rubbish! And then I think, my mother died from cancer and my grandma had it. You start realizing that more and more.

Despite these concerns and her reluctance, Marion, along with most other women, started and/or continued treatment, and they did so even when they felt, in Louise's words that: 'They [the doctors] do not really know much about the effect of this hormonal rubbish in your body'. For one couple, however, concerns about the risks related to hormonal treatments were among the reasons they did not start IVF and for one other couple their concerns stopped them from pursuing an additional IVF cycle. Both women had been concerned about hormonal treatments from the start and had experienced serious side effects in previous treatments (IUI and IVF treatment respectively).[11] Moreover, one of them (Nienke) had had a mammography when she was in the midst of the infertility examinations (as her mother had died from breast cancer). As the initial 'breast photo' had shown irregularities, additional examinations (biopsies and an MRI scan) were performed. Altogether, it had been a long period of uncertainty and that had impacted on the way she and her husband had considered risks. One of the doctors at the Radboud Clinic had told them that IVF could not have any impact on the development of breast cancer, referring to a recent 'good study' that had been conducted on this. Nienke's husband, however, was not convinced of 'the doctor's story' and mentioned this as one of the reasons for not starting IVF.

Besides concerns about the woman's health, several couples also expressed concern about the potential risks for the prospective child, in particular when they were indicated for IVF-ICSI, in which the selection of ova and sperm is done in the laboratory instead of 'natural selection' taking place. In these cases, however, even when they realized that this type of treatment had not been done over a very long period, couples seemed to feel sufficiently reassured by the information the doctors gave them. Some of them knew stories about healthy children born from IVF-ICSI, which also reassured them. On the contrary, knowing stories about less positive outcomes of IVF made people consider twice whether they really wanted this. Anneke and Frits, for example, knew a couple who had a seriously handicapped child who was born after IVF. Initially this had frightened them off IVF, but then they came to know that this unfortunate outcome was just a coincidence:

> Frits: What concerned me most was how high the risk is that your child will not be healthy. But that is not much higher than in a normal pregnancy. That was a relief . . . Those people I know have a multiple handicapped child. But that is not necessarily due to the IVF. That's bad luck.
> Anneke: That bad luck you can simply have. That was initially your big objection against doing the IVF. That scared you off.
> Frits: But at the information evening I learned that the risks are not really higher than in a normal pregnancy.

While such information might change people's views, some continued to be worried. This was the case with Bert, one of the men who – together with his wife Christine – had undergone a TESE treatment abroad.[12] He was sincerely concerned about the quality of the sperm that was directly retrieved from the testicle, despite reassuring statements from the attending doctor in the other hospital. He had agreed to do the treatment; nevertheless, he continued to have his doubts, even after his wife had become pregnant from the treatment. His wife, who was generally much better informed than him, disclosed that she also sometimes felt insecure about the possible impact of the TESE on her child, but then she 'regained trust in the medical technology' by telling herself that:

> These treatments have been done worldwide now for a long period of time [though this is actually not true for TESE] and everybody continues shouting that the number of deformations in children is equal to normal and if not it depends on the age of the woman. So, in that I am a bit the statistician and I think 'it will be okay'. I now fear much more the percentages that are mentioned with regard to miscarriages after some of these prenatal tests you can do. That is what worries me more than that I think that a deformation will develop due to the technology used.

Couples' concerns about risks were thus shaped in context of other experiences, their own or those of others, with IVF and/or related topics, as other studies have also shown (see, e.g., Becker 2000). Later on in this chapter we will see that trust in medical technology, and in particular in the doctors providing the technology, formed another important element in couples' decisions to pursue treatment, despite their concerns.

Are Twins a Risk?

We can't manage to decide on the number of embryos that we want to have transferred. We are going round in circles with our thoughts: emotionally we prefer two, because we do have more chance of a pregnancy and twins would be more than welcome; rationally, one is probably wiser as the risks are less. In our direct environment we know three cases of twin pregnancies that went wrong, among them my parents – my brother was one of twins, of whom one child did not survive. Therefore, it scares me to choose this [two embryos] as it is like tempting fate. We have now decided to let it depend on the quality of the embryos: when it has eight cells we choose for the transfer of one embryo; if the quality of the embryo is slightly less, than we will chose for two . . . Here it is about the chances *and* the possible complications of a pregnancy. The arguments for the transfer of one or two embryos I do know by now, but I am looking for someone who can inform me. What is wisdom in our case? How do doctors see our chances of success? You are sent home with a simple question, though it's hard to decide on.

In a nutshell, Louise described in her diary the ambivalence many of the couples experienced when they had to choose whether to transfer one or two embryos: should they go for an increased chance of success or for fewer risks? Since the results of the study '2x1 versus 1x2 embryos' (Rijnaardt-Lukassen 2005) showed that for women younger than thirty-five years old the chance of conceiving when one embryo was transferred on two occasions was almost equal to the chance when two embryos were transferred on one occasion, women of that age group at the Radboud Clinic were advised to transfer only one embryo, to decrease possible complications and risks for mother and child. Not all couples were, however, fully convinced of the disadvantages of becoming pregnant with twins; and even when they did see the disadvantages, they still found it hard to make a decision. This was primarily because several of the couples would not mind having twins or were even positive about it, as 'your family is then immediately complete' and 'you do not have to go through the hassle of another treatment', while others thought 'it is cute' to have twins.[13] Only a few couples definitely did not want to have twins, either for practical rather than health reasons or because they thought that they already had a 'naturally increased chance of having twins' (as it had occurred frequently in their family) and so were outspokenly against the transfer of two embryos. Secondly, the chances of becoming pregnant in 'one single treatment' were – in spite of above mentioned study results – still perceived as higher if you transferred two rather than one embryo (though they realized that their chances were not doubly high). Thirdly, couples found it difficult to exactly assess the increased risks and increased chances, particularly as both outcomes could not be guaranteed at all but were rather full of uncertainty. As couples found it difficult to make a decision based only on weighing up the increased risks and chances, they employed a third criterion – which was often also suggested by the doctor – namely the quality of the embryos. Couples then agreed with the doctor that if the quality of the embryos was good, only one embryo would be transferred, and if the quality was not good two embryos would be transferred. They agreed on this, even though they were aware that the quality of the embryo does not actually predict the treatment outcome.[14]

While most couples found it difficult to choose between the transfer of one or two embryos, a change in people's standpoint could be seen over the course of treatments: while in the first treatment couples still considered, and occasionally opted for, the transfer of one embryo, they did so much less in their second and third IVF cycles, when they had become less optimistic about their chances of success.[15] Finally, the cost factor – increased health-care costs resulting from twin pregnancies, deliveries and possible complications for mother and children – which is used as an argument against multiple pregnancies by health policy makers and (some) doctors, was not referred to at all by couples when considering the transfer of one or two embryos (probably because these costs were fully covered by Dutch health insurance).

That is Not about Us

José: You think that is an exception to the rule.
Tim: Yes. You think that does not happen to me. That happens to someone else.

Some couples readily admitted – as did José and Tim – that though they were informed about all kinds of potential risks from the IVF treatment, they were inclined to think that this would not happen to them, but to others. Another woman, Margriet, who had her first child as a result of a successful IVF and who had once suffered from hyperstimulation, recalled how at that time she had initially completely neglected the possible risks:

> Apparently, risks were discussed with us then. But then you are like 'My child, my child, my child!' You do not bother about risks. You do not hear the risks. You simply do not hear the risks! Absolutely not important! . . . It does not really enter. At that moment you do not feel it is important. First, you think, this will not happen to us . . . And second, it will not be that serious. That is what you think!

In addition, some couples said that despite the abundant information received about the treatment trajectory and possible risks and side effects, as long as they had not gone through an IVF cycle themselves they did not really understand what the treatment would be like, nor could they imagine what adverse effects or complications they might experience.[16] Therefore, it was not yet an issue of concern for them. Mireille, for example, was very outspoken about this:

> No, you really do not know what exactly it will be like. Yes, you know that you are going to inject yourself. But whether you will experience side effects and how *you* are going to react, that you do not know. So then you think, let us go for it and we will see. And if it is worse than expected, you can always stop.

Couples who in the course of the IVF procedure actually experienced one of the risks they were warned about, like hyperstimulation, a miscarriage or a twin pregnancy,[17] referred to the same way of thinking: only when you have gone through it yourself do you realize that it can also happen to you. One of the participating couples whose IVF ended in a twin pregnancy was confronted with severe complications during pregnancy and delivery; their children were born prematurely and unfortunately one of the children passed away after having lived for a short time. With tears in her eyes, Margriet recounted how she always thought that 'that' would not happen to her, but now she had lost her innocence:

> By now so many things have happened with us that we know that everything can happen to us as well. Even the worst! We are not that naïve anymore. But before that, you think, 'No, this will not happen to us'. No, it was really not our concern.

Thus, women and men in treatment were rather inclined to think that the risks they were warned about would not happen to them.

Moreover, they said – and in particular the men – that if a first IVF treatment showed signs that it was seriously affecting their wife's well-being, either physically or mentally, they would definitely consider stopping treatment. They felt that the woman's health was more important than having a child. In practice, however, as we will see in Chapter 7, once couples had started IVF treatment it was difficult not to pursue further treatment, even if the woman was truly suffering from it.

We Have No Choice – We Want a Child

Whether couples were seriously worried about the possible risks or not, in the end several of those participating in this study claimed that in fact you do not have a real choice: if you want to have a child and you cannot manage to conceive on your own, you simply have to accept that risks will be involved as well. This is clearly illustrated by the reaction of a couple that became pregnant with twins as a result of their IVF-ICSI treatment:

> Johan: I was not scared by that information. We will see what happens.
> Iris: They have told us that there is a chance that our son might have the same problems as Johan ['bad quality sperm']. They have not been doing this treatment [ICSI] long, so they still do not know that exactly. But that might be. That information is not very helpful for me now! I do have a wish for a child now. If he – my son – later on might have the same problem as Johan, I will certainly advise him to undergo the same treatment. But now, I cannot do anything with it. I do have a wish for a child now.

This couple was apparently not too concerned about possible risks, as they felt that they might be resolved for their son as they were for them, reflecting a high confidence in the 'triumphant march of medical progress' (Layne 2003: 94). Some others, though more preoccupied with risks, reached the same conclusion: you do not really have a choice if you want a child. Marion, for example, who had experienced strong adverse effects during the second IVF cycle and whose mother had died from cancer, was really worried and upset about all the hormones that had to be injected into her body. Still, she also felt she did not have a real choice:

> We knew it [the risks] already, by reading. I had looked at the site. You [to husband] have also read it. We knew a lot of friends who were in treatment as well . . . If you think logically, you know it. If you count one and one it makes two. These are hormones, which

> you inject in your body. Of course, risks are connected to that . . .
> But you know you want it [a child] and this is the only way. Yes, you
> have little choice. You simply have to do it. Or better: if you want it [a
> child], you have to do it.

José, another woman who was very much aware of possible complications, also left no doubts about the limited choice she felt she had:

> You are reading so many things. Like for example about the follicle
> puncture – about the risk of infections. You come across so many
> things. You know what it is? You want it, so . . . you hear all the pros
> and cons or the risks. Because you want it, you have to put that aside.
> You can inform yourself, but still . . . even when there is a certain risk
> involved, you have to put it aside, because this is your last chance.
> You do not have any other choice.

Moreover, knowing examples of successes from nearby children
born from IVF – as illustrations that perseverance may be rewarding
– made it even more difficult to say no to (further) treatment.

In sum, while almost all women and men participating in this
study considered it important to receive the information on risks
in IVF, they found it difficult to assess exactly what these risks
could entail and to apply them to their own situation. Their risk
perceptions were clearly shaped in the context of previous experiences (e.g., with regard to the impact of hormones) or informed by
their wish for more children, which made it difficult to see a twin's
pregnancy as a risk.

Beyond Facts: Uncertainty and Trust

Couples thus interpreted differently the information about success
rates and risks they received, partly depending on their own and
others' experiences with IVF and/or related issues, and this affected
their thoughts about further treatment. In addition, as I will show
in the remaining part of this chapter, their considerations about
further treatment were shaped by dynamics and aspects of care
beyond the provided information.

Trusting the Doctor

In couples' considerations about potential risks, trust in the expertise
of the staff seemed to play an important role. Several couples said
they were convinced that the hospital would not offer this treatment if the doctors thought it irresponsible or too risky. Sometimes,

I also heard doctors explicitly saying this to couples when they uttered their hesitations, for example in the following case:

> It is not that we think this [ICSI] is not a responsible treatment. If we thought so, we would not offer it to you. We think it is responsible, but I can imagine that emotionally it is different for you. (Doctor, pre-IVF consultation)

Occasionally, study participants expressed their doubts about the trustworthiness of the doctors' judgements (as we saw in the above case of Nienke and Jos on the impact of hormonal treatments). However, most couples were happy and also felt that they were well monitored. Anne, who had had negative experiences in another IVF clinic but fully trusted that she was in good hands now and that the doctors kept an eye on her, explained:

> Concerning the risks, you are kept monitored. Whatever happens, they intervene! That is based on my experiences [in this hospital], not only with IVF. I don't see that as a problem . . . This time they had adapted it [the hormonal doses]. If you know that beforehand, then you are not too worried about that. That was clearly agreed by our gynaecologist and the IVF doctors.

Couples realized that serious side effects may occur, but at the same time they trusted that the doctors would intervene in time if necessary. They also felt well prepared to recognize signs of risks. In particular, they had learned to be aware of signs of hyperstimulation and they were advised to contact the hospital immediately if they suspected anything might go wrong. Some of them stressed the importance of regular monitoring during the period that the woman was injecting herself with follicle stimulating hormones. Tim and José, for example, who were seriously concerned about the fact that she had to take hormonal medicines for such a long period of time, at the same time felt some form of relief because they knew that José was being intensively monitored, as Tim told me before they started their first IVF treatment:

> Yes, that is what I hold on to. During a certain period she often has to go for checks and I think that has to be monitored well. If there is any indication that things are not going well, we will have to stop, I think. That gives me confidence. That gives me more confidence than if they would say 'Do it on your own, and come back for a check-up once a week'. But that is not how it goes.

While in couples' decisions to start treatment and accept possible risks, trust in doctors' expertise apparently plays an important
role, some couples also realized that they were not in the best position to judge the doctors' expertise. How could they know whether
the doctor had given them the right information or made the right
decisions? Henk, an organisation advisor by profession, was quiet
explicit about that:

> That is typical about specialists, about their expertise, you do not
> know it. That is where you have to trust them.

Louise made a similar remark about her capacity to judge a doctor's
expertise or skills:

> That [a doctor being empathic] is a very strong component and based
> on that you can say if you like a doctor and think she is okay. But in
> fact that does not make any sense at all, because whether someone
> performs a good follicle puncture or not, I really cannot say.

As the women and men visiting the clinic with fertility problems
were (generally) lay persons in this area, they did not have the
means to assess the 'truth' of the information provided by the clinic.
They largely depended on the doctors' selection and interpretation
of information. Of course, women and men visiting the clinic could
and did search for information elsewhere (mainly on the Internet)
and some of them brought their ideas about alternative treatment
options and procedures – like, for example, assisted hatching or
different medicine routings – to the clinic. However, as I noticed
when observing consultations in which such alternatives were discussed, doctors and patients (however well the latter were educated
and informed about the topic) were not equal discussion partners
about medical matters. In practice, couples – when they suggested
an alterative to the normal regime – first listened to the doctor's
explanations of why the clinic had chosen one option over another;
subsequently the women and men could come up with another
question or concern, but then the discussion generally ended. As
lay people simply have not read all the literature and/or are limited
in their ability to really assess the information provided, they have
no other choice than to trust their doctors' skills, expertise and
judgement. This trust in the doctors seems to be enhanced by a
number of factors, such as the appreciated patient-centred practices,
which created an ambience in which (most) couples felt well treated
and their questions duly answered. Doctors' openness about the

limitations of their knowledge, medical science in general, and IVF in particular, and the risks and uncertainties involved, was another factor that seemed to enhance trust (cf. Franklin and Roberts 2006). The latter aspect – the impact of sharing uncertainty – will be further discussed below.

Sharing Uncertainty

> I think that if a doctor shows his limitations, that gives me a lot of trust. Much more than if they pretend that they know everything and that they can accomplish everything. If he is saying, 'We are not yet sure about this or this and that is not yet quite clear'. Yes, if you recognize your own limitations that enhances my trust.

The study participants were profoundly aware that the doctors performing the IVF treatments did not have everything under their control and thus could not make predictions about the occurrence of risks or the outcome of treatment. They could not, for example, predict how women would react to the hormones injected to stimulate the growth of the follicles. A small difference in the amount of hormones injected may make an enormous difference in a woman's reaction. Prescribing too high a dosage may lead to OHSS, which was considered a serious risk; prescribing too few entities, though, may lead to a poor reaction. Both OHSS and too poor a reaction may lead to the cancelling of a treatment cycle and thus a lost chance. The decision about the exact amount of hormonal medicines was based on several factors, including the woman's FSH level, her age and her former experiences (if any) with stimulation of follicle growth. A final decision was made the moment the woman visited the clinic for the first ultrasound control. The ultrasound showed small black spots: the follicles that might develop later on. It was not rare to see an IVF doctor hesitating about the exact amount of hormonal medicines to prescribe or hearing her say that she wanted to consult her colleagues before making a final decision. Doctors shared this uncertainty with the women and men in treatment; sometimes it was even said explicitly that the first treatment was a kind of 'try out' to find out how the woman would react to the treatment. But even then, doctors frankly admitted that this did not predict how the next treatment would go, as women did not always react in the same way. Hence, most couples were aware of the uncertainty involved in this part of the treatment, as well as in other parts.

In the interviews, I spoke with the couples about how they felt, being confronted with this and other uncertainties they came across during the treatments. Most of the participating women and men said they preferred to hear that things were not a hundred per cent sure rather than have the doctors pretend that they knew everything. Sharing the uncertainty increased their trust, several of them said. One of the couples recalled in detail how positive they felt about the doctor's hesitation regarding the amount of hormonal medicines to prescribe:

> Anneke: It should have been a 200 dose[18]. Dr [name of gynaecologist] had advised that. And then Dr [name of IVF doctor] finally decided to go for a 150 dose.
> Frits: Yes, that was nice to see. Suddenly she did not say anything and then we saw her thinking. I thought, 'What is she doing now?'
> Anneke: Yes, she was really thinking.
> Frits: I liked that. I did not have any problems with that. I thought, 'Oh, well, she is really thinking about what she is doing. She is not uncritically accepting it [the gynaecologist's advice]'. And on the other hand it flashed through my head, 'Apparently, there are no norms for that. That is just weighing pros and cons'. That is what flashed through my head. 'Imagine she gives too low a dose and then the first round is already given away!' But they have always told us that the first round is a bit of fine tuning, so to say.
> Anneke: Yes, you don't know it in the first round . . .
> Frits: Someone is just thinking, 'What shall I do – 150 or 200?' That flash I had. And maybe it is a bit naïve, but I do trust people then.

Several research participants shared similar experiences. The quotes below illustrate what some of them said about uncertainty and trust:

> I rather prefer that doctors do not pretend as if they are 'half gods in white'.[19] I think it is realistic when doctors show that they do not know and cannot accomplish everything. It makes them more human. I would not like it if they pretended that they had everything under control.

> I think it is okay when they present themselves as vulnerable at such moments. Because if they said that they know everything, then you are thinking that they have everything under control. And if it fails, then you can reproach them: 'How is this possible? You knew how everything had to be done and still it is not successful'.

Thus, doctors sharing a certain level of uncertainty and unpredictability with their patients seemed to strengthen rather than diminish the trust couples had in them. Franklin and Roberts (2006: 132–38), in their ethnographic study of PGD in the UK, found a similar pattern:

openness about the many uncertainties of PGD technology among medical staff strengthened the feeling among potential patients that they were in good hands. In the clinic where they conducted their study, couples in the intake were not only amply informed about the limited efficacy of PGD, but they also had to prove able to discuss the drawbacks of the treatment. Couples were required to 'think very seriously about what they're going to put themselves through', including reflecting on how they would react after treatment failure (this approach thus goes further compared with what happened in the Radboud Clinic). Apparently, couples' hopes were 'pruned' to such an extent that 50 per cent of them did not return for PGD after having received this first sobering information. While such a procedure might be expected to lead to disappointment, Franklin and Roberts found the opposite to be true: for the couples who returned, these intake sessions raised their hopes and expectations of both the PGD team and the technology, and increased their confidence in their own ability to cope with the treatment's requirements. The authors describe the initial consultation as a *rite de passage*, through which a bond was established between the team and the prospective patients. In their attempts to understand this unexpected pattern (sharing uncertainty increases the trust in the staff and the technique, makes them – so to say – more accountable) the authors discussed two hypothesis. The first hypothesis – linking to notions of the 'risk society' Beck (1992) – was that that when professional experts admit inadequacies 'they *convey accountability*, and thus strengthen the sense of being treated with respect' (ibid.: 201). Admitting uncertainties and risks – admitting the "blunt truth" – is more valued than 'unreliable spin and irresponsible hype' (ibid). Such sociological arguments, according Franklin and Roberts, are contested by people who see them as 'expressions of postmodern pessimism', such as the philosopher and parliamentarian O'Neill. The second hypothesis Franklin and Roberts put forward, building on O'Neill, sees trust as built up 'through openness to critical interrogation' (ibid.: 202). In this line of thinking 'increased trust can be generated both through acknowledgement of uncertainties that are by definition partly unknown *and* through explanation of them in terms of what is known'. O'Neill (quoted in Franklin and Roberts 2006: 203–4) emphasizes the importance of providing layered information and interactive communication, enabling people to critically interrogate the information provided, in order to built trust – which takes time to develop. Franklin and Roberts argue that the lengthy initial conversations and the follow-up thereof over time in the PGD clinic where they did their research, offers an excellent example of how this kind of accountability, this trust, may develop. In the Radboud Clinic, the trust, as experienced by several of the research participants, may have been induced by a similar sort of intensive provision of information and committed interaction between staff and couples, where uncertainties and risks were not hidden, but – to a certain extent – mentioned and explained.

However, not all couples involved in my study appreciated this sharing of uncertainties, nor could they all build up such a trust relation. Some became openly fed up with the lack of precision (as we have seen previously in this chapter) and a few others preferred not to be confronted with the doubts of the doctor as it made them feel uncertain as well. Only one couple could not recall the doctors sharing any uncertainty at all with them. Rather, they were just very much impressed by the achievements of technology and together they reflected on how they were impressed by the medical technology offered at the clinic, even when this technology had not been successful in their case:

> Birgit: No, on the contrary [a reaction to my question about doctors sharing uncertainty], I was impressed about what they have done.
> Harry: I really think it was a nice piece of work.
> Birgit: I made a picture of the embryo, from the Digitale Poli. He [Harry] has enlarged it. Then I thought, 'How are they able to make something from nothing?!' The transfer – artificially – making a pregnancy artificially! In fact that is what it is. It is all made. I then think, 'How clever of all those people who contribute to that'. No, I do not have any . . . On the contrary, I am impressed about what they have managed to achieve.
> Harry: Yes, it really is a great job they do!

A Case of Distrust

The significance of trust in clinic staff is underlined by the experience of one of the couples participating in the study who, over the course of the treatment, became extremely dissatisfied with the clinic staff's attitude, which resulted in a relation of distrust. First, the woman (Liset) felt that her complaints about the side effects of the hormonal medicines were not taken seriously:

> When I had to take the injections [she did not refer to one of the medicines specifically], I got really anxious. I did not dare to go to the supermarket on my own anymore. I waited until my child returned from school and then we went together. In the hospital they

denied that this could be due to the treatment, [saying] 'You do not get anxious from hormones'. I am upset that they deny this. In alternative circles it is generally recognized that hormones [oestrogen] and anxiety can be connected. That also happened to a friend of mine.

Second, the way the (young) doctor had performed during the ova pick-up – she had not been able to find her blood vessels and had then started to curse – had worsened instead of lightened her pain. Third, she and her husband were not only disappointed about the treatment result (only a few ova were fertilized), they had also perceived the evaluation conversation about this treatment as unprofessional and annoying and felt that it complicated informed decision-making on further treatments. Finally, they were worried about the continuing bleedings Liset had had for a prolonged period after the IVF treatment, but were of the opinion that these concerns were not duly responded to by the clinic staff. Liset once summarized in a single sentence how she felt about the IVF treatment: 'You have to go through a lot to achieve very little'.

The combination of these negative experiences with the clinic, in addition to the bad treatment results, made Liset and her husband decide to decline further treatments. Moreover, if they decided to do another treatment, they told me, they would consider doing it in another clinic, even though this would imply that they would have to travel much longer distances to visit the clinic. For them, and this was thus opposite to the overall experiences of the other couples participating in this study, the lack of adequate support and care – of a trust relation – at the Radboud Clinic had worsened rather than diminished the burden of IVF treatment.

The next chapter further examines how the technology involved in IVF and the way it is presented to its users further affects the way people perceive the treatment.

Anticipatory Regret and Ambivalence

If we do not do it [the next IVF treatment], wouldn't we regret it later on? (Various study participants at different occasions)

Couples realized very well that there were risks involved in IVF. At the same time they did not know whether the treatment would ever bring them what they so dearly desired – a child of their own. They did not know whether the first treatment would be successful or whether any treatment in the future would ever be successful. The only thing they knew was that most probably, given their diagnosis, they would not get a child of their own if they did not do IVF. This made all of them, at one or another moment during the course of the study, pose the following question: 'If we don't do the (next) IVF treatment, wouldn't we later regret that we had not taken all available chances?' Fear of 'anticipatory regret', as this feeling has been labeled by Tijmstra (1987), was obviously one of the guiding thoughts when women and men had to decide on doing a first, a second and/or a third treatment, despite the possible risks, despite the limited success rates and despite the pain and emotions the treatment involved for some of them.

In one of the evaluation sessions I attended with Louise and Erik (who at that moment had done twelve IUIs and two IVF cycles), an interesting conversation about anticipatory regret and shifting boundaries arose:

> Louise: We have decided that we want to do one more treatment, though not immediately, because it feels good not to be involved in treatment for a while. . . . I have already invested four years of my life in it. Once you have to stop, at least then I will have the feeling that I have done everything possible! But you never know. Maybe I will shift my boundaries after the next treatment.
> Doctor: A clever sociologist from Groningen [referring to Tijmstra] has put the label 'anticipatory regret' on the idea that you must do everything to avoid regretting later that you did not do everything. But you have to bear in mind that your ideas about 'having done everything' may change over time – you must be aware of that.
> Louise: At least we want to try it once more; but not immediately.
> Erik: But not immediately and Louise has to indicate when she is ready for it.
> Doctor: I would say think it over again. Think again about whether you want to do another treatment and if so, when you want to do it.
> (Observation, evaluation session)

The above conversation addresses a crucial issue: while anticipatory regret may explain couples' inclination to pursue further treatments, inevitably the question arises as to where to draw the final line. When have you reached the moment that you have done *enough*, so that later on you will not regret that you did not do another treatment? To answer this question, the notion of 'the imperative of three' is again helpful. Several of the study participants were aware that the desire to have a child could become an obsession and they wanted to avoid becoming obsessed. For them, 'having done enough' became equal to 'doing three treatments': if you do three treatments you have done your best, without overdoing it and without becoming obsessed. A few couples participating in this study considered or actually did one more IVF to assure themselves (and maybe others as well) that they really *had* done everything possible – they even paid for it themselves – but then they stopped. Pursuing further IVF (thus beyond three or four) might bring them into the danger zone of obsession, while deciding to stop showed good common sense, since 'you cannot continue forever' and 'at one point you have to stop'. It is noteworthy that when couples considered the option of doing a fourth treatment they often added that the money was not the issue: they were able and prepared to pay for a treatment themselves. Rather, the question was whether it was 'wise' to do another treatment. Yet when a self-paid treatment failed, remarks about the money spent were made (this also applied to the TESE treatments abroad) and a treatment failure gained a cost element as well. While during the first three IVF cyles costs were never raised as a consideration in decision-making (in contrast to many places worldwide),[20] based on these remarks, I would assume that cost became an issue for most couples and may have been a reason to withhold them from going beyond four treatments.

While for many couples the notion of 'anticipatory regret' was important in decision-making, one couple, Nienke and Jos, turned this argument the other way round. They felt that their chances of success were low and they did not feel good about the potential risks involved (as Nienke's mother had died from cancer) and this feeling had been enhanced because Nienke had strongly felt the bodily impact of the hormonal stimulation during three IUI treatments. Many a time Nienke and Jos explicitly reflected on the question of whether and to what extent they wanted to medicalize their wish for a child – they felt ambivalent about it and thoroughly discussed the pros and cons of various options. While their views changed over the course of time, one question kept returning, Nienke said:

> Will I regret later on that we have put a lot of energy into it [treatment], while at the end it still will not have been successful?

Nienke and Jos went through the examination phase and did three IUIs, but when they were confronted with the option of IVF they decided definitively – with this question and the previously mentioned concerns in mind – not to further medicalize their wish for a child. They feared that later on they would regret having spent so long allowing medical technology to determine their lives, instead of accepting their childlessness. In addition, they felt that they themselves had to bear the responsibility of not having a child, as they had postponed the realization of their wish for a child until later in life. This couple also raised broader ethical questions about the limits of a 'makeable society'. Finally, while they both would have loved to have a child – and they found the decision not to pursue IVF extremely difficult – they could also imagine living 'a good life' without a child of their own.

While most couples in this study finally chose to do one or more IVF cycles, many of them expressed – as did Jos and Nienke – ambivalence about their choices. They demonstrated ambivalence about wanting and not wanting to do (another) IVF, about taking more or less risks versus more or less chances (e.g., with regard to the transfer of one or two embryos) and many of them shifted between optimism and pessimism, between hope and fear. This ambivalence has also been found in other IVF studies (see, e.g., Sandelowski 1993; Franklin 1997), with one of Franklin's respondents referring to it as the multiple 'shades of grey' in between two extreme poles (Franklin 1997: 155). It was related to the unpredictability of the outcome and the many uncertainties involved in the treatment, but also with the flow of the IVF trajectory, an issue that will be further addressed in the next chapter.

Conclusion

The provision of realistic information about success rates and risks involved in IVF constitutes a crucial aspect of patient-centred practices. Couples at the Radboud Clinic were certainly not provided with false hope; on the contrary, they were highly aware of the lack of guarantee of success and they enormously appreciated this. Still, the presentation of the clinic's average success rates was criticised for being far too general to say anything about their individual situation. Being aware of several personal factors that could influence their personal chances of success, couples tried to assess their own chances, comparing themselves with others and with general statistics, though this was not felt to be satisfying. The presentation of more personalized success estimates in the Digitale Poli is a step forward in the practice of patient-centred medicine, as it enhances informed decision-making and increases a couple's ability to negotiate with staff about further steps in treatment.

IVF success rates were generally considered to be discouragingly low. However, comparison of their chances of conceiving with or without IVF or when using low-tech treatments, made couples think more positively about the presented success rates (cf. Sandelowski 1991). In addition, the lottery-like features of IVF – its unpredictability – and feelings of 'anticipatory regret' made them more inclined to pursue IVF treatment(s), despite the fact that they did not see the presented success rates as particularly encouraging.

Couples also found it difficult to assess exactly what the presented risks could entail in practice for their own situation. Multiple pregnancies, in particular, were an issue that people found difficult to think of in terms of risk. Overall, their risk perceptions were shaped through a number of experiences and influences, some from beyond the actual treatment process (cf. Becker and Nachtigall 1994; Becker 2000). In the course of IVF treatments – when some women actually did experience 'the risks' – their views changed. In particular, they came to question the long-term impact of hormonal treatments on their bodies, also reflecting the overall Dutch societal discourse about the 'danger of hormones'.

In the Radboud Clinic's presentation of risks, two features stood out: couples were reassured that the risks were not 'irresponsibly high' and that risks were largely kept 'under control', e.g., by transferring a maximum of two embryos. Trust in the doctors providing the technology reassured the couples and helped them accept risks. Patient trust in doctors seemed to be strengthened by doctors' transparency about the possible risks, limited success rates and uncertainties involved in reproductive technologies (cf. Franklin and Roberts 2006). This finding reflects notions from O'Neill (quoted in Franklin and Roberts 2006: 203–4) regarding the importance of providing layered information and enabling people to critically scrutinize the information provided, in order to built trust relations and improve accountability. Being open about uncertainty may be more positively valued in contexts where patients are generally satisfied with other aspects of patient–staff interaction, as was the case in the Radboud Clinic (see also Gerrits 2014). In addition, the positive assessment of the doctors' openness by couples using IVF may have to do with their long-term relationships with the clinic's doctors, under which circumstance it is easier to discuss uncertainty (as suggested by Gordon, Joos and Byrne 2000).

In conclusion, the ample provision of information on the drawbacks of IVF – as a crucial element of patient-centred practices – is important to enhance deliberate decision-making. However, the decision to pursue IVF is not purely based on a rational weighing up of the information on risks and rates. People's individual risk perceptions, the lottery-like features of IVF, feelings of anticipatory regret, couples' strong wish for a child and trust in the medical staff all contributed to the fact that most couples in this study were inclined to start and continue IVF. In Chapter 6 I will discuss how IVF technology – the way it works and how it is presented to the couples using it – strengthens people's inclination to use it; while in Chapter 7 I will show how actual experiences with fertility treatments may diminish this inclination.

Notes

1. For discussions of these issues by social scientists see, e.g., Greil (1991); Sandelowski (1993); Franklin (1997); Becker (2000); Inhorn (2003); and Franklin and Roberts (2006).
2. Another issue that is debated among social scientists as well as among medical doctors concerns the limited evidence of the efficacy of IVF based on proper randomly controlled trials (see, e.g., Becker and and Nachtigall 1994; Ten Have 1995; NVOG 1998; Buitendijk 2000; De Joode and Fauser 2001). Only for women with clearly obstructed fallopian tubes can it undoubtedly be assumed – on biological grounds – that IVF treatment gives better results than 'doing nothing' (NVOG 1998). This group, however, constitutes only a minority of the women undergoing IVF. For all women/couples with other types of fertility problems (such as male infertility and hormonal dysfunctions) the decision to start IVF treatment is not really evidence based. Recently a series of studies have been undertaken in the Netherlands to assess the cost efficiency of a number of fertility treatments (ZonMw 2005). In one of these studies the chance of a pregnancy of couples on the waiting list was compared with the chance of a pregnancy for couples following IVF (Lintsen et al. 2007; Eijkemans et al. 2008). The lack of randomly controlled studies on the efficacy of IVF for the majority of indications for which it is currently being used has formed one of the grounds for various scholars to criticise this medical intervention in the past decades (see, e.g., Buitendijk 2000). This makes it hard to determine what the appropriate use for these reproductive technologies should be (Ten Have 1995) and thus also complicates the provision of accurate information on the efficacy of IVF to potential users.
3. From 2003 the number and percentages of single, twin and triplet pregnancies per IVF treatment centre in the Netherlands have been recorded (LIR 2004).
4. When I expressed my curiosity about how this percentage of 50 per cent had been calculated, as not all couples do three treatments, Prof.

Dr J. Kremer explained that the figure was based on the success rates of a cohort of couples starting treatment and doing one, two or three treatments.

5. Interestingly, this man – a highly educated technical professional – and a few other highly educated men were particularly eager to discuss figures, which parallels Rapp's finding of men 'fighting with numbers' (2000: 109).

6. It is striking that none of the study participants referred to the IVF outcomes being in 'God's hands' (Inhorn 2003: 102), as has been observed in IVF studies in contexts where religion is more central to people's life, such as Egypt and Ecuador (see, e.g., Inhorn 2003; Roberts 2006 and 2012).

7. See Woldringh et al. 2011a and 2011b.

8. These were the same two women who also preferred not to know about the limited success rates.

9. This is related to the sampling method. Sixteen of the nineteen couples participating in this study, and that underwent IVF, had already decided to start treatment the moment they started participating in this study; the other three couples entered the study at the point of starting their initial examinations, and made the decision to do IVF during the period in which they participated in the study.

10. Concerns about side effects will be discussed in Chapter 7.

11. These are the same couples mentioned previously in this chapter; both were also rather negative about their individualized chances for success.

12. This treatment they did in collaboration with another Dutch hospital.

13. Franklin (1997: 83) in her study in the UK noted a similar positive attitude to having twins, remarking that her informants 'viewed such a prospect as a bonus'.

14. More about the assessment of the quality of embryos in Chapter 6.

15. Interestingly, the two couples who did TESE treatments in Germany, where they were offered the possibility of having three embryos transferred, also struggled with this decision, using exactly the same arguments pro and con.

16. In the same vein, Franklin (1997: 110) speaks about the 'unanticipated demands' of the IVF treatment 'regime' her respondents felt confronted with, despite being well-informed in advance.

17. These experiences of OHSS, miscarriage and twin pregnancy are discussed in Chapter 7.

18. The number 200 refers to a dose of 200 milligram.

19. This is the translation of the German expression 'Halbgott in Weiß' used by the study participants who originally came from Germany. It refers to a paternalistic doctor-patient relationship, in which the doctor is the one who knows what is best for the patient.

20. See for example Sandelowski (1993); Franklin (1997); Inhorn (2003).

References

Beck, U. 1992. *Risk Society: Towards a new modernity.* London: Sage.

Becker, G. 2000. *The Elusive Embryo: How women and men approach new reproductive technologies.* Berkeley: University of California Press.

Becker G. and R.D. Nachtigall. 1994. '"Born to be a mother": The cultural construction of risk in infertility treatment in the U.S.', *Social Science and Medicine* 39(4): 507–18.

Buitendijk, S.E. 2000. 'IVF Pregnancies: Outcome and Follow-up'. Ph.D. dissertation. Leiden: University of Leiden.

De Joode, S. and B. Fauser. 2001. 'Keuzes, verantwoordelijkheden en dilemma's van een gynaecoloog', in S. De Joode (ed.), *Zwanger van de kinderwens: Visies, feiten en vragen over voortplantingstechnologie.* The Hague: Rathenau Instituut, pp. 84–102.

Eijkemans, M.J.C., A.M.E. Lintsen, C.C. Hunault, C.A.M. Bouwmans, L. Hakkaart, D.D.M. Braat, and J.D.F. Habbema. 2008. 'Pregnancy chances on an IVF/ICSI waiting list: A national prospective cohort study', *Human Reproduction* 23: 1627–32.

Fauser, B. 2002. 'Publicatie van de resultaten van alle Nederlandse centra voor in-vitro fertilisatie: Een belangrijk stap naar verbetering van de doelmatigheid van de behandeling', *Nederlands Tijdschrift voor Geneeskunde* 146(49): 2335–38.

FertEndo. n.d. *In Vitro Fertilisatie (IVF). Patiënten Informatie.* FertEndo, Polikliniek voor vruchtbaarheidsstoornissen, UMC St. Radboud.

Franklin, S. 1997. *Embodied Progress: A cultural account of assisted conception.* London: Routledge.

Franklin, S. and C. Roberts. 2006. *Born and Made: An ethnography of preimplantation genetic diagnosis.* Princeton: Princeton University Press.

Gabe, J. 1995. 'Health, medicine and risk: The need for a sociological approach', in J. Gabe (ed.), *Medicine, Health and Risk: Sociological approaches.* Oxford: Blackwell Publishers, pp. 1–17.

Gerrits, T. 2014. 'The ambiguity of patient-centred practices: The case of a Dutch fertility clinic', *Anthropology and Medicine* 21(2): 125–35.

Gordon, H.G., S.K. Joos, and J. Byrne. 2000. 'Physician expressions of uncertainty during patient encounters', *Patient Education and Counseling* 40: 59-65.

Greil, A.L. 1991. *Not Yet Pregnant: Infertile couples in contemporary America.* New Brunswick, NJ: Rutgers University Press.

Inhorn M.C. 2003. *Local Babies, Global Science: Gender, religion and in vitro fertilization in Egypt.* New York: Routledge.

Inhorn, M.C. and F. Van Balen. 2002. Infertility around the Globe: New thinking on childlessness, gender and reproductive technologies. Berkeley: University of California Press.

Kremer, J.A.M. 2007. *Patient-power in vruchtbare netwerken. Oratie.* Nijmegen: Radboud Universiteit Nijmegen.

Kremer J.A.M., W.Beekhuizen, R.S.G.M.Bots, D.D.M.Braat, P.A. van Dop, C.A.M. Jansen, J.A. Land, J.S.E. Laven, R.A. Leerentveld, N. Naaktgeboren, R. Schats, A.H.M. Simons, F. van der Veen en P.M.M. Kastrop et al. 2002. 'Resultaten van in-vitro fertilisatie in Nederland, 1996–2000', *Nederlands Tijdschift voor Geneeskunde* 146(49): 2358–62.

Layne, L. 2003. *Motherhood Lost: A feminist account of pregnancy loss in America.* New York: Routledge.

Lintsen, A.M.E., Eijkemans, M.J.C., Hunault, C.C., Bouwmans, C.A.M., Hakkaart, L., Habbema, J.D.F., and Braat, D.D.M. 2007. 'Predicting ongoing pregnancy chances after IVF and ICSI: A national prospective study', *Human Reproduction* 22: 2455-2462.

LIR [Landelijke Infertiliteit Registratie]. 2004. 'Landelijke IVF-cijfers 1996–2003', Stichting Landelijke Infertiliteit Registratie. Retrieved 1 March 2015 from www.lirinfo.nl.

NVOG. 1998. *Richtlijn indicaties voor IVF.* Retrieved 1 March 2015 from www.nvog.nl.

_____ 2001. *Patiëntenvoorlichting. Afwegingen bij de keuze voor ICSI.* Retrieved 1 March 2015 from www.nvog.nl.

Rapp, R. 1999. *Testing Women, Testing the Fetus: The social impact of Amniocentesis in America.* New York: Routledge.

Rijnaardt-Lukassen, M. 2005. 'Single embryo transfer: Clinical & immunological aspects.' Nijmegen: UMCN (Ph.D Dissertation). Retrieved on 23 March 2016 from http://repository.ubn.ru.nl.

Roberts, E.F. 2006. 'God's laboratory: Religious rationalities and modernity in Ecuadorian in vitro fertilization', *Culture, Medicine and Psychiatry* 30(4): 507–36.

Roberts, E.F. 2012. *God's Laboratory: Assisted reproduction in the Andes.* Berkeley: University of California Press.

Sandelowski, M. 1991. 'Compelled to try: The never enough quality of conceptive technology', *Medical Anthropological Quarterly* 5: 29–47.

_____ 1993. *With Child in Mind: Studies of the personal encounter with infertility.* Philadelphia: University of Pennsylvania Press.

Slovic, P. 1992. 'Perception of risk: Reflections on the psychometric paradigm', in S. Krimsky and D. Golding (eds), *Social Theories of Risk.* Westport, CT: Praeger, pp. 117–52.

Ten Have, H. 1995. 'Letters to Dr. Frankenstein? Ethics and the new reproductive technologies', *Social Science and Medicine* 40(2): 141–46.

Tijmstra, T. 1987. 'Het imperatieve karakter van de medische technologie en de betekenis van geanticipeerde beslissingsspijt', *Nederlands Tijdschrift voor Geneeskunde* 131(26): 1128–31.

_____ 2003. 'Zwanger tot iedere prijs. Dilemma's in de voorplantingsgeneeskunde', *Medisch Contact* 58(4): 144–46.

Turiel, J. 1998. *Beyond Second Opinions: Making choices about fertility treatment.* Berkeley: University of California Press.

Van Dijck, J. 1995. *Manufacturing babies and public consent. Debating the new reproductive technologies.* Hampshire and London: MacMillan.

Weymar Schultz, W.C.M. 2000. *Fertiliteit en ethiek, een kind voor (w)elke prijs?* Symposium WPOG, 10 November. Groningen: Instituut Wenckebach.

Woldringh, G.H., Horvers, M., Janssen, A.J.W.M., Reuser, J.J.C.M., de Groot, S.A.F., Steiner, K., and J.A.M. Kremer, 2011a. 'Follow-up of children born after ICSI with epididymal spermatozoa', *Human Reproduction* 26(7): 1759–67.

Woldringh, G.H., Hendriks, J.C., van Klingeren, J., van Buuren, S., Kollée, L.A., Zielhuis, G. A., and J.A.M. Kremer, 2011b. 'Weight of in vitro fertilization and intracytoplasmic sperm injection singletons in early childhood', *Fertility and Sterility* 95(8): 2775–77.

ZonMw. 2005. *Vruchtbaarheidsstoornissen. Kansen voor doelmatiger zorg.* The Hague: ZonMw.

Chapter 6

THE BODY AND VISUALIZING
TECHNOLOGIES

Roos and Henk have undergone six IUIs and three IVF treatments.
Until now these treatments have not led to the desired result, a child
of their own. Roos became pregnant once, but unfortunately this
pregnancy ended in an early miscarriage. Today, Roos and Henk are
visiting the clinic for the first time after their third failed IVF treatment to evaluate their situation and reflect upon plans for the future.
During the consultation the doctor talks with them about their disappointment after the last failed treatment. Roos and Henk tell the
doctor about the steps they have taken in the adoption process, but
also say that at the same time they are still considering doing a fourth
treatment. Together they look back at what went well and what did
not go well in the treatments they had. After a while, the doctor
winds up the conversation: 'Let us summarize the situation: the age
of the woman – you are thirty-four, so that is neutral. Once your
FSH [Follicle Stimulating Hormone] level was high, which we cannot
really explain. You reacted moderately to high stimulation, so that
is a set-back. The quality of the embryos was reasonably good, with
the exception of the last time. You have been pregnant once, so that
is good. You are not pregnant at this very moment and that again
is not good. So, some factors are okay; other factors are not okay. If
you want to try once more, we can agree to that. I suggest, for the
time being, that we can do one more treatment and then discuss the
situation again. If you want to start, you should not wait too long'.
Roos indicates that that is exactly what they thought as well. The
conversation continues for a while about payment of the fourth treatment, about the medication and so on. Then they leave the room.
(Observation, consultation)

When people make use of medically assisted conception, they come to view their bodily functioning and conception differently. They come to see conception as a process that is split up into many small steps, which can be followed and 'seen' by means of visualizing medical technologies, namely the microscope, the ultrasound, the X-ray, the laparoscopy, the hysteroscopy and further laboratory technologies. In this process of conception, several instances of success or failure can be distinguished, as the doctor's summary in the above observation shows. After having visited the clinic over a period of time, couples become familiar with all sort of factors, related with bodily processes and substances, that play a role in conception and they are able to follow doctors' reasoning about the – visualized – outcomes in the process of medically assisted conception.

Visualization of the body interior and bodily processes is a central feature of modern Western medicine and modern medical technologies. Various social science scholars have considered the meaning, implications and complications of visualization in medicine (see, e.g., Van der Geest 1994; Berg and Mol 2001). While health professionals are often thought of as being in charge of these visualizing medical technologies, the opposite is found to be equally true. In fact, according to Van der Geest (1994: 4–5), there is a dialectic relationship between individuals and technology: medical technology seduces the health professional or patient to see 'reality' in a certain way. Visualizing medical technologies thus steer the way health professionals conceptualize diseases, what they focus on, and subsequently inform their diagnosis and proposed interventions, while non-visual signs are considered less and less. When visiting clinics, Van der Geest further states, lay persons are inclined to take on health professionals' way of looking at their body and diseases.

Several social scientists working in the field of (assisted) reproductive technologies have discussed what these visualizing technologies mean to lay people, and how they change their perceptions, when they are confronted with them in clinical practices.[1] Building on the work of these scholars, in this chapter I first discuss how couples visiting the Radboud Clinic, while undergoing fertility examinations, were initiated into the medical world of infertility and got insight in their bodily functioning regarding conception, which insight, I argue, increased their 'medical gaze' (Foucault 1973). The second part examines how the couples – with this newly acquired knowledge in mind – experienced and assessed the various steps in IVF

cycles and how this coloured and shaped the further use of reproductive technologies.

Gaining Insight into the Reproductive Body and its Flaws

Fleur and Simon are visiting the Radboud Clinic for the very first time.
The attending doctor first carries out an extended medical history,
which is followed by bodily examinations of both. I am sitting on the
other side of the curtain and follow the conversation. While Fleur is
undressing, the doctor is already checking Simon's penis and testicles.
The doctor observes that the left testicle is positioned rather high. She
asks whether it has always been like this, a question that Simon is
not able to answer as he has never given it any attention. Then Fleur
returns to the consultation room and the doctor turns her attention to
her. First, the doctor does an internal examination using a speculum.
It strikes me how cautious she is when informing and handling Fleur,
who just told her that she has never had such an examination before.
The doctor tells her what she is feeling when she touches her from the
inside and after some minutes she concludes that 'everything looks
fine' and starts preparing for an ultrasound. Once again she carefully
informs Fleur about what she is going to do. She enters the probe into
her vagina and tells her what she sees on the screen: 'Now you see
the uterus. You look at it in little slices. Your uterus is a bit turned'.
When Fleur asks the doctor if that is good, she answers, 'This is what
we see most often. But in this nothing is good and nothing is bad'.
Then she comments on the current thickness of her uterus mucus,
which indicates more or less the seventh day of her menstrual cycle
and she points to small black spots, which are potential eggs. They
continue for a while like this: the doctor comments about what she
is seeing and Fleur asks questions to better understand what she sees
and to check if things are 'normal'. Her husband sits silently next to
her, watching and listening to their conversation. At the end of the
examination, the doctor concludes that, 'In fact everything looks
quite good'. Fleur dresses herself and when she returns the doctor
informs them about blood and sperm tests that have to be done as
part of the initial examinations. (Observation, consultation)

When men and women underwent fertility examinations they
came to know and see all kinds of details about their own body
that they did not know or had not seen before. As with Fleur and
Simon in the above observation, these examinations started with
an extended medical history and bodily examinations. In general,

doctors at the Radboud Clinic used to give lots of explanations about what they did and saw. These first visits to the clinic can be looked at as couples' initiation into the medical world and jargon of infertility.

Anamnesis

Through the many questions asked when their anamnesis (medical history) was taken, the couples became more aware of the type of factors that may play a role in conception, and indications that may possibly explain why conception has not yet occurred in their own case sometimes came up in this very first visit. Obviously, several of the issues raised in the medical history did not come as a surprise to the couples, like for example questions about the woman's menstruation cycle, the frequency of sexual intercourse, the man's ejaculation and so on. Other issues, however, sometimes came as a complete surprise. For example, a man working in a sauna was not at all aware of the fact that frequent sauna visits (as he was used to) might negatively impact on the quality of the sperm, because the testicles were exposed to high temperatures. At times, couples seemed to be surprised to hear about the enormous impact that smoking might have on both the quality of the sperm and the woman's capacity to conceive (while the notion that smoking is bad for pregnant women was widespread). Equally, the impact of alcohol use – and in particular peak load – on the quality of the sperm came as a surprise for some couples. This was the case with Bart, who told me in the first interview that he used to be a heavy smoker and heavy drinker. He said he had not been aware of the possible impact of these habits on the quality of his sperm until he came to visit the Radboud Clinic, even though he and his wife had previously been in treatment for artificial insemination in another hospital. He became upset when he recalled the moment he first found out about this:

> I even asked the doctors in the [other] hospital, 'Could it be because of my smoking or drinking?' . . . I told them, 'If I go out for an evening, twenty glasses of beer is nothing! And as far as smoking concerns, at this moment I have reduced it to one bag of full strength tobacco a week, but before!' But they said 'No, not due to smoking, neither to drinking' . . . When we came to Nijmegen, we also told it. That doctor looked at me like [both Bart and his wife start laughing when they remember the doctor's flabbergasted face]. I was really angry about that. Why did not they tell me two years earlier?

The Body Interior

Bodily examinations also added to the couples' growing insight into factors that played a role in conception. In particular, women got detailed information about the appearance of their internal reproductive organs. Like Fleur above, many women came to know and see for the first time in their lives their interior reproductive organs on an ultrasound screen and they heard the doctors make all kinds of comments about them, like for example:

> I am not feeling anything strange at your ovaries. They have a good mobility. That speaks against endometriosis. (Doctor, consultation)

Women came to know how their uterus was positioned and whether the thickness of the uterus mucus fitted with the current stage of their menstrual cycle. Women were often surprised and impressed by the fact that doctors were able to estimate almost exactly the day of their menstrual cycle, simply by seeing a white line on the screen. The following exchange between a doctor and a woman who was undergoing gynaecological examinations for the first time in her life nicely illustrates this:

> Doctor: You are now in the middle of your menstrual cycle. I can see that by the mucus.
> Kim: Can you really see that?
> Doctor: Yes, clearly.
> Kim: Great that you are able to see that!
> The doctor laughs and says jokingly: Oh yes, doctors can see so many things! (Observation, consultation)

The Hormonal Cycle

A hormonal cycle analysis was a standard procedure for almost all couples visiting the Radboud Clinic.[2] A cycle analysis gave detailed insight into several aspects of the woman's menstrual cycle and also included a post-coitus test. According to the clinic's brochure, the following elements were assessed in a cycle analysis:

- the growth of the follicle;
- the quality of the mucus (around the moment of ovulation);
- the post-coitus test;
- the moment of the ovulation;
- the duration of the second half of the cycle;
- the length of the cycle;

- the hormonal level (progesterone) in the second half of the cycle. (FertEndo n.d.: 8, translation TG)

Results of this cycle analysis were shared with the couples and generally extensively explained. For this purpose doctors often used a book containing colourful drawings of men's and women's reproductive organs, showing how conception normally takes place and at which stages problems may occur. Doctors used these pictures to facilitate understanding of all kinds of issues, as the below example illustrates:

> Let's look at the normal situation [he browses until he finds the picture he needs in the book]. You must imagine the fallopian tubes as baseball gloves partly covering the ovaries. And here [he points to different places] your fallopian tubes can be obstructed, due to the chlamydia or the appendicitis operation. (Doctor, consultation)

In the course of a cycle analysis couples got a fairly good idea of what could be seen and measured in the woman's menstrual cycle and what seemed to be good or bad in their case. Generally speaking – and this is not only with regard to the menstrual cycle – couples seemed to remember very well whether the doctor referred to findings as 'normal' or not. Questions such as, 'Is this normal, doctor?' and 'Should it be like that?' were frequently heard in the consultation room during examinations and treatment processes alike. Clear, affirmative and positive answers from the doctor's side were greedily welcomed and were sometimes proudly recalled in the interviews: 'The doctor told me that my uterus looks really good!' Negative answers were listened to and received with concern. Even when people did not fully understand all medical details and explanations, doctors' judgments – either positive or negative – seemed to be stored in people's mind and were recalled when making future speculations about their prospects.

While the major part of the cycle analysis focused on processes in the woman's body, the post-coitus test also provided information about the interaction between the man's and the woman's body material. When the woman's follicle was found to be big enough – which was monitored by means of ultrasound – the couple was requested to have coitus. The day after, at the clinic, mucus was taken out of the woman's cervix. The doctor immediately looked at the mucus under a microscope (in the consultation room) to assess the quantity of sperm and its movements. The man and woman were also invited to look through the microscope to see, most probably for the first and only time in their life, how the man's sperm was moving (or not) in his partner's body material. Men and women might experience this as a nerve-racking moment, because it gave them their first indication about their capacity to conceive as a couple.

The Uterus

As part of the initial examinations, some women also underwent a hysterosalpingogram (HSG), an examination in which a contrasting liquid is injected into the uterus. By means of this liquid, the uterus and the inside of the ovaries were made visible by means of X-rays and projected on a screen, which both the doctor and the couple could see. Though some women remembered the HSG as a painful event, some were also excited to have seen this part of their body which 'you normally do not see' and which looked like 'a picture in a biology schoolbook'. A first interpretation of the HSG was given immediately when it was made, but the couple also had an appointment with the doctor to talk through the results in more detail. The HSG pictures were then once more shown to the couple on the computer screen at the doctor's desk and the doctor explained what could be seen in the pictures. This was another opportunity for the doctor to give detailed information about the interior of the female body, as the following observation shows:

> This looks really good [the doctor points to the picture on her screen]. Here you see the uterus. Around the uterus things seem empty [it is white]. That is the uterus wall, which is very thick. It is a muscle. These are the ovaries. They are comparable with 'deep-pile carpet'. The liquid is going through the ovaries and subsequently runs over into the belly. (Doctor, consultation)

Blood

In the same period that the hormonal cycle analysis was carried out, women's blood was tested. Women found out that their blood could tell different stories that might be related to their fertility problem. One purpose of blood testing was to find out whether they had been infected with chlamydia, a sexually transmitted infection that can and does go easily unnoticed but which may seriously affect the ovaries and cause fertility problems. Not all of the female study participants were aware of the possible effect of chlamydia, though some had heard about it before. For some of the study participants it was a complete surprise to find out that they had such an infection;

and for a few of them it was an unpleasant reminder of an event they had gone through in another period of their life. One woman, for example, who knew that her ex-partner had also suffered from a chlamydia infection, was still very angry with him and blamed him for her fertility problems:

> Yes, that is really terrible! Especially because in that relationship he always beat me up. For years I have been burnt out because of that. And he [she points to her current husband] helped me to overcome that . . . And then you think you have found the man of your life, everything is going perfect and you want to start with kids and then you get this. That puts a dampener on you! This is a remainder from your former relationship. You don't expect this at all! I found that really, terribly difficult. I have sometimes thought 'I am going to shoot him!'

Another purpose of testing the blood was to obtain information about women's hormonal values. Through the outcome of this test, couples were introduced to the concept of 'biological age'. The 'biological age' referred to the woman's FSH (Follicle Stimulating Hormone)[3] level, which gives an indication of the woman's capacity to stimulate the growth of a follicle.[4] Women who had an FSH value of below ten were not expected to have a problem conceiving (as far as FSH hormones are concerned); for women with an FSH value between ten and twenty, conception was still possible, though it might become more difficult; and women with an FSH value higher than twenty were not given any chance for conception – even with medical assistance – for their 'biological age' was said to be too high.

'Biological age' appeared to be an appealing concept. Almost all couples participating in the study referred to it at one moment or another during the study and they seemed to recall the number referring to their biological age as easily as they recalled their age in years. Marion, for example, who was thirty-seven years old when starting her first IVF treatment, proudly compared her own low FSH level with that of her younger friend:

> Yes, she [her friend] will be thirty-three in September and she has an FSH of eleven. And me, I have 3.3. So, yes, that was okay!

Semen

For men, besides the initial examinations of their penis, testicles and epididymis, the semen test was the most important part of the diagnosis. Men also learned to assess and judge the product of their ejaculation according to clinical criteria. They came to talk about their sperm in terms of quantity, mobility of sperm and normally or abnormally formed sperm. This was what one couple heard from the doctor when the man's sperm was tested for the first time:

> The semen examination shows some distortions. It is not bad, but it could be better. You do have lot of sperm, but they do not move well. They swim, so to say, in rounds, not neatly up, as you certainly may know from television pictures. But in itself the sperm is of good enough quality to cause pregnancy. (Doctor, consultation)

Men became aware of the enormous amount of sperm that is involved in 'normal' conception: one does not talk about sperm in terms of thousands, but in terms of many millions. Couples were quick to integrate this newly gained insight into their considerations, as the following dialogue between Fleur and Simon shows:

> Fleur: Your volume was higher the second time.
> Simon: Yes, that increased, the doctor said. But at the same time the percentage of abnormal sperm also increased. That went from 92 per cent to 98 per cent. So, 2 per cent was okay. He said, 'Two per cent of fifteen million spermazoids is still a lot'. I said 'Yes, I do understand that'. Then he said 'So the chance to conceive naturally is always there, but that chance is very low, if I am honest. Since many of them die on their way, you must be really lucky if exactly that one is to get there, but it may happen'.

In addition, men found out that both the quantity and quality of their sperm might vary substantially over time, which might be due, for example, to the physical condition of the man (a serious fever, for example, can drastically decrease the amount of sperm) or due to changes in the man's drinking and smoking patterns.

Increasing the 'Medical Gaze'

At the end of the examination phase couples had absorbed an enormous amount of information and they had an idea of the manifold factors that, from a biomedical point of view, are involved in successful conception, information that made some couples remark, 'You sometimes wonder how it goes well so often!' They also got insight in what may cause failure to conceive. For some couples the examinations lead to a clear diagnosis of their infertility, for others their infertility problem remained 'unexplained'. Most of the couples at the Radboud Clinic, after the examination phase, first went through a phase of low-tech treatments, in which phase they continued acquiring insights about reproductive processes.

Obviously, not everything they heard was new. They added newly gained insights to their already existing understanding – sometimes very basic and sometimes more 'advanced' – of how human conception occurs. The clinic was also, of course, not the only source of information for these couples; quite a few searched on the Internet, consulted books and/or spoke with friends or relatives who had been in similar situations. The level of understanding was highly divergent among the men and women visiting the clinic.[5] Yet, however low or high the exact level of their understanding was, at this stage all of them came to see and acknowledge new biological processes and entities that they had not been aware of before (cf. Becker and Nachtigall 1991; Franklin 1997). They underwent a rapid learning process in which they became increasingly sophisticated in their understanding of how doctors think and the modalities they use – they learned to judge their own reproductive parameters as 'good or bad' and as 'normal or deviant'.

This increased knowledge enabled the couples to better understand their own diagnosis and proposed steps in treatment, which in turn allowed them to be actively engaged in decision-making and – in some cases – to even negotiate with doctors about further treatments, as other scholars have found as well (see, e.g., Becker and Nachtigall 1991: 883). At the other hand, though, I argue that by getting accustomed to and impressed by all these medical insights, examinations and procedures, they became more and more inclined to see themselves, their bodies and their habits – like drinking, smoking, sauna visits – through a 'medical gaze' (Foucault 1973). They thus came to look at their infertility problem and solutions more and more in medical terms and to see themselves as patients, which, in turn, increased their ability to behave as such (cf. Lupton 1997). By acting as (good) patients, and here I follow the arguments as presented by Thompson (2005) and Pasveer and Heesterbeek (2001), most of them were well prepared to follow complex medical instructions and to endure demanding treatment trajectories, as was required when doing IVF.

In Vitro Fertilization in Eight Steps

An IVF cycle can be seen as a trajectory consisting of several steps; at the Radboud Clinic an IVF cycle normally involved eight steps.[6] At the end of each step another visualized criterion defined whether this step had been passed successfully or not (see Table 6.1).

TABLE 6.1 Visualized Outcome Criteria in Steps of IVF

Steps in IVF	Visualized Outcome Criteria
First ultrasound	Small black spots
Ultrasound controls	Number and size of follicles
Follicle aspiration	Number of eggs retrieved
Production of sperm	Quantity and quality of sperm
Fertilization	Number of eggs fertilized
Embryo transfer	Quality of embryos; number of cells
Pregnancy test	A blue line[1]
Foetal ultrasound	A ticking heart; size of foetus

Note:
1. This is the positive sign of a frequently used pregnancy test. Other tests show different signs.

In the first step, the woman's own cycle was suppressed by the use of triptoreline (Decapeptyl®), a GnRH agonist that suppresses the production of FSH and LH (luteinizing hormone)[7] in the pituitary gland.[8] After that the growth of follicles was stimulated by (recombinant) FSH (Puregon®). In this period the follicle growth was monitored by regular ultrasound controls. Once follicles were big enough, women had to take an injection of Pregnyl®, which is a (urinary) HCG (human chorionic gonadtropin) that stimulates the ovulation and supports the luteal phase. The following day, the follicle aspiration (ova pick-up) took place and the retrieved follicles were immediately brought together with the man's sperm. In the laboratory, fertilization was then supposed to take place, which should lead to the development of a number of embryos. Three days later, one or two embryos were selected and transferred to the woman's uterus (embryo transfer). If the remaining embryos were of good quality, they were frozen (cryo preservation) for use in a potential next treatment. A period of two weeks of waiting started, during which the woman took progesterone (Progestan®), a hormone that also supports the luteal phase. After this period of two weeks – and if the woman had not yet started her menstruation – a pregnancy test was done. If this test showed a positive result, couples visited the hospital, after another three weeks of waiting, for a foetal ultrasound, which was the last step. The total period from starting the first hormonal injection up to the foetal ultrasound took about nine weeks (about 60–65 days).

In theory, each step thus should lead to the next step, but in practice each step might also result in a failure, and could become an 'obstacle' (cf. Franklin 1997: 107). Louise, who kept a detailed diary of her experiences throughout the IVF cycles she underwent, was very much aware of these steps and obstacles; she described an IVF cycle as going from 'milestone to milestone'. Excerpts of her diary illustrate clearly how she experienced the different steps and 'milestones' (see Case Study: Louise's Diary). In the section that follows I discuss how she and other study participants experienced the different steps in an IVF cycle and how they interpreted, in constant interaction with clinic staff, their achievements at each step.

Case Study: Louise's Diary

Louise and Eric first underwent twelve IUIs before they started IVF treatments. The first IVF treatment, which was almost cancelled due to a threatening hyperstimulation (Louise had 'produced' thirty eggs), initially lead to a pregnancy but unfortunately ended in a miscarriage, which they found out at the moment of the foetal ultrasound in the hospital. The second IVF treatment also ended in a very early miscarriage. In total Louise has had four miscarriages. Because of these repetitive miscarriages, the clinic performed a habitual miscarriage examination before starting the third and – as they felt at that moment – last IVF treatment. This 'habitual abortion examination', however, did not provide any insight into the reason for the frequent miscarriages.

Louise is one of the women who kept an extended diary on behalf of the study, from the moment she and her husband started their first IVF treatment. Below I present some excerpts from her diary. We enter her story when she has just visited the clinic for the first ultrasound of their *third* IVF cycle. The excerpts show the ups and downs during the various stages in one treatment cycle and how the outcomes at the visual milestones of conception affected her mood and expectations.

Day 1 – First ultrasound
The starting ultrasound. Everything is okay. But I was not afraid of this anyway. At this stage things have always been okay . . . Next week Friday, on the eighth day, I have to come back to see how many follicles are growing.

Day 8 – Ultrasound check-up 1
Friday the thirteenth. What a day for such a thrilling ultrasound! I am extremely anxious about this ultrasound. On the one hand I fear that again I will have too many eggs. On the other hand I am afraid that there are not enough [eggs], because I am feeling very well and I do not at all

have the feeling of being 'filled' . . . Luckily, the ultrasound shows that things are going fine . . . In the afternoon I was phoned [by someone from the clinic] and they told me that we can stimulate one more day, to allow the small follicles a bit more time to grow.

Day 9 – Ultrasound check-up 2
That extra day of stimulating was helpful: both on the left and on the right side small follicles are doing a pursuit race. It looks good, as far as I can judge as a lay person. . . . They phoned me to say that the follicle aspiration will only take place on Tuesday. One more day for the small follicles to grow! Everything looks super fine this time. I hope this is a precursor of a good ending of this (last!) attempt.

Day 12 – Follicle aspiration
The day of the follicle aspiration. I am really super relaxed and do not fear the treatment. I have slept fine, without tranquilizers. The only thing I am worried about – each and every time – is that I have had an ovulation in between and that they cannot find any follicles anymore . . .

Immediately after the follicle aspiration (in the restroom) we are informed that twelve eggs have been found. This is the same number as during the second treatment in October. At that time only four were fertilized. Then we were disappointed, because the average fertilization rate is sixty or seventy per cent. Why would it be that much lower with us? I so much hope that it will be better now. In the first place I hope that more eggs will be fertilized and in the second place that they [the embryos] will divide as well. The last time they transferred two embryos, both of 4 cells: one of moderate and one of reasonable quality. Everything has to be perfect this time; this has to be the one!

Day 14 – Phone call about the number of embryos
Five years married. Our first lustrum. I so much wanted to get good news on this day, but no: only three out of the twelve eggs are fertilized. Twenty-five per cent instead of the average of sixty to seventy per cent. I could cry. And did so, I have to admit. . . . I am convinced that after this news [the realization of] our wish for a child has come to an end.

Of course, tomorrow it might be that the embryos are of good quality, but how big is that chance? In the first attempt only two [embryos] out of nineteen were okay. In the second treatment none of the four were optimal. How naïve you have to be to assume that these three [embryos] will be good? And I do not want to give up hope. But from where can I get some hope? I simply don't know . . .

Day 15 – Embryo transfer

From eight o'clock I press the 'refresh button' on the Digitale Poli page until data about the transfer appear. A bit before nine it is there: one embryo of 'quality two' and one of 'quality three' will be transferred (on a scale of one to four, of which one is bad, two is moderate, three is reasonable and four is good). I am relieved. I was already convinced that all three would be of the first category. The site also shows pictures of our embryos! Great! Suddenly I see things much less negatively than yesterday. We try to decipher how many cells they have, but we do not manage. Apparently that needs a more trained eye.

In the afternoon during the embryo transfer we hear that the moderate embryo consists of five cells and the reasonable one of six. We are not unsatisfied! In the former treatment we only had embryos of 4 cells. So, if you look at it like that, we can count on our cards this time. And that time we also became – though very briefly – pregnant. We keep hoping!

Day 16 – First day of the waiting period

I am getting mad with all that well meant advice around me . . . Of course, everybody wants the best for me. But, if there is one person who wants to stick to those two tiny tots, it is me!

Day 18

Working again. I rather would have stayed at home . . . But of course, during a fresh pregnancy you normally do what you are used to do. So you may work as well. Who knows if anything has already nestled. Or it happens today. Or tomorrow . . .

Day 22

I am pregnant. I simply know it for sure. I feel it. Of course I do not dare to be happy, but if I am honest, I think it is okay this time. Without any doubt my breasts are bigger, they are very sensitive and it simply feels good.

Day 24

The last days I had sensitive breasts, but that feeling is slowly passing away. A bad sign? I know I had it during the first treatment as well . . . It does not look to be a good sign, but what do I actually know about pregnancies?! I am not really an expert in that. I am surfing like a fool on the Internet about whether this is normal, but it does not give me too much.

Day 24 until Day 28

In the five days before the testing day as proposed by the clinic, Louise does four pregnancy tests. In her diary she describes nuances in how the test results looked exactly, how quickly or slowly they disappeared, and her interpretations of all this. She also pictures the feelings of uncertainty that arose because of the different signs her body gave, which confused her. She kept wondering whether the changes in her body were a side effect of the hormonal treatment or signs of an ongoing pregnancy.

Day 29 – Pregnancy test day

The formal pregnancy test day. The whole night I was awake because I was afraid that the test would not be positive anymore. At two o'clock in the morning I do a test. It feels as if it takes ages, but at the end the test really shows a second line. But I am frightened that it is less convincing. I am not really reassured when I return to my bed . . . At six o'clock I do another test. Very clear and quickly positive. That is encouraging! I phone the hospital to inform them about the result . . .

Day 31

Again I am afraid that it is not okay . . . [She describes in detail how bodily signs change again]. I phone to make an appointment for the foetal ultrasound . . . We have set a date, but I am afraid that I will have to cancel it because of a loss of the pregnancy [before that date].

Day 32

I am so terribly sick!!!! Great! How weird that you can so much enjoy feeling so terribly sick . . .

Day 32 to Day 52

Louise describes the bodily signs she is confronted with and how she interprets them. Slowly, she becomes convinced that she is pregnant, though she has strong moments of uncertainty as well. One night she panics completely and dreads it is all over. Then she phones the clinic and manages to move the appointment for the ultrasound from Friday to Monday (four days earlier). The day before the ultrasound she feels absolutely nervous. She writes: 'The idea that our future regarding our wish for a child depends on tomorrow's ultrasound. This is unbearable!'

Day 53 – The foetal ultrasound

I thought there were two possible scenarios for our ultrasound visit:
1) I come extremely happy out of the hospital, because we have seen a ticking heart and so I am really pregnant with one or two growing embryos;

2) It becomes one of the most difficult days of my life because I will not carry to term this pregnancy because there is no viable foetus.

I had not reckoned on a third option: uncertainty again. We had the ultrasound, the heart is ticking and the foetus is of the size that fits with the duration of the pregnancy. But still, we have to return in two weeks for an extra check-up. Why is that now? . . . A reason for the extra check-up has not been given. We can only guess. I am angry with myself: why did not I ask more questions? . . .

Day 53 – Day 62
Louise describes how tired she feels and how her mood affects her work. She does not enjoy her pregnancy. She does not feel sick anymore and that makes her feel uncertain and worried again. She phones the hospital and asks whether she cannot come a day earlier for the second foetal ultrasound, but they do not allow her because her situation is not really acute. She very much realizes that she only wants to be reassured.

Day 63 – The second foetal ultrasound
Finally, the ultrasound! With another doctor this time. Immediately it becomes clear why we had to return for a second ultrasound. The other doctor had jotted down a different date for the follicle aspiration . . . In his perception the foetus had growth retardation at the moment of the first ultrasound. Why did not he simply tell us? . . . Now we have been uncertain for two weeks, while there was no reason for that. [Though very upset about such an error, they also enjoyed extremely seeing the images of the second foetal ultrasound]. What we see cannot be described. The small [her family name] is already 2.5 centimetres and has a head, arms and legs. Incredible. We both got silent about it . . . Our mini-person, of Erik and me. And it grows in my belly!

First Ultrasound: Small Black Spots

Fourteen days after women started to inject Decapeptyl®, which – as they had learned – suppresses the woman's hormonal cycle, they returned to the clinic for the first ultrasound. Based on this ultrasound the doctor decided whether a couple could start treatment. The doctor checked for the absence of cysts and measured the thickness of the mucus. Moreover, she looked at the number of 'small black spots' in the ovaries, which gave an indication of the number of follicles that potentially might grow when stimulation with hormones was started. Couples were sometimes surprised to see these black spots, as they thought that suppressing their hormonal activity meant that nothing would be seen at all. More than once I heard the doctors explain that suppressing a woman's hormonal cycle meant that, although the follicles did not continue growing, they were still there. Rarely did people exhibit much worry about this first ultrasound. Apparently, they did not consider it to be a very decisive moment in terms of continuing or not continuing treatment, probably due to the fact that it was seldom couples were not allowed to continue treatment at this stage of the first ultrasound and therefore it was apparently also not emphasized by clinic staff as a critical moment. However, in the interviews some people did refer to this moment as the point at which 'we were allowed to start', indicating that they were aware that it could have turned out differently. Others recalled exactly the comments made by the doctor when she saw the number of black spots and how they interpreted this. Marion, for example, understood from the first ultrasound that things looked very good and therefore she was eagerly looking forward to know the impact of the hormonal stimulation, as she had high expectations for this as well:

> Marion: Yes, she [the doctor] was really surprised to see five already
> – she called them 'bubbles' – on one side.
> Kees: And on the other side even six or seven!
> Marion: That many! I could not see it that well. So the doctor said, 'We are going back to a 125 [milligram] dosage [instead of the standard dosage of 150 Puregon®]'. Yes, I am curious to know it [the result]. I am thirty-six now, but apparently I am still in my fertile period.

Seeing a high number of black spots – potential follicles – and having the planned doses of medicine lowered, was here interpreted as a good start for the IVF trajectory. Theoretically, a limited number of black spots could occasionally have raised people's concerns, but I did not come across such a situation.

Control Ultrasounds: Growing Follicles

Yes, and she [the doctor] is very clear ... She did that first measurement – yes, it was like that – and then there were only four follicles on the left side. And then she said, 'That is really disappointing'. That was because of the high doses I got. Yes, they were big, but she [the doctor] had thought that there would have been much more and also some on the right side. But there were none at all.

Immediately after the first ultrasound, women started to inject hormones stimulating the growth of the follicles (Puregon®). I heard the doctors tell the men and women in treatment that ideally five to fifteen follicles should grow in the woman's uterus in a stimulated cycle. In practice, however, this did not always happen. Women reacted differently to hormonal stimulation and this was not only dependent on their personal FSH level or on the amount of hormonal medicine injected. Nobody could predict how a woman would react. Sometimes couples – and the doctor, as we saw in the introductory case above (which refers to Christine and Bert) – became disappointed because the reaction was lower than expected. Production of a low number of follicles gave reason for concern for the ongoing treatment cycle, but also for a couple's future treatment opportunities. Before starting the treatment, couples were informed about the fact that if they produced less than three follicles with maximum stimulation (i.e., 300 entities of Puregon®) and did not become pregnant as a result of that treatment cycle, they would not be allowed to do another IVF treatment. In particular, older women whose FSH level was relatively high and who injected the maximal dosage of Puregon® feared that scenario. Birgit, for example, expressed her worries about that before starting her first IVF treatment:

> I really was shocked when I heard from that doctor [during the pre-IVF consultation] that if no eggs get 'released' then it is over and finished. That is what I am really worried about. Imagine you have the bad luck that you do not produce any eggs! Then it is finished and nothing can be done anymore! . . . I am really concerned about that, the more so because with the check-ups of my ovaries I regularly had cysts.

Unfortunately for Birgit and her partner, Harry, they indeed had the bad luck that Birgit only 'produced' a few eggs in their first IVF treatment cycle. When I met them in the clinic at one of their ultrasound controls, Birgit told me that she had had a nervous breakdown over the weekend because she had only produced two eggs. She had really been panicking that this would be the end of their IVF story. Yet the day I met them at the clinic the doctor had just told them that the follicles were big enough now to plan the ova pick-up, meaning that they were 'allowed' to continue treatment. Birgit and her husband were pleasantly surprised to hear this, as they had understood that a minimum of three eggs had to develop for an ova pick-up to take place. Unfortunately for them, the treatment did not result in a pregnancy, so for them their first IVF treatment was also immediately their last one as they were not allowed to do a further treatment. Birgit, however, tried hard to convince the doctors to give her one more chance (she also asked me if I could try to influence the doctor). Finally, as she told me in the second interview, she stopped her resistance to the doctors' decision when the head of the department convinced her, by showing her that she really did not have any more eggs:

> Birgit: He made one more ultrasound. He examined me again and everything and he then said, 'There is nothing left'. And if there is nothing left, then . . .
> Harry: You are fooling yourself if . . .
> Birgit: Yes, you are fooling yourself.
> Harry: That is what he [the doctor] also said.
> Birgit: Okay, it is difficult. I have now heard it from all the doctors.

This case underlines the ideas about the pivotal role of visualization in the production of authoritative knowledge, as put forward by George (1996) and Layne (2003).[9] These authors claim that the authority of imagining technology primarily rests on its ability to create a straightforward sense of reality. Birgit could not be convinced by explanations alone, but once the doctor had *shown* her that her eggs were finished she was convinced, though actually she fully depended on the doctor's interpretations of the pictures. In general, lay people need doctors to interpret what they see, as 'the objects of scientific and medical scrutiny must be rendered, they are rarely perceived or manipulated in their "natural" state' (Rapp 1999: 119). Doctors were thus in charge of the visualizing technologies, as they were the ones who interpreted the pictures (which are not always incontestable or clear). In addition, they could decide to be flexible in the application of clinic criteria, which added to their authoritative position (as in this case the couple was allowed to pass to the ova pick-up with 'only two' instead of the required three follicles).

In the above case, the production of only a few follicles was reason for stress and concern. In other cases where the production of follicles was found to be good or better than expected given the amount of black spots seen at the first ultrasound or the FSH level of the woman involved, this clearly enhanced hope. Yet at other times a high number of follicles was reason for concern and stress: some women participating in the study dreaded that they would react too strongly to the follicle stimulating hormones and that this might lead to the risky situation of hyperstimulation. Women who had once been close to hyperstimulation or had actually had to stop a treatment cycle were clearly more conscious and scared of this in a following treatment cycle. We can see this in the case of Louise, who had once produced thirty follicles and only narrowly escaped a hyperstimulation, but also seriously suffered from side effects after the aspiration.

Not only was the number of follicles an indicator of successful or unsuccessful stimulation, but follicles should also be of a certain size. On the patients' form (on which IVF doctors kept a record of the growth of follicles during the stimulation period), a bold line distinguished between the follicles that had the right size, i.e., everything above fifteen millimetres, and those that were still too small. Often, doctors had to decide whether to continue stimulation (which allowed the smaller follicles to grow, but possibly at the expense of some of the larger ones which could snap before the aspiration took place) or to stop stimulation (which saved the bigger ones, but implied that the small ones would still be small when 'harvested' in the aspiration). As the IVF doctors often reflected loudly on this decision in the presence of the couples, they became aware of this kind of consideration. Regularly, I heard couples make remarks about both the size and number of follicles. These numbers became part of the information which they used to assess their chances in a given treatment cycle and they also compared them with other cycles.

Follicle Aspiration: Number of Follicles

> I am entering the recovery room, a small room next to the room where the follicle aspirations take place, to see Jeanet and Karel. Jeanet has just undergone the follicle aspiration and is now recovering from it. I ask her how she felt about this aspiration and she answers that it went okay – 'much better than the other time'. They know there were 'many eggs', but do not yet know how many. At that moment the laboratory technician knocks on the door and enters the room. She has good news to tell. 'We have found sixteen eggs and the sperm is also good for ICSI'. Karel and Jeanet are visibly pleased to hear this. The laboratory technician asks if they have any questions at that moment. As they do not have any she wishes them all the best and leaves the room.
> (Observation, recovery room)

Counting the number of follicles during ultrasound controls was one thing; knowing the exact number of eggs retrieved in the aspiration was another. Over the course of the treatment trajectory couples came to know that the number of eggs was generally a bit lower than the number of follicles seen at the last ultrasound control. Partly, this could be explained by the fact that some of the developed follicles were empty, so did not contain any eggs at all. It could also be partly due to the fact that some of the follicles – in particular the bigger ones – might have snapped before the aspiration took place. Finally, it might be that not all follicles were punctured: the doctor may have overlooked one or more follicles, or may have decided not to puncture them all because the aspiration was difficult. At times, I heard IVF doctors making remarks like, 'That one is too difficult to get. I will leave it where it is'. Occasionally, when doctors saw that the aspiration was becoming too painful for the woman, I heard them consider or suggest that they should not retrieve the very last one(s), although the women did not always agree; they would rather suffer a bit longer than lose one or more eggs, which they saw as diminishing their chances.

Even when couples had consciously followed and counted the number and size of the follicles during the ultrasound checks, the exact number of eggs retrieved in the aspiration was still a surprise. Couples were anxious to know the number of eggs that were punctured and they were told this almost immediately after the follicle aspiration; generally it was the laboratory technician who came to bring the news.[10] At the same moment, s/he gave feedback about the sperm that the man has handed in the same morning. Thus on the day of the aspiration, couples left the hospital fully informed about the number of eggs that (maximally) would be fertilized. As Louise wrote in her diary when she had the aspiration in her second treatment cycle:

> We drive home [after the follicle aspiration]. We had thirty eggs and twenty-five million spermazoids. That looks really good! Let us now hope that fertilization will take place.

Production of Sperm: Quality and Quantity

Men whose sperm in the examination phase was of good quality and quantity were generally not concerned when they handed it in on the day of the aspiration (though producing it on the spot, or bringing it on time to the clinic might be a point of concern). This was different, however, for men whose sperm in former tests was of low quality and/or quantity. If the sperm was shown to be of too bad quality to expect fertilization to take place in 'normal'

IVF procedures, it was often decided that ICSI should take place. In ICSI, the laboratory part of the treatment is different: for each ovum one sperm is chosen and injected into it. For ICSI to be possible, a certain minimum number of motile sperm has to be available. So for couples undergoing IVF-ICSI, this added an extra critical moment to the treatment trajectory. I sometimes found that couples were visibly relieved when they heard that the man's sperm was found to be good enough for ICSI to take place.

For couples undergoing IVF-PESA things were even more stressful, as seen in the following observation of Christine and Bert, the only couple participating in this study that underwent PESA.[11]

> I meet Christine and Bert in the recovery room, where Christine is recovering from the follicle aspiration (this is their second IVF-PESA treatment). I also attended the aspiration, which has apparently been a painful event. After the aspiration Christine almost fainted. Her face became pale and her heartbeat went down. She got some more atropine, a medicine used to enhance her heart beat, as the doctor explained. After having rested for a while in the aspiration room, she needed a wheelchair to go to the recovery room to fully recover. About fifteen minutes later I enter and by then they have already received aspiration results. They proudly tell me about it: 'Sixteen eggs. That is much more than the other time. I injected the Puregon® one day longer than the other time. So that might explain it'. Then she continues, a bit worried, 'I hope they will find enough sperm to fertilize all the sixteen eggs. I am not saying that all sixteen eggs will be of good quality, but at least twelve to thirteen, I hope'. She is referring to the fact that her husband's sperm still has to be retrieved through a PESA procedure (on the same day). As his sterilization could not be undone, there was no option left other than to obtain his sperm by retrieving them directly from the epididymis. (Observation, recovery room)

Ideally, when a couple underwent IVF-PESA, the man's sperm was retrieved before the IVF treatment started, in order to know whether sperm was still available and indeed could be retrieved from the man's epididymis. If so, the sperm was frozen and used for fertilization the moment the woman had the follicle aspiration. Couples then did not need to be concerned, because they knew there was sperm available. If, however, as in the case of Christine and Bert, after the first failed IVF-PESA treatment no sperm was left for a second treatment, a so-called 'acute' PESA had to take place. Acute here means that it took place on the same day as the woman underwent the follicle aspiration. In these cases the couple did not yet know whether there would be (enough) good quality sperm to fertilize the retrieved eggs. Unfortunately for Bert and Christine, the PESA did not give the desired result. After a painful PESA, performed by an urologist in the presence of a laboratory technician from the fertility clinic, who searched for sperm on the spot under the microscope (which process I could follow in an adjacent room), the couple heard that sperm was found, but that further laboratory tests were needed to check whether there were any *moving* sperm. When the urologist informed them about this, the laboratory technician added:

> We hope for the best. We will try hard to find them. Later today you will get a phone call to inform you about the number of spermazoids and whether they are motile. (Observation, PESA)

As they had received a similar comment when they did their first PESA, the couple did not seem too worried. I told Christine and Bert that I was curious to know the result and asked them to keep me informed. Christine first laughingly questioned whether 'the researcher was not becoming too involved' (she pointed to the fact that I had been with them for the whole day and I had seen them both suffering from their interventions, so indeed I had become engaged in their situation) and then she promised to inform me. The next morning I found a short message in my e-mail box, saying: 'Dear Trudie, no moving sperm was found. Kind regards, Christine'. I did not need any more explanation to understand what impact this message must have had on the expectations of the couple. In their case this was not only an abrupt end to the treatment cycle, but also the end of any form of treatment at the Radboud Clinic.[12]

Fertilization: Number of Eggs Fertilized

Two days after the follicle aspiration had taken place, couples were called and informed about how many of the retrieved eggs had actually been fertilized. During these lab procedures the couples were 'transferred' to the side-lines: there was nothing they themselves could contribute other than waiting for a phone call from the clinic. The phone became 'a dreaded source of potential disappointment' (cf. Franklin and Roberts 2006: 146). Several women and men told me that they were nervously waiting for this phone call, in particular – but not only – when it was their first treatment and they did not yet know whether fertilization would be possible at all.

When I left the clinic [after the follicle aspiration] the doctor said, 'I will phone you on Wednesday between one and two and then you will hear how many eggs are fertilized'. I purposefully planned to go to the hairdresser on Wednesday morning; I do have all kinds of mechanisms for myself [she laughs]. If the entire morning you expect to get that phone call, of course you go mad. Then you get all kinds of ideas into your head. So, I had better sit at the hairdresser's, for relaxation, for distraction. But then, just when I was paying my bill at the counter – I had my mobile phone with me – my phone rang. 'Oh, that is not good, if they phone now'. That is your first thought! Later on they phoned me again, I was in a small side road nearby. Then she told me that of the four eggs only one was fertilized.

Louise, who suffered from serious side effects from the hormonal stimulation, also nervously waited for such a phone call. She wrote in her diary:

We should be phoned between 11.00 and 14.00 and I was afraid that they wouldn't call until just before two. Fortunately doctors understand how stressful this is, because the doctor phoned at only 11.15: There are sixteen fertilized eggs! Fantastic! They are possibly our future kids. What a wealth to reach at least this stage.

Louise referred here to sixteen embryos – which had not yet been transferred to her body and were not visible to the eye (they are smaller than the point of a needle) – as her potential 'future kids', while women who become pregnant in a 'normal' way are not even aware at this stage if fertilization has taken place at all. This case demonstrates how, by means of assisted reproductive technologies, 'hidden' aspects of conception become exposed to the eye and to the consciousness (cf. Sandelowski 1993), and shape people's expectations as well as their connection with the embryos. Referring to similar cases[13] Tjornhoj (2005: 86) distinguished between 'what is shown' to women and men undergoing fertility treatments and 'what is seen'. She argued that what is seen is a question of interpretation, depending on the perspective of the spectators: their life worlds, knowledge, desires and hopes. Louise referring to her fertilized eggs as her future children indeed very much reflected her desires and hopes. Thus, when couples are going through IVF 'the social construction of their baby' may already begin before implantation (cf. Layne 2003: 83).

While Louise expressed anxiety about the outcome of this step in treatment, for most couples in IVF treatment this stage did not form a major obstacle. One of the two couples who did an IVF-TESE treatment, however, had the following bad fortune.[14] The woman wrote me an e-mail about this:

> The next day we could phone [the doctor in the other hospital] to hear whether fertilization had taken place. He told me that something was going on, but it was not yet clear. So, I had to phone again the next day. I was a bit worried, but okay, when Theo [her husband] calmed me down, I could bear it. The next day, on my birthday, the doctor phones me that there had been five useful eggs, but that NO [her capital letters] fertilization had taken place. What a disappointment!!!!! The more so because the chance of fertilization is eighty per cent . . . This time I cried quite a lot . . . because you are losing hope. This [no fertilization] is a possibility as well, so this stage becomes more stressful. The stress is increasing.

For some couples, in particular when it was their third IVF treatment, such a phone call could suddenly mean the absolute end of their attempts to conceive with medical assistance.[15] For others, as with the number of eggs retrieved, the number of fertilized eggs – that is, the number of embryos developed – increased or decreased their hope. Annelies, who heard that she had only one fertilized egg in the second treatment, sadly illustrated this when I spoke with her on the telephone:

> The second treatment only gave me one embryo and that one also developed badly. But when we started, they really gave me lots of hope: 'It looks as if you are a woman of twenty to thirty years old'.

Embryo Transfer: Quality of Embryos

Before starting their first IVF treatment Sylvia and Bob talk with me about what they think will be different in an IVF cycle compared to the IUI treatments they have had. They have heard stories from good friends who have also done IVF treatments.

Bob: In any case, you then know that fertilization has taken place. Whether you have 'top embryos' or 'less [quality] embryos'. Yes, that is the kind of terms they use to talk about it.

Sylvia: Yes, they [their friends] had top embryos. At least, that is what they made of it. Very nice ones! [All laugh]

TG: Very nice ones!

Sylvia: Of nine cells. Apparently, those are very nice ones.

Bob: . . . At this moment I think that in the cycle we will encounter the same kind of problems as we had with IUI: stressing about whether it has been successful after two weeks and such things. Yes, I think that I have to expect the same; but maybe it is different if you have top embryos. That is going to play differently on your mind.

Two days after the fertilization couples came to know over the phone how many eggs had actually been fertilized, but at that moment they were not yet informed about the quality of the embryos. They came to know this one day later, when they visited the clinic for the embryo transfer. According to what I learned from my visit to the IVF laboratory, there were two basic types of criteria used to assess embryos. The first one referred to the partition of cells and the second to the quality of the embryos. Regarding the partition of cells, the embryo was supposed to consist of four cells on the first day and seven to eight cells on the third day (the day of the embryo transfer). The quality of the embryos was judged by the laboratory technician and s/he also decided which embryo to transfer:[16] when no distortions were noted at all, the quality was good (*goed*), less than 10 per cent of distortions meant reasonable (*redelijk*), 10 to 50 per cent of distortions was moderate (*matig*) and more than 50 per cent was bad (*slecht*). The laboratory technician who gave these explanations immediately added, however, that the quality judgement was 'a bit subjective'. To illustrate this he showed me how he filled in the laboratory form of the first patient for that day: '8c m/r' (the *m* refers to moderate and the *r* to reasonable). Subsequently, however, on the form to be used by the doctor he had written in full 'reasonable', as, he added, this sounds friendlier for the couple concerned. This well-meant practice once more shows the malleability of the interpretation of treatment outcomes at different stages, which is in the hands of clinic staff.[17]

Two different types of judgements thus existed. I heard doctors explain to couples what cell partition entailed (and this cell partition was also visible on the pictures of the embryos which couples participating in the Digitale Poli could see – see below); but I never heard any couples receive an explanation or any details about the percentage of distortions. Almost all couples could tell me, though, when I asked them, about the quality of the embryo(s) transferred, either by recalling the exact number of cells and/or by mentioning the quality judgement. As indicated by Bob and Sylvia in the above interview excerpt (when they referred to the 'top embryos' of their friends), knowing the quality of the embryos transferred definitely played a role in the way people assessed their own chances. Good quality and many cells sometimes made people feel as if they had won at least half the battle. Contrarily, 'bad quality embryos' decreased people's hope, as was illustrated by Mireille, who described herself as more pessimistic in the second treatment compared to the first treatment and clearly linked this to the quality of the embryos:

> The first time, I felt something like, 'Everything is okay. It cannot go wrong'. But now, I do not know . . . Also because you know the embryos were moderate. That sounds different than reasonable. Yes and then you think – I thought – according to me it will not.

A number of times I heard clinic staff saying that they were not too pleased about mentioning the quality of the embryo, as they were well aware of the hope or despair it might create (and they might also have been aware that there is a level of subjectivity involved in the quality assessment, although I never heard any of the clinic staff actually mention this). Therefore, in a staff meeting they agreed to first ask couples whether they wanted to know the quality of the embryo(s). The reason behind this question was sometimes explained to the couples: they stressed that a good or bad quality embryo did not predict a good or bad outcome and it certainly did not say anything about the 'quality of the child' that might be born from the treatment. Still, and notwithstanding these reservations, couples showed contentment when they heard that their embryos were of good quality or consisted of eight or more cells. Sometimes couples were extra pleased to have good quality embryos, as former steps had not been very successful:

> It looked as if things went very badly because we had very few eggs and only three were left for the aspiration, of which only two were fertilized. But then, finally, these two embryos were so nice.

Couples participating in the Digitale Poli proudly told me that they had seen a picture of the embryo(s) on their personal file and added comments such as, 'this you normally do not see', 'it is very special' or 'so nice'. Apparently, seeing the picture of an embryo that you normally do not see at that stage and which in reality is smaller than a pin head, made people speak and feel differently about an embryo than when conception is not medically assisted. It is as if seeing the embryo made it more tangible and in a way confirmed its existence. Seeing pictures of the embryo was clearly a 'record of achievement' and a 'visual document of almost offspring' as has also been described by Franklin and Roberts (2006: 153). The embryos were ascribed qualities that more readily refer to babies than to embryos, which is similar to what Layne (2003) found regarding parents' interpretations of foetus ultrasounds. Women (and men) used the pictures of their embryos 'to enlist others in the social construction of their baby' (cf. Layne 2003: 85).[18] For example, one of the couples (Anneke and Frits), who had seen the embryos on the screen and who indeed became pregnant from that same IVF, shared the picture of the embryos with their colleagues:

> We want to do something with it on the birth card . . . It is one of the two. We do not know whether it is 'a' or 'b', but okay. [Both laugh]. We have forwarded the picture to many people at my office. They say, 'In fact you cannot see anything', but they still found it very special to see.

Anneke here points to an interesting contradiction regarding the embryo pictures on her screen: on the one hand they are considered as highly personalized pictures – one of the embryos is 'their baby'; at the same time, though, the picture does not show that much, and they would certainly not have noticed if they had received the picture of another embryo at the same stage of development. The pictures are in fact 'interchangeable', and this, as Layne has argued regarding ultrasound pictures, increases their 'iconic power' (cf. Layne 2003: 98). The pictures only get their meaning because of the medical authority attached to them.

Embryos that were not used in an IVF treatment and which were of good quality could be preserved (cryo preservation) to be used in a (potential) next IVF treatment. At the Radboud Clinic this was said to occur in about one out of six or seven IVF treatments. When the remaining embryo(s) were of good enough quality to be frozen, this immediately implied that the transferred embryos were of very good quality as well, as the best ones were always selected for immediate use. Obviously, couples in the study that could freeze one or more embryos were extremely satisfied about this, as this gave them good hopes for the current treatment cycle, plus an extra chance in the future. This was literally an extra chance, as the Radboud Clinic did not count or charge the treatment with preserved embryos as an extra treatment, but saw it as part of the IVF treatment cycle in which the embryo(s) developed.

Couples were thus optimistic because they had reasonable or good quality or even preserved embryos, or contrarily worried because the quality of their embryos had proved to be low. Still, several of them were, rationally, fully aware that this did not give them any guarantee of success or predict failure. Regarding this, the experiences of friends or relatives were at times recalled as evidence that 'bad quality embryos' could lead to good results and the other way round. As Marion commented, for example, when the doctor made a positive comment about the big follicles she had noticed:

> You never know! A friend of mine got pregnant from two moderate
> ones [embryos]. Twins! One of them did not survive though.

At this stage of the IVF treatment, knowing the quality of the
embryos clearly increased or decreased people's expectations, while
at the same time feelings of uncertainty were also expressed.

Next to knowing the quality of the transferred embryo(s), reaching the stage of the embryo transfer impacted on people's expectations. Many told me that they 'had not been this far before'. They
were very much aware 'that you really have something in your
body then', or as one woman enthusiastically put it, 'Then you
have a mini baby in your belly. That is great!' Probably, most of the
women had indeed never been this far before; a number of them,
however, might have been without being aware of it, as normally –
when people try to conceive without medical assistance – they are
not aware of a fertilization (conception/pregnancy) that lasts just a
few days.

In particular, actually seeing the transferred embryos seemed
to affect couples' perception of this very early stage of pregnancy.
When I started the fieldwork, embryo transfer at the Radboud
Clinic was done without the use of ultrasound, which meant that
the doctor – and the couple alike – could not see the actual transfer
on a screen. Once the woman had been prepared for the embryo
transfer, the laboratory technician was called to bring in the 'cane'
containing the embryo(s). Often, they then showed the 'cane' to
the couple and said something like, 'Here they are, but you cannot
see them with the naked eye!' The couples could not do anything else but believe it was true. The doctor would transfer the
embryo(s) and when she thought she had done so, the laboratory
technician took the 'cane' back to the laboratory and put it under
the microscope. Within a few minutes someone from the laboratory
phoned the room where the embryo transfer had taken place to say
that the 'cane' was empty (I never attended a session in which the
'cane' was not found to be empty). This was the only check which
the doctor and the couples had to be sure that the embryos had
really been transferred.

At a certain moment the transfer procedure changed: from then
on the embryo transfer was accompanied by ultrasound, as it had
been proven elsewhere that this would lead to better results. So
from that moment the doctor and the couples could see on the
screen a small white spot at the place in the uterus where the doctor
had placed the embryo(s). Couples in my study who had undergone

both methods of embryo transfer said they appreciated this change. They perceived it as positive that they now 'really saw something', even when it was just a vague spot which would not have any meaning at all without the doctor's interpretation. As one woman said, 'It was just a small spot, but she [the doctor] could move it'. Another woman recalled that, 'It was just a small white spot and you wonder whether it was not there before. But it is rather vivid compared to the rest'.

Being aware that one or two embryos had been transferred into the woman's body and having seen this 'with your own eyes', thus made people feel that they were coming closer to their goal than most of them had ever been. In addition, the couples participating in the Digitale Poli saw their own increasing expectations also translated into increasing percentages. Medically assisted conception and the way it was visualized at the Radboud Clinic thus added a consciousness to this stage of 'pregnancy', which almost inevitably gave hope to the couples involved. At the same time, while their hopes increased, they felt that their hopes should not become too big, as they were informed and rationally knew that the chance that things could go wrong in this stage was still bigger than the chance it would go well. Most of the couples, if not all, were fully aware that the implantation which has to take place at this stage is the major obstacle in IVF treatment. Karel, for example, described very clearly what he felt about this stage, when I spoke with him and his wife after their first failed treatment:

> We knew very well that it is only a small percentage [for success], but still! Look, they replace the embryos and then you really think like 'that has most probably not happened to us before'. So, then you have much more hope than you in fact can have . . . And I think we indeed had too much hope. And maybe that is not bad, but then it falls harder afterwards.

On the one hand people had hope and felt that they should do, because 'if you do not have any hope you better not start'. But on the other hand they knew that their hopes should not become too big, because in case of failure the disappointment will be big as well. Some of the couples described the period after the embryo transfer as a constant swinging 'between hope and fear' and this feeling of ambiguity dominated people's mind and mood in the two week period of waiting that follows the embryo transfer. Christine described her ambiguous state of mind after the embryo transfer, which she thought was due to the use of hormones:

Before and during the treatment the hormones were not a problem for me. I did not feel any side effects. But after the transfer suddenly things became different. The hormones pull your leg. Even if you – between your ears – realize very well that it can all be negative, you are almost floating on a pink cloud. The image of how it could be with your child is almost constantly in your mind. Bert [her husband] let himself go as well, after some initial reservations based on realism. Dreaming together, great! Even if there is always that warning voice in the background.

Normally, when people have sex in the hope of conceiving, they also have to wait a couple of weeks before they can do a pregnancy test. While this may also lead to anxiety and disappointment, the major difference between 'normal' conception and conception through IVF in this stage is that in the latter case the couple *knows* that one or two embryo(s) have been transferred. Couples undergoing IVF at the Radboud Clinic had even seen these embryos on a picture or as a white spot on the screen. Knowing this affected the way they experienced this stage of the pregnancy, as José and Tim pointed out when they told me how they felt after their first failed IVF treatment, having come so far in the treatment trajectory:

Tim: Yes, disappointed.
José: Disappointed.
Tim: Because you have gone through the whole process from the beginning to the end. At the moment of transfer you are aware that after a few days it is going to nestle and that you are possibly pregnant. While someone who is not undergoing IVF, when things go in the natural way, is not aware of anything at all in those two weeks, or at least not that consciously. You are living that very consciously.
José: Yes, there is really something in you. You know that beforehand. Something has been placed in you, so to say. So you know, 'Something is there'.
Tim: Yes.

Seeing and interpreting visual images – at all stages of the IVF cycle – can thus be reassuring and exciting, but may also have the contrary effect of producing hope, anxiety and ambivalence (cf. Franklin 1997).

Pregnancy Test: A Blue Line

Once the embryo transfer had taken place, couples went home in the hope that implantation would occur. In that period they had to take Progestan®, hormones that are supposed to stimulate the implantation of the embryo. After fifteen days of waiting and if the woman's menses had not yet started, they were supposed to do a home pregnancy test. Almost all couples described the weeks between the embryo transfer and pregnancy test and in particular the second week, as hard to get through. The nearer they got to the end of it, the more stressful it became.

> Birgit: Those two weeks! Whatever I felt, I immediately went to the toilet to have a look. Until the day before I had to do the test, nothing happened. I told my sister-in-law who called me, 'Nothing is happening'. 'You could do a test now' [her sister-in-law had suggested]. 'No, I'm not going to test'. I had said this in the morning and in the afternoon my period started heavily. That is still possible and the doctors said 'You can still do a test'.
>
> TG: While you were menstruating. They still advised you that?
>
> Birgit: Yes, so I did. But, no [not positive].

Another couple, Iris and Johan, also recalled very well the moment they did the pregnancy test. The night before they were supposed to do the test Johan could not sleep well. Early in the night he asked her to do the test, to 'get rid of the trouble'. They did not have any hopes that she was pregnant, as she had gone through a period of confusing symptoms. Iris, however, did not want to do the test in the middle of the night. Finally, at around seven o'clock, she did it, to put an end to her husband's requests. She did the test and left it at the bathroom, without watching it. Her husband went to the bathroom and he saw a blue line. Then he asked her 'Is this what it should be?' They watched it together, took it up and immediately went to her parents. There they concluded that, after all, she was pregnant. Initially, they could hardly believe it.

Aside from the ambiguous feelings described above – between hope and realism – while the women were waiting they were often confronted with a number of bodily symptoms which they found hard to interpret and which added to their feeling of uncertainty. In this stage, women were very much aware of each and every bodily sign that was different from normal and their interpretation of these symptoms jumped from positive – 'my breasts are very sensitive, this is a sign of pregnancy' – to negativity and pessimism – 'I feel as if I am getting my period'. They found it hard to interpret all the different bodily signs. Some realized that the hormones they had taken might have an impact on what and how they felt: 'It does not feel like my own body anymore', some women said. Moreover, at that point they were still taking Progestan®, which – as they were told – postpones the onset of their menstruation. Finally, some women said they did not know how to interpret the changes in their body as they did not know how it should feel to be pregnant, 'Since I have never been pregnant before!' While women were thus consciously watching their own body during these two weeks, their partners, who in this phase were fully dependent on them for information, attentively watched their wives. Several men told me that they were anxiously observing their wife's face each and every time they saw her return from the toilet.

Whereas the couple's stories about the weeks of waiting followed more or less the same lines, their stories about the end of these two weeks varied enormously. A few could not wait to do the pregnancy test and therefore did it before the formal test day indicated by the clinic. A good example of this is Louise, who wrote in her diary that she did five tests before the formal test day. This is the most extreme case I encountered in terms of testing, though it clearly shows the extra uncertainty that testing in this early stage may lead to. Instead of bringing more clarity, it increased doubt. Some couples did not reach the test day, as the woman's menstruation set in clearly days before the pregnancy test should be done. For most of them this implied a sudden and clear end of any hope for a pregnancy in that treatment cycle and they did not even do a pregnancy test. Others did a pregnancy test even when they were menstruating to be fully sure, 'as you never know'. This was also the case for Mireille, who started bleeding slightly a number of days before the actual testing day. But, she told me, she felt confused about how to interpret the body signs ('It was not yet like a real menstruation'), which meant that she and her husband continued doubting and hoping for some more days:

Mireille: You start thinking . . . Maybe . . .
Chris: Should it then . . .?
Mireille: Yes, I continued using the Progestan®. I think, 'I can do two things: call the hospital, but they will say that I have to wait until Friday to do the test. Or I just continue and I will see'. But it [the menstruation] did not come. Because of the Progestan®, of course . . . And then you think 'maybe I have a little bit of luck then'. Then on Friday we did the test and I said to Chris, 'You may look at it' and then I did not hear him and I did not see him flying back, so I thought, 'That is not good'. And it was not.
Chris: And then it was over . . .

Mireille: But then you have hope until the end, that maybe one of the two [embryos] is still there or whatever . . . You hear all kind of stories of other people, that they had bleeding in between and so on.

When the woman's menses did *not* start before the test day, a pregnancy test was of course always done. For some the test result was clearly negative, for others clearly positive. But results were not always so unequivocally clear: sometimes test results did not immediately give the much wanted clarity.

The first scenario – a clearly negative result – put a quick end to all hopes of a pregnancy in that treatment cycle. People felt disappointed and sad, but at least the period of anxious waiting and uncertainty about the outcome of that cycle had passed. However, for them new uncertainties about what to do in the future may soon follow. When couples knew the treatment outcome – either negative or positive – they were supposed to call the clinic to inform them about the result. Almost all couples – mostly the women – did this on the same day or within a few days' time. Several women told me about the conversation they had with the nurse on the phone. Some of them recalled exactly how the attending nurse had reacted when they told her that the pregnancy test was negative or that their menses had started. Generally, the nurses were felt to be very considerate and compassionate. Some women quoted the nurses who made remarks such as, 'What a pity, you were so close!' or, when the nurses looked at their files or remembered their case, they sometimes commented, 'While overall your picture is so good!' or 'Your embryos were so nice!' At times I heard doctors or gynaecologists say similar things when they were evaluating the failed treatment(s) with couples and the outcomes at certain treatment steps had looked very promising. When the women or men recalled these sorts of remarks, it was as if they saw it as a kind of confirmation of their own thoughts that they had been very close to success. This kind of reaction actually seemed to influence the way people looked back at their treatment. Mireille, for example, who shared her doubts about doing another treatment after her third treatment failure (as she had suffered from painful side effects), recalled exactly what the phone call with the nurse did to her:

During the last treatment I thought, 'I will never do it again' . . . Then you have the test result. And when you phone the clinic about it you have a conversation with the nurse. And she said to me, 'You were so close!' She [the nurse] was also present at the transfer. So she said, 'Things looked so good, but just that last part!' And then you get hope again and you start thinking, 'What now? Shall we do it a fourth time?'

While a negative treatment result put an end to the uncertainties of that cycle, couples had to think about the possible continuation of treatments (though they did not need to decide immediately). This brought new ambiguities and more so after the second and third failed treatment than after the first failed treatment. Several considerations played a role in this decision and the successes and failures within the past treatment cycles, plus the reaction of clinic staff, definitely affected these considerations.

The second scenario concerned the couples whose pregnancy test result was not unequivocally clear: the test was not really negative, but also not convincingly positive. Quite a few couples told me about test results that were initially vague and in combination with bodily symptoms left space for multiple interpretations and a situation of ongoing uncertainty. Sylvia and Bob recalled the period of testing after their third IVF treatment, which in the end proved to be successful. The dialogue between them, below, which took place when they knew that she was pregnant, illustrates perfectly the confusion they and other couples felt:

Bob: Yes, that pregnancy test, that wasn't one-two-three-positive either.
Sylvia: That means ... Yes, we saw something which we thought, 'Is this positive or is this not positive?' So, we phoned – you have to phone then – and then that person [the nurse at the clinic] said, 'Yes, it can be, but . . .' And also because I was losing blood constantly. If I had not had that loss of blood and then you see such a vague spot, then you think 'It will be it'. But now, the combination of such a vague spot and the loss of blood, then you think, 'Is this as it should be?' Then she [the nurse on the phone] said, 'You better do it again, tomorrow'. Now, that was the same thing . . . And then she said, 'You better wait one week'.
Bob: And then we did another test, with three different tests.
Sylvia: A spot, a spot, a line and a cross, or something like that.
Bob: Yes, we had to do three of them . . .
TG: And how did you feel in that period?
Sylvia: I thought, 'We will never do this again. This is really terrible! This is really nothing! Terrible!'
Bob: That uncertainty, yes.
Sylvia: What a hassle!

For this couple, the pregnancy test after this protracted period of doubt finally indicated a positive result. Other couples were less fortunate and after some stressful days they saw themselves confronted with a negative test result. They had to consider anew, after having felt for a while so very close to pregnancy, whether they wanted to continue with another treatment.

Finally, the third scenario regards couples who immediately saw a positive test result: a clearly blue line, (or whatever sign the test should show according to its instructions). Clearly positive pregnancy tests of course lead to happy and enthusiastic reactions, though at the same time it struck me how many reservations several of the couples initially had. Several of the men and women who had a positive test result told me that they were very pleased with the good result, but at the same time they did not dare to believe it. Such comments refer to the notion of 'tentative pregnancy', as introduced by Rothman (1986), pointing to the felt need to maintain a distance from it, as it still may go wrong (cf. Rapp 1999). Marion, for example, who became pregnant in the third treatment cycle, is one of the people who could hardly believe it was true:

> From the moment I was pregnant, it has been unrealistic. I have constantly looked at that test. I made a picture of it. But it is unreal. It is extremely nice.

So, despite being happy with the positive results, these women and men also were concerned that it still might go wrong and dreaded that their pregnancy would not last. The more treatments they had undergone, the stronger this feeling of hesitation or reservation seemed to be. Couples were told that IVF pregnancies had a higher chance of ending in a miscarriage than normal pregnancies, so this might have contributed to their reserved feeling as well. For some, these reservations were based on their own experiences (if they had had a miscarriage before) and for others on stories they had heard. Moreover, throughout the whole process couples learned to temper their hope and to think of negative scenarios as well, meaning that they simply could not feel fully certain, relieved and happy immediately. That is what Roos told me after her second failed IVF treatment, in which the pregnancy test had been positive but the foetal ultrasound showed that she was not pregnant anymore:

> Yes, I think because you have gone through all these medical things, because you have been busy with it for such a long time, you are much more careful. I mean . . . and probably you do it out of self-protection

as well . . . [You are] not too happy, as it will only be more disappointing then later, I think.

Roos' cautious attitude to not having too much hope was shared
by several other participants and has been found in other studies
on reproductive technologies as well (cf. Franklin 1997; Thompson
2005; Franklin and Roberts 2006). This rational form of emotional
protection against the potential devastating costs of failure has been
described as a form of control that belongs to the complex 'ontological choreography' that IVF requires (Thompson 2005; Franklin
and Roberts 2006: 138).[19] People need to mould their subjectivities,
bodies and lives to the demands of the treatment (cf. Pasveer and
Heesterbeek 2001).

Thus, most of the couples who had a clearly positive pregnancy
test result appeared not to immediately and fully trust that things
were really okay. This lead to a continuation of uncertainty, or,
as some couples called it, 'a continuation of the waiting period';
as Sandelowski et al. (1990: 279) put it: 'Their passage from not-
pregnant to pregnant [became] ambiguous'. A pregnancy test, in a
way, was perceived to be a limited form of evidence of pregnancy,
or, in the words of one of the men, 'A pregnancy test is . . . is a
bit strange, because you cannot really see something'. Apparently,
what was shown in a pregnancy test was felt as too abstract – or
not straightforward and real enough to be perceived as a proof
(cf. George 1996). Couples eagerly wanted to see their pregnancy
confirmed in a different way, which of course may also be related
with past experiences (one or more miscarriages) and the warnings
that couples received from clinic staff. Consequently, most of them
eagerly looked forward to having their pregnancy confirmed by
means of an ultrasound.

Foetal Ultrasound: A Ticking Heart

For couples who had undergone IVF, the foetal ultrasound was the
'moment of truth'. After a positive pregnancy test result at home,
they had to wait another three weeks before they could go to the
clinic for the foetal ultrasound. In the course of these weeks, though
most women got more and more 'convinced' by bodily symptoms
that they were really pregnant, almost all couples continued to have
some kind of reservations or even moments of serious doubts and
uncertainty, as 'you never know'. Again, Louise's diary clearly illustrates this (Day 32–52). From what I have seen and from what the
couples told me, most of the couples were absolutely nervous when

visiting the hospital on the day of the ultrasound. They dreaded that their dream might fully collapse within a few moments. The observation below of Anne and Joost's ultrasound session clearly illustrates this tension:

> I meet Anne and Joost in the corridor. Today they are visiting the clinic to have their foetal ultrasound. When I ask them how they feel, Anne answers, 'Nervous. We have had this before. The other time I miscarried within eleven weeks. So I really think this is very stressful'. Then the gynaecologist calls them in and I enter the consultation room with them. Briefly, the doctor talks with the woman about how she feels, about the fact that she is 'still smoking' and about her medicine use. The doctor then quickly prepares things to make the ultrasound, in order to relieve the couple from the stress. Immediately, a foetus with a ticking heart can be seen clearly on the screen. Joost and Anne look at each other, obviously relieved. The gynaecologist tells them what she sees, makes a print of the foetus and continues looking to see if there is another foetus. The couple follows meticulously all the movements the doctor makes. After a while the doctor concludes that there is not a second one. Anne comments that the other time she had not seen the heart ticking like this. They are visibly happy. The doctor measures the foetus and its size exactly fits the stage where it should be today (seven weeks and three days). The doctor explains that they calculate the duration of the pregnancy from the day of the follicle aspiration plus two weeks. Then Anne heaves a deep sigh of relief and says, 'So, it is simply good. This diminishes my burden'. The conversation continues for a while about several different things. Finally the doctor says, 'Then I think I may congratulate you now' and adds with a friendly voice, 'You know what can go wrong. I cannot give you any guarantees. But if you are this far, there is very little chance that things go wrong. Very little. The heart is ticking. You are on schedule.' Not long after that they leave the consultation room.
>
> Some weeks later I meet Anne at the corridor. I am surprised to see her at the clinic and she tells me that she has come for another ultrasound. Because of her background – a miscarriage at eleven weeks – she still felt insecure about her pregnancy and therefore she had asked for an extra ultrasound, which she will have today. She tells me after the ultrasound that everything looks good. About seven months later I receive a birth card, announcing the birth of their child. (Observation, pregnancy ultrasound)

An ultrasound confirming pregnancy is *the* moment that couples have been hoping for for many years, and in particular have been working towards during the few last months. Visualizing medical technology showed them whether the foetus' heart was beating and whether the size of the foetus conformed to standards. I cannot think of any other consultation at the Radboud Clinic in which the ambience was so full of tense expectation than in the consultation in which the foetal ultrasounds are made. I became aware of this early in my fieldwork period, when I was attending a full afternoon of consultations with one of the doctors, during which she did several foetal ultrasounds. Another couple would come in, eagerly and anxiously looking forward to having the ultrasound done; and once it was done and the result was clear there was that sudden change of mood, from anxiety to relief, or occasionally from anxiety to deep sadness.

Foetal ultrasounds – and other electronic monitoring instruments – have been the subject of feminist critiques arguing that: 'they have contributed to an increasing medicalization of pregnancy, the attendant diminution and devaluation of the mother's role in pregnancy and birth, and an earlier conceptual separation of the fetus from the mother' (Layne 2003: 89). Layne, however, in her book on miscarriages, nuances such criticisms, as she argues that they may affect people in different ways, depending on their specific situation. She suggests that some women may indeed resent the use of these technologies on the grounds mentioned by the feminist critiques, while others may really enjoy 'reading and interpreting sonogram screens and fetal monitors' and for others it may increase their 'perception of control and predictability' (ibid.: 90). In particular, she argues, women who have undergone one or more pregnancy losses are very well aware that 'technologies that bring joy on one doctor's visit may bring grief on the next' (Layne 2003: 91).

This was very true for the informants in my study as well. While the above case of Anne and Joost illustrated a change from anxiety to relief and joy, the case below shows how differently the consultation ended when the outcome was not good. Roos told about her enormous disappointment when the foetal ultrasound showed that the foetus was no longer living:

> And yes . . . Then we had the ultrasound with the doctor and then . . . Yes, first I was lying in such an ordinary ultrasound room, but she said, 'I cannot see it very well', so we moved to the aspiration room. 'The ultrasound machine over there is better' [the doctor had said]. So, then I already started thinking, 'This is not good'. And you [to husband] had that as well, didn't you? So, I dressed myself again, we went to that aspiration room and on that ultrasound you could see it very well: you only could see a very small ring, so to say, and

for the rest nothing. 'And yes', the doctor said, 'with eight weeks you must see a ticking heart'. I heard all that and I thought, 'It will be like that'. I did not really register what happened actually until we walked outside.

In a phone call that I had with Roos almost immediately after she had the above ultrasound, she told me how 'duped' she felt by the bodily signs she experienced, even after the ultrasound:[20]

> Awful! You feel duped by your own body. You have painful breasts. I also just then started to feel sick . . . When I came home on Tuesday [the day of the ultrasound] I did a pregnancy test. I was curious to see what it would show. That was really weird: the test was still positive!

A diagnosis of a forthcoming miscarriage that is based on technology (i.e., an ultrasound), Layne (2003) has argued, impacts on the mechanics of pregnancy loss as it cuts it up into three moments, namely: 'the moment of the demise, the moment of learning the demise, the moment of the surgical removal' (Layne 2003: 86). This may thus create the 'surreal situation', exactly as Roos indicated, in which a woman still feels pregnant and walks around knowing that she is carrying a child that has passed away.

While for Roos and her husband the foetal ultrasound put an end to their dream, for most other couples this ultrasound confirmed the pregnancy. For the latter, this moment was the beginning of the end of their uncertainty, but definitely not yet the absolute end, as several couples told me in the interviews after they had become pregnant. Feelings of uncertainty often persisted or returned for a while. Couples needed some time to become convinced, to dare to trust that this was a pregnancy that would last. For the women who had miscarried before, the duration of their former pregnancy became another step to be passed. Unfortunately for one couple participating in this study, the worst case scenario became reality: the woman miscarried in the twenty-second week of her pregnancy, at a moment when she and her husband had already felt convinced that it was a pregnancy that would stay. The emotional impact of a miscarriage after an IVF treatment – and of other mishaps – will be described in the following chapter.

Trying Once More? Compelling Technology

Results at different steps in IVF thus informed couples about their chances in a treatment cycle, which increased or decreased their hopes in that specific cycle and thus affected their mood. However, the results did more than that. When results at a certain stage were bad – for example when few eggs were 'produced' – this could have implications for the couple beyond the actual treatment cycle. In these cases, as we have seen, a step could suddenly turn into an endpoint, not only for the current treatment, but also for any fertility treatment at all (at least at the Radboud Clinic). An IVF treatment cycle can thus also be considered as a process of ongoing diagnosis (and doctors also presented it as such), as it provided detailed insight into possible obstacles in conception and informed doctors and couples about future treatment options. The treatment results showed exactly at what stage things went wrong. Doctors, on the basis of treatment results in a cycle, sometimes suggested doing another type of treatment (e.g., ICSI instead of IVF in case of 'bad quality sperm'); in other cases they decided to stop further treatment because, according to the clinic's medical guidelines, treatment results – and subsequently the couple's prognosis – were considered too bad to expect IVF to increase the couple's chances to conceive. In these cases it was the doctor who decided; little or no choice was left to the couples.

Research at the Radboud Clinic showed that after the first failed IVF, 5.6 per cent of couples did not continue treatment – on the doctor's instigation – because they had a bad prognosis, and this applied to 4.6 per cent of couples after a second failed treatment (Verhaak et al. 200;2 Smeenk et al. 2004). In my study, of the nineteen couples who started IVF, three couples were not allowed to do a further treatment. Couples could and did (sometimes) argue against such a decision, but they had relatively little agency in this as the Radboud Clinic proved to be rather strict in the application of their clinical guidelines.

Bad results at the in-between steps thus meant that doctors did not allow couples to undergo further treatments. The situation, however, changed completely when results at milestones had been good or reasonably good, but pregnancy had still not yet occurred. In such cases doctors could generally not explain fully why the past treatments had not been successful. In particular, as I heard the doctors say regularly, they could not explain treatment failures at the end of the treatment cycle, after the embryo transfer. One doctor even referred to this stage as 'the flaw of IVF treatment'. Doctors were not able to predict whether another treatment cycle might lead to the desired result or not and thus they did not have a medically sound reason to withhold further treatment. Another treatment might still give another chance. When biomedical criteria could not (fully) explain the treatment failure and ambiguity prevailed, it was up to the couple to decide whether or not they wanted to continue treatment. How then did couples go about these decisions while confronted with this ambiguity?

When reflecting on future treatments, I noticed that the couples actively considered the insights they had gained at the milestones in former treatment(s). When looking back on treatment failure(s), they not only took into account the negative end result (not being pregnant), but reflected on all the steps in treatment: what went well and what went wrong. The results in between gave them food for thought and formed part of their considerations regarding future treatments. While the IVF cycle thus far had not brought them the desired end result, they knew exactly up until what point things were going fine; and having reached a certain step, or having produced a certain amount of fertilized embryos, was often interpreted in terms of 'gain' (cf. Sandelowski et al. 1990: 280). They might have felt that they were very close to pregnancy (or might have actually been pregnant for a short while), a feeling that was sometimes reinforced by nurses' and doctors' reactions when talking through treatment failures. Franklin and Roberts (2006: 166) refer to this as similar to the dynamics in gambling: a 'near miss' may make it harder to stop than a 'nowhere near', exactly due to the disappointment of the near miss. One way of dealing with failure is trying it again. Thus, I argue, knowing and seeing the results at the different treatment steps formed an incentive for couples – seduced them into trying one more treatment, even when they were simultaneously ambivalent about it.

This argument reconfirms the way Sandelowski (1991: 31) has looked at the 'nature' of reproductive technology and 'how it operates' to grasp why these reproductive technologies are so compelling for many couples with fertility problems. She has firmly argued against locating the compelling character of reproductive technologies exclusively in pronatalist values and patriarchal agendas, as radical feminists previously did. Rather, she starts from the position that in order to understand the persistence in the use of reproductive technologies, these technologies should be known both from the inside and from the outside. Viewed from the outside, cultural values may indeed push couples and doctors to use these technologies; viewed from the inside, she argued, reproductive technologies also had their own pull. When taking this latter perspective, the fragmenting character of the technologies used in IVF treatments is one aspect which makes these technologies 'compelling' as 'it segments the normal, biological process of conception, transforming it from an inchoate event into consciously lived stages of achievements and failures' (Sandelowski 1991: 39). Women in her studies in the USA felt that achievement at one stage compelled them to move to the next (see also Williams 1988; Sandelowski et al. 1990).

This is also what happened to the majority of the couples in the current study: even though they felt ambiguous about the first IVF, they did not really hesitate starting for a second time.[21] Some did start to hesitate about doing a third IVF after a second treatment failure, as they had become pessimistic about the in-between results or because of intensive suffering during the treatment. And yet still none of the couples actually stopped at that stage on their own initiative (the only two couples who stopped after the second treatment did this at the doctor's instigation). Continuing was still considered more obvious than stopping. This was, however, completely different after the third failed treatment, at which point some of the couples who had not yet become pregnant firmly decided to stop ('Now we have done everything possible') or were at least strongly hesitant about continuing.[22] For a few of them – knowing the variable and sometimes contradictory results at different steps throughout the three treatments, as we saw in the introductory case in this chapter – their feelings about treatment rendered strongly ambiguous. Still, they were inclined to give it another try.

Conclusion

In the patient-centred Radboud Clinic couples received plenty of information, including on the process of conception and where it may go wrong. This increased medical insight turned them into better-informed patients whose capacities to make informed decisions and negotiate with their doctors increased. On the other hand, I have argued, their sharpened 'medical gaze' also affected the way couples assessed – medicalized – their own situation, their bodies and possible solutions.

Splitting up the process of medically assisted conception into various steps and being amply informed about the visualized outcomes at each step had several implications. Couples ended up in an almost continuing flow – lasting around two months – of uncertainty and ambivalence. As soon as one moment of uncertainty had been successfully passed, another moment started, making people feel that they were repeatedly swinging between hope and fear. This became stronger when couples progressed further in a treatment cycle, but also when they underwent more than one IVF treatment. In addition, throughout the IVF cycle – and especially after the embryo transfer – they became more and more aware of being close to a pregnancy. This awareness by couples undergoing medically assisted conception forms a major difference compared to couples who try to conceive 'normally' by just having sex at the proper time. Knowing and seeing the in-between results, I have argued, formed an incentive for couples to try one more treatment.

The findings in this study are remarkably similar to what other scholars in this area – in the UK and USA – have described (see, e.g., Williams 1988; Sandelowski et al. 1990; Sandelowski 1991; Franklin 1997). Yet the continuing expansion of the visualization of outcome results at different treatment steps, as happened in the Radboud Clinic, for example, in the form of pictures of the embryo on the Digitale Poli, or the white spots seen on the screen after the embryo transfer, seems to intensify these processes and reinforce the sense of imperative couples felt to continue treatment. Visualizing the various outcome steps of conception, as George (1996) has argued regarding foetal images, thus strengthens a 'feeling of reality' of what is going on in all treatment stages.

For the interpretation of the images, however, couples remained dependent on clinic staff, which gave them 'authoritarian power'. This is the more so as the doctors are the ones who can decide over exceptions of the clinic rules. The conflation of medical technology and power – and this is most explicit in case of conflicting views between the doctor and the patients – thus confirms the idea that 'medical technologies give power to the ones possessing them', as 'the technology makes their knowledge authoritative, their intervention indispensable and their word law' (Van der Geest 1994: 11; my translation). Thus, while the provision of extended and visualized information in the patient-centred clinic is empowering in decision-making, it may not make couples less dependent on clinic staff and thus does not fundamentally change power relations in clinical contexts (cf. Mayes 2009).

Notes

1. These include: Williams (1988); Sandelowski et al. (1990); Becker and Nachtigall (1991); Sandelowski (1991); George (1996); Franklin

(1997); Rapp (1999); Pasveer and Heesterbeek (2001); Layne (2003); Thompson (2005); Tjornhoj (2005); Franklin and Roberts (2006).

2. When a couple's need for medical assistance has an obvious reason, for example when one of the partners has been sterilized or the man's sperm is frozen, a full cycle analysis is not always indicated.

3. The FSH is the pituitary hormone that makes the ovaries and egg cell develop into a follicle.

4. At the moment of fieldwork the Radboud Clinic did not yet offer Anti-Müllerian Hormone (AMH) tests, to estimate the ovarian reserve. AMH is a hormone produced by reproductive tissues; the concentration of AMH present is related to a woman's likely responsiveness to IVF treatment.

5. Rapp (1999) observed that in her study among couples being counselled about amniocentesis, 'nonscience speakers get less scientific information than their more privileged pregnant peers', which, she argues, increased their disadvantaged position in decision-taking (ibid.: 66). This might have been true for the couples visiting the Radboud Clinic as well.

6. These steps can differ slightly in different clinics.

7. See Glossary for explanation of medical terms.

8. From here on I refer to the hormonal medicines by their brand names, as study participants also did.

9. In their studies they spoke mainly about foetal imaging, but the principle is similar.

10. I was told that the reason why laboratory technicians normally provide this information was because it was believed that this direct contact with patients enhanced their involvement in the treatment process. Only when the amount of eggs retrieved was very low did the doctor come to inform the couple, as clinic staff were aware of the sensitivity of this kind of message and doctors were supposed to be better trained in bringing bad news.

11. PESA was at that time only allowed in Radboud and two other fertility clinics in the Netherlands (see Chapter 2).

12. This couple went for further treatment to another Dutch clinic which collaborated with a fertility clinic in Germany, where TESE was allowed. TESE involves retrieving sperm from the testicles, which at that time was not yet permitted in the Netherlands (see Chapter 2).

13. She illustrated this with an example of a woman in her study who saw two fertilized eggs and thought 'Those are my twins' (Tjornhoj 2005: 86).

14. This refers not to Christine and Bert, but to the only other couple participating in this study who did an IVF- TESE in another Dutch clinic in combination with a German clinic.

15. This was not the case for the above couple, as their next TESE treatment was successful and led not only to fertilization, but also to the birth of a healthy child.

16. Couples were thus not involved in the selection of the embryo(s) to be transferred, as was the case in the clinic conducting PGD in the UK, where the couples themselves had to choose between the genetically or morphologically best embryo(s) (Franklin and Roberts 2006: 152–53). Being actively involved in the decision-making, the authors argued, contributed to their confidence that the right decision had been made, even when the treatment failed afterwards. This level of patient involvement required staff that were highly committed and had excellent communication skills.

17. In a similar vein Rapp (1999), in her study on amniocentesis, speaks about the creation of laboratory results as an 'informal interpretive craft'. She shows how laboratory technicians constantly construct 'stable interpretations in the face of material ambiguity' (ibid.: 208).

18. Layne (2003) referred to the social construction of a child in a later phase of embryonic development by women who got pregnant without medical assistance. In addition, though, she observes that in case of IVF-induced pregnancies women may already start the social construction before implantation, thus 'personifying follicles' (ibid.: 83).

19. Thompson (2005) speaks about the complex 'ontological choreography' that is needed to make a viable embryo in an IVF cycle, which requires various actors, including clinic staff and patients, to perform a complex and precisely timed set of actions (like injection of hormones, ejaculation of sperm, fertilizing eggs, and so on), both in and beyond the clinic.

20. If a miscarriage is identified by an ultrasound and the foetus has to be followed by a curettage, a woman remains chemically pregnant (though not physiologically pregnant) for a period of time until her hormonal levels drop (Layne 2003: 86).

21. Only one of the couples in my study strongly hesitated about doing a second IVF treatment and ultimately decided against it. They felt that the results of their first IVF treatment cycle were too discouraging to go once more through the agony of treatment, even when, according to clinical guidelines, their in-between results would have allowed it.

22. The 'imperative of three' thus helped them to decide this at this stage.

References

Becker, G. and R.D. Nachtigall. 1991. 'Ambiguous responsibility in the doctor–patient relationship: The case of infertility', *Social Science and Medicine* 32(8): 875–85.

Berg, A. and A. Mol. 2001. *Ingebouwde normen. Medische technieken doorgelicht.* Utrecht: Van der Wees.

FertEndo. n.d. *In Vitro Fertilisatie (IVF). Patiënten Informatie.* FertEndo, Polikliniek voor vruchtbaarheidsstoornissen, UMC St. Radboud.

Foucault, M. 1973. *The Birth of the Clinic.* Routledge.

Franklin, S. 1997. *Embodied Progress: A cultural account of assisted conception.* London: Routledge.

Franklin, S. and C. Roberts. 2006. *Born and Made: An ethnography of preimplantation genetic diagnosis.* Princeton: Princeton University Press.

George, E. 1996. 'Fetal Ultrasound imagining and the production of authoritative knowledge in Greece', *Medical Anthropological Quarterly* New Series 10(2): 15–75.

Layne, L. 2003. *Motherhood Lost: A feminist account of pregnancy loss in America.* New York: Routledge.

Lupton, D. 1997 'Foucault and the medicalisation critique', in A. Petersen and R. Burton (eds), *Foucault, Health and Medicine.* London: Routledge, pp. 94–110.

Mayes, C. 2009. 'Pastoral power and the confessing subject in patient-centred communication', *Bioethical Inquiry* 6 (4): 483–93.

Pasveer, B. and S. Heesterbeek. 2001. *De voortplanting verdeeld. De praktijk van de voortplantingsgeneeskunde doorgelicht vanuit het perspectief van patiente.* The Hague: Rathenau Instituut.

Rapp, R. 1999. *Testing Women, Testing the Fetus: The social impact of amniocentesis in America.* New York: Routledge.

Rothman, B. 1986. 'Reflections on hard work', *Qualitative Sociology* 9: 48–53.

Sandelowski, M. 1991. 'Compelled to try: The never enough quality of conceptive technology', *Medical Anthropological Quarterly* 5: 29–47.

———— 1993. *With Child in Mind: Studies of the personal encounter with infertility.* Philadelphia: University of Pennsylvania Press.

Sandelowski, M., B. Harris and D. Holditch-Davis. 1990. 'Pregnant moments: The process of conception in infertile couples', *Research in Nursing and Health* 13: 273–82.

Smeenk, J.M.J., C.M. Verhaak, A.M. Stolwijk, J.A. Kremer, and D.D. Braat, 2004. 'Reasons for dropout in an in vitro fertilization/intracytoplasmic sperm injection program', *Fertility and Sterility* 81(2): 262–68.

Thompson, C. 2005. *Making Parents: The ontological choreography of reproductive technologies.* Cambridge: The MIT Press.

Tjornhoj, T. 2005. 'Close encounters with infertility and procreative technologies', in R. Jenkins, H. Jessen and V. Steffen (eds), *Managing Uncertainty: Ethnographic Studies of Illness, Risk and the Struggle for Control.* Copenhagen: Museum Tusculanum Press, pp. 71–91.

Van der Geest, S. 1994. 'Medische technologie in cultureel perspectief. Inleiding', in S. van der Geest, P. Ten Have, G. Nijhof and P. Verbeek-heida (eds), *De Macht der dingen. Medische technologie in cultureel perspectief.* Amsterdam: Het Spinhuis, pp. 1–19.

Verhaak, C.M., Smeenk, J.M.J., Kremer, J.A.M., Braat, D.D.M., and Kraaimaat, F.W. 2002. 'De emotionele belasting van kunstmatige

voortplanting: Meer angst en depressie na mislukte eerste behandeling'
Nederlands Tijdschrift voor Geneeskunde 146(49): 2363–66.
Williams, L. 1988. '"It is going to work for me". Responses to failure of IVF',
Birth 15: 153–56.

Chapter 7

GENDERED SUFFERING AND SUPPORT

The day before the embryo transfer in their first IVF cycle, I call
Christine and Bert to hear how they have experienced the treatment thus far. Christine first briefs me about what is freshest in her
memory – the ova pick-up: 'They did not manage to place the infu-
sion, which in itself was annoying. But still, they handled that in a
rather nice way and in the end they managed'. When I ask her how
she felt about the injections she replies, 'In hindsight it was not too
bad. Everybody always says that that is so terrible. It hurts – as the
ova pick-up hurts as well – but it was not that bad. I was tired and
I have slept a lot. For the rest that was not too bad either'. Some
weeks later I call them again (knowing already that their first treatment has failed). Christine tells me that the embryo transfer had been
easy, but the waiting period up to the pregnancy test had been terrible. 'Waiting is the worst thing! Even compared to the ova pick-up
– which is painful – waiting is the worst thing. And now we have to
wait again before we can start the next treatment cycle'.

About three months later, when Christine and Bert are at the end
of their second IVF treatment cycle, I speak to them again over the
phone. Christine tells me about the injections. This time Bert has
been injecting her, because when she did it herself the first time she
was always bruised. Bert feels bad about his wife having to undergo
all these injections, even more so because he knows that it is because
of him that she has to undergo all this, as he has was sterilized a long
time ago, after having two children with his former partner. He thinks
that in this cycle the injections were even more painful for his wife
than in the first treatment cycle, something that Christine confirms.
'[It was] as if they had to pass through two layers; and it was bleeding

more often'. When I ask her if she felt any side effects, she mentions hot flushes, although she thinks that they might have been partly due to the weather, as 'it was exactly in that very hot period'. As regards changes in mood, she thinks that she was hardly affected by the medicines. Her husband, however, thinks that she was moaning more than normal, though he questions whether this was due to the injections or rather due to her concerns about the treatment in general. Looking back at the ova pick-up, Christine tells me that this time it was worse compared to the first time: 'It was much more painful than the first time. But I had more follicles this time. I had ten follicles . . . I had to be rolled out of the treatment room on a stretcher. Many women had that on that day, as it was a hot day. I saw one woman coming out on a stretcher and another in a wheelchair'.

Whereas Christine had experienced the ova pick-up as more painful the second time, the waiting time was in fact less stressful. At the beginning – shortly after the embryo transfer – her body had felt different and she and her husband had immediately got the feeling that this time it would be positive. But that feeling had turned by the end of the waiting period. Christine tells a lengthy story about confusing bodily symptoms and unclear test results, which rendered them uncertain and stressed about the outcome of the treatment. One week after the phone call they did one more test. Unfortunately, the test proved to be negative again: their second IVF had thus failed as well.

It is not difficult to imagine a more pleasant way of conceiving a child compared to IVF. The couples in this study undergoing IVF treatments had many stories to tell about how these treatments affected them – their bodies, their minds, their lives, their relationships and decisions. Most of these stories were, as with Christine and Bert above, about pain, anxiety, uncertainty and hope.

It is generally acknowledged that both women and men suffer from IVF; but that women bear the major part of the treatment burdens, in particular the physical burden (see, e.g., Greil 1997; Hardy and Makuch 2002; Verhaak et al. 2005; Greil et al. 2010). Women's bodies are more affected by IVF than men's bodies, even when the cause of the couple's fertility problem lies with the man.[1] For (feminist) social science scholars this gender inequality – women putting their healthy bodies at risk for the sake of procreation – has been a major element in their critiques of the new reproductive technologies (see, e.g., Van der Ploeg 1998). Inhorn, however, has criticised these feminist writers (including herself in earlier work), arguing that under-privileging men's role in the infertility treatment process is an ideologically driven idea 'in order to make an important feminist point, but which also ignores the lived realities of many infertile men's lives' (Inhorn 2003: 188).

This chapter provides in-depth insight into both women's and men's bodily and emotional involvement throughout the IVF cycle. Their stories reflect how reproductive technologies both affect and are affected by gender, as enacted in conjugal relationships in contemporary Dutch society (cf. Greil 1991; Becker 2000; Inhorn 2003, 2012; Thompson 2005). Further, throughout the chapter I show and discuss how the daily patient-centred practices in the Radboud Clinic, while supporting couples in bearing the burdens of treatment, simultaneously have the effect of 'disciplining' the couples to adhere to treatment requirements and clinic routines and 'normalizing' the hardship of treatments (cf. Pasveer and Heesterbeek 2001; Thompson 2005).

The Gendered and Unequal Burdens of IVF

Hormonal Injections

When I visit Annelies and Bart for the first interview, they have already started with the daily injections. Bart is injecting Annelies, as she absolutely refuses to inject herself. Annelies' mother joined them at the pre-IVF consultation and received injection instructions as well. She will substitute for Bart in case he cannot be at home to inject his wife. I ask Annelies how she has experienced the injections thus far. She answers in an agitated voice, 'Now it is reasonable, but in the beginning I did not like it at all! That needle I did not like at all – it [the liquid] is biting. You feel that liquid enormously! Now it is okay. The first days I was thinking, "Do I really have to do this again and again?" I stopped thinking that. That new one [the Puregon® pen] is much better – you hardly feel it'.

Setting Daily Injections

The first phase of an IVF cycle focuses solely on women's bodies. Women in treatment at the Radboud Clinic had to take four different hormonal medicines, all of which they could administer themselves at home.[2] During the pre-IVF consultation hour IVF nurses instructed the couples on how to inject the hormonal medicines and couples also practiced injecting themselves. Nurses encouraged the couples to do these injections themselves at home and not to depend on a health professional. Most women participating in this study indeed injected themselves; in only a few cases did the man inject his wife and only rarely did a third person give the injections. Before starting the IVF treatment almost all women dreaded administering and/or receiving these injections, which Iris clearly expressed:

> I got the medication already in December. Big bags! . . . I have put it all in the fridge. For a month or so I did not look at it at all. I only looked at it once I felt I was ready for it. The first thing I noticed was that big needle. My father has told me 'If you cannot do it yourself, I will do it'.

Several women told me that though they initially feared the injections, once they had received instructions from the nurse and practiced it, they felt in a way relieved. Still, despite well-received injection instructions and former experiences, most women disliked injecting themselves. In particular, several women commented negatively about the needle used to inject the Decapeptyl®. Louise was explicit about this in her diary:

> Today I have taken the first Decapeptyl® injection. What a drama! I have been sitting half an hour with the needle in front of my belly and I simply did not dare to do it. In the end I succeeded, while the tears were running over my cheeks. I am even saying that I will stick to this one IVF treatment only. I really do not know whether I can do this. Maybe I will get used to it, but I cannot imagine that right now.

Women's experiences with the injections differed from day to day. One day they might have sucked up blood or the injection may have caused a bruise; another day there were no problems at all. One day they felt everything went quickly and fine; another day they hesitated about injecting themselves and hardly managed to do it.

While the focus in this stage is on the women's bodies, women highly appreciated their partners' involvement. Most women said that they wanted to have their partners around when they injected themselves. They were positive about the practical support (preparing the needles) and the emotional support they got from their partners at this stage of treatment, saying things like, 'I just want him to be around', 'He calms me down' or 'We joke a bit about it, which helps me'. Christine, for example, was clear about this right from the start of her first IVF treatment:

> It is a threshold to put that needle into my belly. If he [her husband] had not been here when I did the first injection, then I would have felt very bad. It is a threshold. Not a pleasure at all. But you have to do all these things for it. Compare it with diabetes: then you have to

do it as well. And if you *have* to, then you *can* do it. Of course, I do not have to – it is our choice to do this now. But if I want to achieve this goal, then I will have to do it.

Women said that in a way they got used to the injections: giving themselves the injections became part of their daily routine. But even then, obviously, none of them liked to do it. They simply endured it, saying – like Christine – things such as, 'Even if I do not like it, I have no choice'. Setting the daily injections is part of the process through which infertility patients become 'bureaucratic objects' (Thompson 2005: 1999): they get used to all sorts of clinic routines and requirements. While this bureaucratization potentially threatens patients' individuality, Thompson argues, being good at it also facilitates their flow through the clinic and treatment, an insight that also applies to the women in the current study.

Women also made relativizing remarks about the injections, like Mireille, who said, 'It is just four weeks'. Louise, who had lots of injection experience as she had undergone twelve IUIs (most of them including hormonal stimulation) and who regularly sucked up blood when injecting herself in the second IVF treatment cycle, in hindsight still did not perceive the injections as a major issue. For her the annoyance of the injections was not what bothered her most. She suffered – as many other women also claimed – much more from the anxiety and stress throughout the treatment cycle and in particular in the waiting period after the embryo transfer.

Experiencing Side Effects

The IVF nurse informs Johan and Iris about the medicines Iris has to take during the IVF treatment and about possible side effects that may occur. She starts with the Decapeptyl®: 'The Decapeptyl® is meant to stop your own cycle, to prevent the ovulation coming too early. You may get menopausal complaints like sweating, hot flushes, etc. The most annoying is often – for both of you – that the woman can become irritable. It does not *have* to happen, but it *may* happen. And if it does not happen, you are one of the few for whom it does not happen'. (Observation, pre-IVF consultation)

Before starting the first IVF treatment cycle, couples were informed about the medications they had to take and the possible adverse effects that might occur. With regard to Decapeptyl®, menopausal-like complaints such as perspiration, hot flushes and its impact on the woman's mood were mentioned as the most disturbing and most often occurring side effects. Regarding Puregon®, Radboud fertility staff advised women to carefully watch their bodily reactions as hyperstimulation may occur, while for Progestan® and Pregnyl® no side effects at all were mentioned in the pre-IVF sessions I attended. Both doctors and nurses emphasized again and again that women should warn them immediately if things were becoming too painful and that they should not hesitate to phone the clinic with any doubts or concerns. The pre-IVF consultation was not the only source of information about possible side effects, however, as women's reactions to the medicines were also frequently discussed on the Digitale Poli and the Freya website.

About half of the women participating in the study and undergoing IVF expressed at one moment or another during the treatment that they had an aversion to the idea of taking hormonal medicines. They had different reasons for this. Among them were the women who had previously taken hormonal medicines and they dreaded reacting in a similar way as they had in the past. In particular, women referred to their strong reactions to Clomid®.[3] Almost all of them remembered substantial changes in their mood or psychical function in the period they had taken the Clomid® and they dreaded that this would happen again while taking the medicines for the IVF treatment. Annelies, for example, said that she had become confused because of these medicines: 'I could not find my own things anymore'. Anneke, who had undergone six IUIs with hormonal stimulation, recalled that she 'was very emotional in that period'. While these women mainly expressed their concerns about the short-term effects of the medicines, other women were more concerned about possible long-term risks, specifically their association with cancer. In particular, women who had a close relative that suffered from breast or cervical cancer strongly expressed these worries. As with administering the injections, there was enormous diversity in the ways women actually experienced the adverse effects, both in the type of side effect they experienced and the extent to which it affected them.[4] Women who underwent more than one treatment often did not suffer from the same side effects across the different treatments.

Regarding actual experiences of side effects, in the first treatment phase, when women injected the Decapeptyl®, menopausal-like complaints were, as predicted by clinic staff, dominant. Women referred to hot flushes, sweating, headaches, dizziness, fatigue and being nervous, anxious, and/or irritable. Liset was one of the women who reported feeling a substantial impact on her mood in the period when she started taking the Decapeptyl®:

> I found it extremely heavy. I got very depressed from it. I did not
> become a nicer person! I became very melancholic and anxious. Here
> in the house they have noticed this!

José represents the other extreme as she was not hindered at all
by the Decapeptyl® injections. After two completed and two interrupted IVF cycles she had not felt any side effects from Decapeptyl®:
'It never bothers me'. Marion was among the women who experienced different side effects from the Decapeptyl® in the different
treatment cycles. While in the first cycle she complained about 'a
gigantic headache' and 'lots of trouble with my eyes', during the
second cycle she felt things become even worse. She then suffered
from typical menopausal complaints such as hot flushes and sweating. The strong side effects in the second cycle made Marion and
her husband have serious doubts about doing another treatment.
Despite those doubts, however, they did do a third treatment after
a break of five months. In that third treatment Marion did not feel
any side effects at all, saying: 'I felt so little of it that I even forgot to
inject myself!'

Several women described themselves as being more emotional
during the period in which they were injecting the Decapeptyl®.
Birgit, for example, pictured herself as follows:

> Emotional. Yes, that I was. Crying . . . When I was looking at the
> Digitale Poli and saw the stories of the other women. When they failed
> . . . One of the women was completely panicking. Then I became
> emotional. Once you are doing such a treatment, everything around
> you is about babies. You only see babies and buggies . . . Emotionally,
> I found that tough.

On the contrary, a few women described themselves as 'in high
spirits' or 'strong'. Some of them explained this as a result of 'finally
doing something'. In general, though, women and men noticed
a negative change in the woman's mood when she was taking
Decapeptyl®. Yet they realized that they could not tell whether
this was due to the medication or just the 'stress' of the treatment. Women's extremely diverging experiences of side effects of
these and other hormonal medicines is striking and may be partly
explained by the fact that the medicines actually affected them differently, physically speaking. In addition, as has been noticed in the
literature about pain, negative emotions such as anxiety may intensify physical pain, distraction or a euphoric mood may alleviate pain
experiences (Helman 2000; Aalten et al. 2008). It is impossible to

distinguish between the physical and psychical components of pain, as these are supposed to be in constant interaction with each other, and for people in different circumstances – such as women in labour or when involved in top-class sport – pain may have a different meaning and people may express pain differently. In addition, previous experiences with pain in health care and interactions between health staff and patients may affect the meaning people attach to pain and how they further react to it (Nettleton 1995; Helman 2000). The experience and expression of pain is thus always socially constructed, resulting from 'a complex combination of causes, influences and consequences of the body, mind and the external world' (Aalten et al. 2008: 10, translation TG). This was also referred to by several couples and clinic staff, when commenting on the divergent reactions of women: it might be a combination of the injection and the tension – or excitement – of treatment that triggered the bodily and psychical changes.

After fourteen days of Decapeptyl® injections, and if the first ultrasound check-up showed that everything went well, women started concurrently injecting the Puregon® (hormonal medicine to stimulate the growth of the follicles). Belly pain, a 'swollen feeling' caused by the growth of a number of eggs, and weight increase were most often mentioned in this stage of the treatment; additional but less-mentioned effects were headache, fatigue and being 'emotional'. Weight increase in particular was a side effect that seriously bothered a number of women involved in the study. When I spoke with Annelies after her second IVF treatment, this was one of her major concerns:

> Annelies: My weight! The increase of my weight. Ten kilos!
> TG: Ten kilos? In the first or second treatment?
> Annelies: In both. I mean in total. Fortunately by now I have lost most of that. And that has nothing to do with eating. You do not eat more. You do not take more sweets. But in one way or another you are swelling.

Again, these side effects were, however, far from equally felt by the women participating in the study. Some women did not feel any of these symptoms when injecting the Puregon®; others really suffered from it. Mireille was one of the unfortunate women who seriously suffered from swollen ovaries in all three IVF treatments and her complaints became worse with each treatment cycle. In the first cycle she had the feeling that her ovaries were 'as big as apples'. The doctor at the clinic had suggested that that might be due to the type of work she did, which involved standing up most of the time. In the second cycle the belly pain had already started in the stage when she was only injecting the Decapeptyl®. Mireille recalled this period:

> And then I had not even started the Puregon®! I felt nothing else than belly pain, cramps and a swollen, heavy feeling, which the other time I had only felt at the end. So, I thought, 'This is not going well – I better stay home from work'. In the hospital I told them about my belly pain, but they could not find anything strange. So, as normal, I started with the Puregon®. And in fact I have spent that entire time sitting on the sofa or lying in bed.

When the second treatment failed again she started a third one and again she suffered from a swollen and painful belly. In the third interview Mireille told me how she experienced this treatment cycle:

> After two days [of injecting Decapeptyl®] I had a filled feeling in my belly. I did not fit in my trousers anymore . . . It became heavier and heavier . . . At the first ultrasound check everything looked fine: I had three ova on the left and six on the right. From that moment I was on sick leave, because I could not manage. I had a swollen feeling; I was tired. I was at home for three weeks – throughout the treatment, so to say.

She continued her story, telling about how her complaints increased, that she had pain in her leg from buttock to calf. She returned to the clinic earlier than planned and the doctor checked her for thrombosis. Nothing alarming was found, so she continued treatment, again spending most of her time on the sofa or in bed. Clearly, Mireille was among the study participants for whom this stage of treatment was extremely burdensome, but even then she did not decide to stop further treatment. She was determined to have a child from her and her partner.

Once women's follicles were big enough for the ova pick-up to take place, women had to take a Pregnyl® injection to facilitate the ova releasing from the follicles. Generally women did not refer to any side effects from this medicine, though occasionally women referred to an 'annoying lump' as a result of this injection. Lastly, some women spoke about the impact of Progestan®, the hormonal medicine taken vaginally over a period of two weeks to promote the implantation of the embryos. In advance the nurses warned the women about the 'dirt' in their vagina that results from the Progestan® capsules. These Progestan® capsules have been designed for oral intake and therefore have a sugared layer, but during IVF treatment they have to be placed in the vagina, as research has shown that this gives better results. Once the capsules are placed into the vagina, the sugared layer dissolves and causes a sticky substance. Several women in the study commented that they detested this 'dirt' and wondered why this medicine could not be prepared differently. Besides this effect, a few women also felt mentally affected by the Progestan® medicine. Sylvia was among those who actually felt hindered in her daily functioning by the Progestan®:

> I do have more problems with the medicines after the ova pick-up than with the Decapeptyl® or Puregon® . . . I am really living in a mist. It costs me lots of efforts to concentrate. Ten days after the ova pick-up I started to feel a big change in my body . . . And that period, that is . . . [deep sigh] that is tough. And it takes so long. You are tired; it is annoying. I manage to follow conversations, etcetera, but it costs me a lot of effort.

Sylvia said that it had even crossed her mind during the next treatment to immediately stop taking the Progestan® when that same feeling came up, however she laughingly concluded, 'but I would never do that'. While couples were not pleased about the daily injections and many suffered substantially from the side effects, most of them proved to be extremely disciplined 'infertility patients' (cf. Pasveer and Heesterbeek 2001: 51–89; Thompson 2005). They became experts on their own bodies and on IVF procedures, including injecting themselves. They simply continued, even when they strongly disliked doing it and the side effects they felt.

Watching out for Ovarian Hyperstimulation Syndrome (OHSS)

> On Sunday I had the first ultrasound check-up. That went fine. On Monday they took some blood, as the ova pick-up could be done. Then my hormonal level [of Estradiol, an oestrogen produced by the follicles] proved to be too high. I had a swollen feeling and problems when walking. My belly was very swollen and I had swollen legs and blood vessels – from under my breasts downward. On Monday they could not immediately tell me what should be done. The entire week I have been under observation. I had to stop injecting myself. Each day of the week I had to go to the hospital [it takes her one and a half hours to get there]. Initially, my hormonal level increased from 2,200 up to 2,400 – then it went down to 1,900. On Thursday it was okay to do the ova pick-up, but I still had complaints – I still

had some liquid under my lungs – so then it was decided not to do the ova pick-up ... I was disappointed about that. But at that moment your own body and your health are the most central. And, probably, that one injection before the ova pick-up [the Pregnyl®] and a possible pregnancy could have increased my hormonal level even more. I did not feel myself anymore! I think they slowly worked towards this decision.

Before starting the IVF treatment, couples were warned that Ovarian Hyperstimulation Syndrome (OHSS)[5] may occur as a result of the hormonal injections. To prevent OHSS, an ultrasound of the ovaries was always done before women were allowed to inject the Pregnyl® and when the woman had produced many eggs their blood was examined for Estradiol, an oestrogen produced by the follicles.[6] Moreover, women were advised to be aware of any alarming signs during the period in which they were injecting themselves.[7] If a certain Estradiol level was reached the doctor decided to cancel the treatment cycle.[8]

Of the forty IVF treatment cycles I followed in this study, one treatment cycle (José's case, described in the above introduction) was cancelled because of a 'threatening hyperstimulation', as she called it. In addition, four women (one of whom in two cycles) were intensively followed because their Estradiol level did not properly correspond with the number of developing follicles observed. In the end, however, these four women were allowed to continue the treatment.[9] The way these women experienced this threatening hyperstimulation varied. Two felt hardly anything at all, while the other three reported serious complaints. Sylvia – who twice had a threatening hyperstimulation – e-mailed me the day after the ova pick-up in her third IVF cycle and wrote:

> Did you already know that after nine days I had to stop injecting Puregon® because my values were very high (Monday 10,000 and Tuesday 14,000)? Fortunately, it stabilized and we could do the ova pick-up. The risk for hyperstimulation is still there, but I feel well and hope everything will go well. I drink and drink and drink . . . and take it easy.

Contrarily, Louise was one of the less fortunate women who really suffered from the threatening hyperstimulation. She wrote about it in her diary:

> Today is the embryo transfer. Last night I did not sleep at all. I felt sick: belly pain, sick. With a 'harvest' of thirty ova hyperstimulation

is a possibility and I am convinced I have it. I even feared last night that I would end up in the hospital – so sick do I feel. Fortunately, the complaints seem less in the morning and we go to the hospital. I mentioned my complaints, but I keep up appearances and do not tell them how painful it is, to prevent them cancelling the transfer. We are now this far. I will not let this chance be taken away!

In her diary she further wrote that on the day of the embryo transfer the doctor warned her about the risk of hyperstimulation and advised her to drink a lot and to slow down. For a couple of days she felt she had no other choice than to take the doctor's advice as she felt really sick and was not able to do anything other than lie on the sofa. Afterwards, at different instances, she told me that her own health had to come first; however, in her diary notes she wrote that at the very moment of the embryo transfer she did not call the doctor's attention to her complaints out of fear that the doctor would cancel her treatment. At that moment her eagerness to get pregnant thus overruled her rational thinking about putting her own health first. She did thus not behave in a 'disciplined' way, but rather put herself at risk.

In general, the women (and their husbands) stressed the importance of their own health and realized that it was necessary to be well monitored. Overall, study participants were well aware of the risks of OHSS and most of them indeed contacted the clinic when they felt concerned. In Chapter 5 I mentioned that being able to contact the clinic for anything and trusting that you are being carefully followed-up and receiving adequate responses from the doctors, enhanced people's trust in the IVF procedure and this seemed to be even more so when potential risks (nearly) became reality. In addition, some couples stressed that you also have your own responsibility to yourself. Anne and Joost, for example, told me about their experiences in the period when Anne was injecting herself with Puregon®. They stressed that the doctor could only react adequately because they themselves had been alert:

> In between I have returned [to the clinic] two extra times. I had headaches and some blood coagulation. Then they adapted it [the medicines]. I could choose between stopping or adapting. Then the Puregon® was adapted. I continued with a dosage of 100 [milligram] Puregon®. Then my problems passed. You must watch yourself carefully. You have to listen to your own body . . . If I do not trust it, I phone them. I have learned by asking.

Anne and Joost, as did other couples, thus also acknowledged that in part it was their own responsibility. Over the course of the treatments women (and men) were trained to carefully watch and become experts of their own bodies (cf. Pasveer and Heesterbeek 2001; Thompson 2005). However, they also strongly felt they were in safe hands. Knowing what to do and trusting that proper monitoring would take place, enhanced the feeling that things – however bad they may feel at that very moment – were kept under control, and this diminished anxiety. The careful preparation and monitoring, I therefore argue, contributes to the trust couples put in the health staff (as discussed in Chapter 5). It shows that clinic staff care for them and take their health seriously: staff would not let them undergo or continue treatments if it would be irresponsible to do so.

Organizing Life around Injections and Hospital Visits

Next to the annoyance of actually administering the injections, couples – and in particular women – explained how they had to plan their life around the injections (cf. Franklin 1997; Franklin and Roberts 2006).[10] Most people chose to take the injections after dinner time, when they were normally at home. Almost all couples told stories about how the timing occasionally interfered with their evening programme, such as birthday parties, meetings or eating out and how they sometimes had to rush to be home in time. Other women told stories about injecting themselves in public toilets, one even referring to it as being like 'injecting yourself as a junky in a toilet'. Taking injections when other people were around, or when at friends' houses, was even more disturbing when couples had not shared that they were undergoing IVF treatment. Christine, for example, recalled how she had to take an injection while a party was going on in the living room, with friends who were unaware of their treatment:

> Yes, that was a strange experience. Because he [her husband] had said, 'Just simply do it upstairs'. But I was really frightened that one of the kids would see me with that injection needle – he might get strange ideas about it. So I chose to do it in the toilet . . . Not really what I like!

A few couples chose to take holidays during this part of the treatment trajectory to avoid any stress around the injections, while others tried to plan the IVF cycle in such a way that it would not interfere with events that they perceived as important.

A number of the couples, and again women in particular, also reported experiencing stress resulting from the frequent hospital visits. In the period when taking Puregon®, when the growth of follicles is monitored by regular ultrasounds, the women may visit the clinic between two and seven times a week (men do not always join their wives at the clinic for the ultrasound checks). In particular, for women who had first undergone a series of IUIs with hormonal stimulation, the frequent hospital visits were experienced as an extra burden. José was among them: she was really fed up with driving to the clinic again and again (it took her one and a half hours to get there), though at the same time she felt she had no other choice but to continue. She said:

> Going there every time and you are only five minutes inside. And every time you see someone else. I hate that. That is the most awful part of it. If it were only the ova pick-up and the embryo transfer. But before that you have to go there a couple of times . . . I told you [her husband], 'It's only because of the hassle that I'd want to stop the treatment' . . . I say that out of resistance, but I still do it! Otherwise you know for sure that you will not succeed. I mean, I can take it, but I really do not like it.

One couple calculated in the first interview (this was even *before* starting IVF treatments) that they had visited the Radboud Clinic over sixty times in the past one and a half years. Couples residing out of town spoke about the stress resulting from traffic jams on the highways when they had to reach the clinic early in the morning for the ultrasound check, to hand in the semen on time, for the ova pick-up or or embryo transfer. Moreover, as almost all women continued working while they underwent treatment, they felt (as did some of the men) increasingly bad about their frequent absences from work or repeatedly arriving late. In particular the higher-educated women put much effort into planning their hospital appointments in such a way that they would disturb their working routine as little as possible. Scheduling and sticking to appointments, and adapting work and private life to clinic requirements, is another element of what Thompson (2005) has labelled as infertility patients becoming 'bureaucratic objects'. They may not like it, but being good at it facilitates the treatment process.

Radboud Clinic staff were also aware of the logistical burdens of the treatment and tried hard to take women's agendas into account.[11] In general, couples were pleased with the staff's consideration for their personal agendas and they were also glad about the limited waiting times at the IVF department. Couples spoke about a 'good flow' or 'an oiled machine' to indicate that IVF procedures generally went smoothly.[12]

Despite the fact that the fertility clinic tried to take people's preferences into consideration, women and men were still regularly absent from work. Some felt that they performed less effectively than normal and a few women had to take sick leave as they felt too sick to work. One of the men who insisted on always accompanying his wife to the hospital even started to work one day less a week because of the stress of the IVF treatment, including the frequent clinic visits. Thus, for at least some of the women and men, the logistics involved put an additional burden on the already burdensome IVF treatment.

The Ova Pick-up: 'A Dreadful Event'

The ova pick-up was terrible. The doctor did not manage to place the needle for the narcosis properly. She had to try it a few times. I think that is strange, as I have been a blood donor for several years and they never find it a problem to find my vessels. Also, the aspiration itself did not go well. The doctor found it difficult to puncture the follicles. That was very annoying, as it was very painful. Moreover, the doctor started to curse a few times . . . I do not know how often she punctured me . . . I left the ova pick-up room in a wheelchair. In the restroom I felt very well treated: somebody kept sitting with us and we were told how many ova were found.

The ova pick-up was the part of the treatment that most women participating in the study and undergoing IVF treatment dreaded the most and for some it indeed became an unpleasant experience. For Liset, whose experience is described above, her bad experiences with the ova pick-up (including her irritation with the doctor's performance and distrust in the staff's advice) turned out to be one of the deciding factors in declining further treatment (her case was discussed in Chapter 5).

In the Radboud Clinic the ova pick-up took place thirty-six hours after the woman had had the Pregnyl® injection. By means of an ultrasound the follicles were made visible on the screen. The doctor put a special needle into the vagina and pricked the ovaries with it, punctured the follicles one after the other and sucked them empty. The point of the needle was constantly visible on the screen. During treatment the woman's heart beat and respiration was controlled and her body was covered with a sterile green cloth. Women were told in advance that the ova pick-up might be painful and that therefore as a standard part of treatment they would be given a painkiller, Rapifen®.[13] In addition, women were offered two tranquilizers (Seresta®), which they might take the evening before and again one hour before the ova pick-up, though not all women opted to take the tranquilizers. Partners were explicitly required to be present at the ova pick-up; during the intervention they sat next to their wives to hold their hand. To create a more relaxed ambience couples were invited to bring a CD with their favourite music to be played during the ova pick-up and many of them did so.

Almost all women dreaded the ova pick-up; in practice though, their actual experiences – again – differed substantially. In about one-fifth of the forty IVF cycles I followed, the women assessed the ova pick-up as 'really very painful' or 'terribly painful'. The other women expressed themselves in less extreme terms, saying that it 'was not a pleasure at all' but they found it 'bearable'. A few women said that they hardly felt anything at all. Birgit was among the latter group, saying, 'No. It did not bother me at all. That went fine!' Marion was also not too overcome by the ova pick-up, as she commented, 'I would rather undergo another ova pick-up than pay a visit to the dentist'. Huge differences thus existed among the different women (partly depending on the number of ova punctured); and the women that underwent more than one ova pick-up could also experience each ova pick-up differently. Sometimes, when women who had not taken a tranquilizer before their first ova pick-up had experienced it as fairly painful, they would take a tranquilizer in the second treatment cycle as they then feared it even more.

Women referred to different aspects of the ova pick-up as causing pain. The moment that the needle enters the ovary and the follicle is actually punctured was often mentioned as the most painful. Some women recalled being bothered because it took a while before the doctor could find the ovaries or because of the effect of the pain medication. Some other women said that they suffered more after the ova pick-up, at home, than from the intervention itself, making comments such as, 'When you are sitting you feel a bit frail from inside'.

While Liset (in the above case) was complaining about the way the doctor's attitude negatively affected the experience of the ova pick-up, several other women and men commented positively on the attentive care they received during the ova pick-up (which I also often observed in the ova pick-ups I attended), which helped them to bear it. Generally, the doctor or nurse told them in advance that the actual ova pick-up would only take between five and seven minutes (while the remaining time of the scheduled half an hour was used for preparation and aftercare). Many women were relieved when they heard this and this statement was often recalled in the interviews. Some women explicitly stated – such as José below – that clinic staff's support enabled them to bear the ova pick-up, even when in itself it was considered a 'dreadful event'.

> The ova pick-up itself was do-able . . . In retrospect, though, I think in fact it is dreadful. But when I was there and I had to undergo it . . . It was not painful. They were very friendly. Everything went fine. It went super fast. The doctor told me, 'It takes seven minutes'. That I found very reasonable. The helpfulness . . . the care they have for you. You cannot say anything negative about that.

Typically during the ova pick-up, doctors and nurses also complimented the women about the way she was cooperating and standing the pain; as one of the nurses said, for example, 'You did very well – you managed to remain lying quietly'. At times study participants quoted these compliments during the interviews, as Tim proudly said about José, his wife:

> Tim: She is very brave during the treatment. The nurse also said so during the aspiration, 'You are doing great!'
> José: [Laughing] Maybe I did not shout as loudly as some others do!

Women were thus made co-responsible for how the ova pick-up went.[14] At the same time, doctors and nurses were empathetic, they showed the women that they were aware that it was a painful event and doctors tried to minimize the pain. For example, during one of the ova pick-ups I attended, when the doctor noticed that the experience of the puncture was tough for the woman, she apologized for it and reassured the woman that as soon as possible (when starting to prick the second ovary) she would add some pain medication.

Women often compared their own experiences with other women's experiences which they come across when chatting on the Freya site, the Digitale Poli, in the waiting room or among their own circle of friends and relatives. They then sometimes concluded that their own experiences were not too bad compared with what other women went through. Christine, for example, recalled the conversation she had with two other couples when waiting for her first ova pick-up:

> One of these couples came from Amsterdam and the other from Limburg [southern province]. They both told stories that do not really

make you happy. One of them had been pregnant twice, but the implantation was the problem. Twice she miscarried. And after the ova pick-up she really had a lot of complaints. And the other woman had a very swollen belly. Compared with them, things are not too bad for me, though I had pain after the ova pick-up when sitting and standing up.

Despite the pain or stress they felt, they often commented that it affected them much less than they had thought it would do beforehand, as Jeanet remarked:

No, I have not really been ill. Oh well, I was a bit sick, but not really ill. That [being really ill] is of course also possible . . . During the first treatment I was dizzy at night during the first three or five days, but that was all. And now [the second treatment] I felt more sick and tired. When you get really ill from it, things become different, I think. This is still to come.

Knowing that the ova pick-up did not take long, that it could be expected to be annoying or painful and that it 'could have been worse', plus having the feeling that they were well taken care of by the clinic staff, helped women to bear this part of the treatment.

In addition, while men were not physically involved in this part of the treatment, their presence and support was apparently highly valued and helped the women to bear the burden of the ova pick-up. When attending these treatment sessions, it struck me how involved and concerned most men were when sitting next to their wife lying in the gynaecological chair, undergoing this intrusive treatment:[15] they carefully followed all of the doctor's and nurse's actions and watched the screen, but above all they held their wife's hand, reacting to each and every expression of pain on her face and making supporting comments. More than once men and women (somewhat jokingly) told me afterwards that the men had also suffered physically from the ova pick-up: the woman had squeezed her partner's hand so strongly that her fingernails were imprinted into his hand. Several men commented that they felt bad that their wife had to undergo the ova pick-up (in addition to taking all those medicines), while their role was limited to sitting and watching.

In sum, the ova pick-up was clearly the most dreaded, the most intrusive and – for most women – the most painful moment of the treatment. Feeling well prepared and supported by clinic staff certainly helped (most) women to bear the burden of this part of treatment. Looking at this from a Foucauldian perspective, however, the clinic's intensive preparations and support did more than that. First, couples learned that experiencing pain and stress was not exceptional, but – up to a certain extent – a normal part of the IVF treatment. They became fully permeated with the idea that attempting to conceive through IVF should not be expected to come without some sort of suffering. This normalization of pain – both physical and psychical – in the context of IVF, I argue, makes people more willing to accept it when it actually occurs. Further, as has also been argued by Benjamin and Ha'elyon (2002: 677), women tend to consider this pain as meaningful, as it held the promise of motherhood; the pain is part of 'women's commitment to motherhood', which makes it worthwhile to undergo it.[16]

Production of Sperm: Men's Contribution for 'the Good Cause'

Men's major bodily contribution in a standard IVF cycle is 'producing' and handing in sperm, which they normally had to do on the same day as the ova pick-up. The sperm had to be handed in within an hour of 'production', the term generally used by clinic staff to refer to the masturbation and ejaculation involved; a term that was taken up by the couples as well. When couples lived nearby the hospital, the men could masturbate at home and bring the semen to the laboratory; otherwise, they had to do it at the clinic in the seed production room. In Chapter 4 I described how some of the men had an aversion to using this room, as they perceived it as an intrusion of their privacy. Regarding the sperm production itself, men generally said that they were not bothered too much; they disliked masturbating just for the sake of the production of semen and this might require more efforts than usual because of the circumstances under which they had to do it, but none of the men in this study referred to it as a major issue. Rather, they saw it as their only contribution for 'the good cause', as one of the men called it and acknowledged that it was a minor and pain-free contribution compared to the treatment procedures their partners had to go through.[17]

While for most men the 'semen production' was not a painful event, this was not true for all. Men who undergo IVF with PESA or TESE must have their semen retrieved from the epididymus (PESA) or testicles (TESE). At the Radboud Clinic PESA was done by an urologist under local anaesthesia.[18] Bert, the only man in the study group who underwent PESA and whose experiences I referred to in the previous chapter, clearly remembered the painful after effects of the PESA procedures:

Yes and this time it was painful compared to the other time. This
second time they really pinched me. I felt it for a couple of weeks . . . I
cannot say that I could not walk for a couple of weeks, but still, it was
painful . . . I think that lady [the urologist] was pinching a bit hard. It
was as if she had to force the needle into it.

In 'normal' IVF procedures, the treatment only affects women's
bodies, yet the increasing availability and use of new reproductive
technologies such as PESA and TESE affect the way men are physically involved in IVF treatment. These new technologies thus, as
Inhorn claims, render the 'feminist adage that infertile men's bodies
are somehow untouched by these technologies . . . both dated and
untrue' (Inhorn 2003: 188). Still, without intending to downplay
men's involvement in and suffering from IVF procedures, in the
current study women's bodily involvement was much more intensive than men's.[19]

Embryo Transfer: 'Peanuts'
And then you have the transfer . . . You do not feel anything at all.
That is a bit weird. Then you see a small tube; they place it into you
and that is it. Then you have to wait.

Immediately after the ova pick-up the eggs and sperms are brought
together in a petri dish in the laboratory, where the actual in-vitro
fertilization takes place. In the Radboud Clinic the embryo transfer
normally took place three days later, when one or more embryos
have developed.

On the day of the embryo transfer women were requested to
come to the clinic with a half-full bladder as this was supposed
to facilitate the procedures of the actual embryo transfer. For the
embryo transfer the doctor first placed a speculum into the woman's
vagina and cleaned it. Subsequently, she positioned a catheter with
the embryo(s) (which was brought in by the laboratory technician)
into the uterus and injected the embryos into the uterus. The doctor
then removed the catheter and the laboratory technician took it to
the laboratory to inspect whether it was empty.

Women were told in advance that the embryo transfer was not
painful, which is also how all women participating in this study
experienced this stage of the treatment. 'You do not feel anything
at all!' or 'That was peanuts!' were remarks I almost always heard
when I asked the women about their experiences with the embryo
transfer. Still, while the transfer itself was not painful, several
women disliked having to come with a full bladder.

The fact that the embryo(s) had been placed into the woman's uterus made most women feel vulnerable; several told me that they had been afraid 'to lose the embryos'. They felt that they should avoid making wild movements such as cycling on uneven roads[20]. The couples' anxiety about losing the implanted embryo(s) was an issue regularly discussed when they were still in the room where the transfer took place. Doctors and nurses emphasized that the women could behave normally and that they should not be afraid of losing their pregnancy as a result of normal activity. In these conversations, many a time I heard the 'peanut butter story', an apparently convincing image in the Dutch context,[21] invented by one of the doctors to clarify that the embryos would not simply fall out of the uterus:

> You must imagine your uterus as a peanut butter sandwich and the embryo as *hagelslag* (a strand of chocolate). You can imagine that *hagelslag* will never fall out of a peanut butter sandwich. (Doctors, Various observations of embryo transfers)

Ria, for example, one of the women who had been anxious about losing her embryos, remembered how relieved she felt once she had read the 'peanut butter story' on the Digitale Poli. While the embryo transfer itself was not perceived as a painful or annoying event, it made women very conscious that they were carrying one or two embryo(s) and this made them feel vulnerable and anxious about losing it/them. Two long weeks of waiting and watching then followed the embryo transfer.

'Just Waiting' and 'Watching the Woman's Body'

After the embryo transfer the intrusive parts of the IVF treatment have passed. Women at the Radboud Clinic still had to take Progestan® capsules to increase the chances of implantation taking place, but apart from that, the only things they could do were wait, watch and keep their fingers crossed in the hope that things would work out well. They did not have any other means to influence the course of events. This period of 'just waiting', however, was what several couples experienced as extremely difficult. Some of the women had suffered substantially in the previous stages, yet almost all couples described this waiting period as the most difficult phase of the treatment. Roos, for example, who hardly experienced any physical effects in the entire treatment, had a hard time in this waiting period. She – as did many other women – checked her underwear keenly for any sign of having started menses, each and every time she went to the toilet, as she noted in her diary six days after the embryo transfer:

> Today we had a family day . . . It was a nice day, lovely weather. We enjoyed cycling. My sister-in-law asked me a lot about the treatment and she told me how she had felt when she was pregnant and how it is to have children. I do not dare to think of that. Worse even, every time that I go to the toilet, I am watching more anxiously if I have not already started to lose blood. Yah! Those waiting weeks are really awful!

While the waiting period was experienced as stressful, for most couples the stress and anxiety did not start with the embryo transfer but long before that. All men and women participating in the study said that they were emotionally affected along the course of the IVF treatment. When expressing their experiences about the treatment most of them used words/expressions such as 'tough', 'heavy', 'heavier than expected', 'burdensome', 'awful', 'stressful' and so on. Yet an enormous diversity existed among the couples' emotional experiences, between women's and men's experiences, along the different stages of treatment and between the different treatment cycles. About one-third of the study participants (women and men) felt that they were not too heavily affected by the treatments: they said that they managed to 'function quite normally' or that 'the treatment did not fully take over our life'; though even these couples had their tough moments, either in the waiting period or when confronted with treatment failure. Personality traits, the way women (physically) reacted to the hormonal treatments, and the number of IVF cycles they had undergone, may explain these different reactions. In addition, women and men who already had a child (and in particular when a couple already had a child together) tended to feel less tense. While they would (obviously) love to have another child together or a child with their new partner, and they were prepared to go through the IVF procedures to achieve that goal, they said that at least they already had a family and that fact, in a way, diminished the tension they felt.

In this period they did not visit the clinic and only the couples who were participating in the Digital Poli interacted with clinic staff. While some women and men commented that they missed having contact with the clinic staff, many of them stressed the importance of being able to talk together with their partner and to share their ambiguous feelings of hope, anxiety and uncertainty.

Few couples had the luck of their first IVF being successful;[22] and even when a treatment was successful, some couples were confronted with 'loss' at different stages of the pregnancy. While, again, women were more physically involved in these losses, both men and women were highly emotionally affected by these losses, as will be discussed in the next section.

Sharing the Grief of Loss after IVF

Miscarriages

Miscarriages can take place at various stages of pregnancy. It is widely known – and couples undergoing IVF treatment at the Radboud Clinic are explicitly warned about it – that pregnancies resulting from IVF treatments more often lead to miscarriages than normal pregnancies (because, among other reasons, couples undergoing IVF treatment are aware of their pregnancy in an early phase). At the time the study took place at the Radboud Clinic one out of five pregnancies confirmed by a pregnancy test ended in a miscarriage before the tenth week, when the pregnancy was supposed to be confirmed by a foetal ultrasound.[23] For four couples participating in this study, an initial pregnancy ended in a miscarriage: three came to know of this at the moment of the ultrasound and for the fourth couple the miscarriage occurred in the twenty-second week of pregnancy. How did these couples experience these miscarriages? Louise's diary notes provide good insight into how deeply affected she felt when she had a miscarriage after the second treatment:

> So my hunch was correct: no baby is coming. An empty foetal bag, no ticking heart. I am broken. I do not know where to find any relief. It is so dishonest, so mean! Why? Why am I not allowed to get this child? Why do I deserve this? Why did I just not get my period as normal? Why am I first kept in the belief that things are fine? So many questions, so few answers. I am carrying an unviable foetus. I cannot grasp it. This child was so much more than wanted; it already had a place in our life. It was living: in our dreams, in our future . . . I do not know how to get over this grief. The doctor is friendly, but she cannot console us (who can?), but she shows that she realizes the impact of this message on us. After all, it is she who is throwing us from a pink cloud into a deep black hole. Keeping hope is not allowed anymore; it is not good. Those words are hard (tough), but clear. We have to get over the fact that we will not have a baby. Though I do not know how I will ever work through this.

Having been so very close and then being confronted with the news of failure, made Louise and her husband feel deeply grieved. This is also a feeling that the other couples expressed when they learned that they were no longer pregnant. In the back of their minds they had known and had been afraid that it might not be going well, but at the same time they had deeply hoped that it would be okay. I spoke with José one day after she had heard that she was not pregnant anymore. Both she and her husband experienced the miscarriage as an enormous setback:

> José: The ultrasound was on my birthday. I had done that purposefully. Tim took a day off. Nothing indicated that it would not go well. Finally, after three and a half years! We were fully confident . . . You take into account that it might not be good, but still. It was strange . . .
> TG: And what about Tim? How did he react?
> José: He is completely down. Even more than I am . . . Tim is in a dip. He was so glad and cheerful over the last period. He was busy at work, but he was so happy that finally it had been successful . . . Last week, Thursday [after the foetal ultrasound], he immediately phoned the office that he would not come to work on Friday. And over the weekend he completely collapsed. He was apathetic. You sometimes hear from others how much impact it has, but now we are living that ourselves as well.

Men and women felt sad and gloomy when confronted with treatment failure at this stage. Moreover, as they only came to know about the miscarriage at the moment of the foetal ultrasound, they still had to go through the actual miscarriage. The actual miscarriage might start spontaneously or – if that did not happen within a week – the woman would have to undergo medical interventions again (either a curettage or induction of the miscarriage by injections). Though their actual experiences of this varied, all of the couples were confronted with the painful loss of a foetus that signified the end of a precious pregnancy. Louise wrote about it in her diary:

> It has gone . . . Yesterday it was aborted while I was under full narcosis. It is a double feeling: on the one hand I needed this to be able to continue, on the other hand it is definitive now – the end of my first real pregnancy. I thought I would be able to focus my attention on the future and muster up the courage to do a next attempt, but I am falling – in as far as is possible – into a deeper hole than before. It is over – our dream has broken up into pieces. Very definitive. No child will be born in February 2005. Sometimes I do not know what to do out of misery. I cry, I scream or I am lying absolutely silent in my bed.

This grief is more than I can bear ... The operation itself went fine. Everybody was friendly and it was all small scale. That's just as well, as when undergoing an intervention like that, you do not want to be treated as a number. In the operation room a friendly man was standing next to me and said before I fell asleep 'I will care well for you'. I found that very special. Such a small phrase, but I remember it. It showed for me that they are involved and that they realize they have to deal with people.

Clearly, miscarriages in the early stage of pregnancy strongly affected the moods of women and men who had been so delighted that their treatment had been successful. While miscarriages after a normal conception are already often an intensive emotional experience (cf. Layne 2003), the grief the couples in my study experienced was clearly connected to their previous experiences of having been a couple with fertility problems, some of whom had had several miscarriages, and whose IVF treatment had finally been successful. They lost their 'precious pregnancy'. Further, as Layne (2003: 89) has suggested, being aware of the pregnancy and actually seeing the foetus in an early stage of development (long before the woman can feel its movements) strengthens the attachment, the prenatal bounding, of parents – both mothers and fathers – with their child. In infertility treatment, as we have seen in the previous chapter, the personification and bonding can even begin in an earlier (embryo) stage. Consequently, Layne argues, as the feeling of attachment and love may thus be expected to be greater, the feeling of loss may be greater as well.[24]

The experience of a miscarriage in the twenty-second week of pregnancy after a successful third IVF treatment, as experienced by Marion and Kees, was probably even more emotional, as they had by then become convinced that it was 'a pregnancy that would stay'. As soon as I heard about the miscarriage I called them (though formally we had already closed their participation in the study) and it was one of the most difficult and emotional calls I made during the entire study. Kees picked up the phone, but as he found it hard to find words to talk about the experience he handed the phone over to his wife. Marion told me their story, from the moment she started to loose amniotic fluid, about the visits to the midwife and the clinic and the infection that was detected, up to the delivery of their daughter: 'A beautiful girl who has lived only half an hour'. She also told about her contentment that they could take their daughter home, that they had been able to 'hold our little girl and caress her' and how they had given her a proper and warm farewell ceremony on the day of the cremation, surrounded with relatives and friends. For the ceremony Marion had written and read aloud a farewell letter in which she expressed her and her husband's contradictory feelings: happy and proud that they had had a beautiful daughter ('We have been mum and dad') and sad because they lost her ('We will miss her. Now we know what it is like'). The performance of a ritual like this confirmed both 'the uniqueness and individuality of their baby' (cf. Layne 2003: 100), but also confirmed their own identity as parents, for themselves as well for others, which enabled them to act and be seen and supported as bereaved parents.

The Loss of a Child

Deep grief and feelings of being overwhelmed by loss was also the fate of Margriet and Hein, another couple participating in the study. Their first foetal ultrasound had shown that Margriet was pregnant with twins, though at the same time it was observed that one of the foetuses was smaller than the other. This first foetal ultrasound proved to be the starting point of a complicated and risky pregnancy, which led to a cumbersome delivery and the birth of two premature babies, one of whom tragically passed away after having lived for almost three months. As said before, twin pregnancies resulting from IVF treatments are nowadays considered as a risk, as they potentially entail risks for both the pregnant woman and the babies to be born. Unfortunately for Margriet and Hein, those potential risks became hard reality. Their story, which I describe below, gives in-depth insight into a scenario that nobody wants to think of when implanting two embryos in an IVF treatment.

Three weeks after that first foetal ultrasound, Margriet and Hein returned to the clinic for a second ultrasound, which confirmed the initial observation. Because growth retardation at that foetal age may point to a chromosomal distortion – and because of Margriet's advanced age (thirty-nine) – a nuchal translucency measurement was done at ten weeks. This measurement showed that they indeed had an increased chance of having a child with a chromosomal distortion. To be sure of this, Margriet and Hein were then offered the option of doing an amniocentesis at sixteen weeks. They hesitated about doing this prenatal test, firstly because they both felt that a child with Down's syndrome would be more than welcome (though they felt they would like to know beforehand, to be prepared for it) and secondly because they feared that the amniocentesis could do harm – inducing a miscarriage, causing an infection or 'damaging something' (cf. Rapp 1999).[25] The doctor informed them about the

possible risks involved in amniocentesis, which were, as they interpreted his words, 'minimal'. Moreover, Margriet felt reassured by
what she had seen in her own environment:

> All my friends became mothers at an older age and nothing ever hap-
> pened. And I just wanted to have confirmation that everything was
> fine – because that was what I still thought.

Thus, they went for an amniocentesis; the same afternoon she
started to loose amniotic fluid. Months later, when I spoke with
her, she still felt guilty that they had decided to do the amniocentesis. A period of leaking and not leaking amniotic fluid started,
and after four weeks the leaking stopped completely. In the meantime, they were informed that the smallest child would indeed be
born with Down's syndrome; moreover – and this they felt to be
worse – it was suggested that the child might have serious cerebral
problems and several other physical distortions. When I then spoke
with Margriet over the phone she told me that she was extremely
worried and 'absolutely not sitting on a pink cloud'. Weeks later
(the foetuses were twenty-six weeks at this point) she started to
leak again. Margriet received medication to stop the contractions.
This medication decreased her own blood pressure drastically, thus
she was urgently put under coronary care at the intensive care unit.
The four weeks that followed she moved from the cardiology ward
to the gynaecology ward. At thirty weeks the babies were delivered
by a C-section full of complications: Margriet suffered from heart
rhythm defects and it took a long time before the spinal puncture
was effective; and the children were positioned in an 'awkward
way' so that the doctor had to pull hard to get them out. Both children then needed intensive care. The child with Down's syndrome
was indeed lighter than the other child and he had a hole in his
heart and kidney problems; but to their relief he did not have the
feared-for cerebral defect.

The babies stayed in the hospital for about two months. Both of
them had hard times, going through pneumonia and other viral
infections. At a certain moment the condition of the child with
Down's syndrome deteriorated and he apparently suffered from a
lot of pain. He was operated on, but it did not lead to any improvement in his condition and his situation became worse and worse. His
lungs were damaged and it became clear that he would have a life-
long dependency on oxygen machines. After an intensive period of
deliberation the doctors decided that further treatments would not
be helpful and that the artificial respiration should be stopped. So

it happened. Margriet and Hein held their child in their arms when the respiration stopped, then they took him home, as they wanted him to be in their home before they definitely had to say goodbye to him. The same day that their son was cremated, they received a call from the clinic telling them that their other child had become sick again. They feared for his life as well. Fortunately, he recovered from this illness and after some setbacks he could finally go home.

The moment I spoke with Margriet and Hein (they insisted on remaining in the study) the child had been home for about four weeks. Though he still needed extra attention and medical care, his parents were by then more trusting that things would turn out fine with him. They were of course happy that they had got and could retain this child, but they were also filled with grief for the child they had lost. In hindsight, they said the following:

> Margriet: If we had known all this before, we would never have done this IVF. Our grief is enormous. Look: *now* we know our children and we do not want to lose them – even when we lost [name of deceased child]. *Now* you cannot say anymore that you rather would not have done it . . . But if you had known all the sorrow beforehand.
> Hein: And also the risk for your [Margriet's] health . . . No, that risk I would not want to take.
> Margriet: Then you would not have been pregnant, you would not have known them and you would not have loved them. But I am very cautious to say this to others, as it may sound as if [name of the child that survived] was not worth all the trouble. But that is not the issue.

Margriet and Hein, who had experienced an enormous turmoil of intense emotions and enormous grief over a long period of time – starting with the IVF – kept emphasizing how important it was for them to 'do this together'. Despite all the anxiety and grief, they felt it had brought them closer together, a feeling that was expressed by several other study participants as well. How can we understand this and other gendered dynamics between women and men?

Essentializing Genetics and Gender Dynamics

Genes Matter: 'We Want a Child of the Two of Us'

Without any doubt, all women and men in this study agreed that the physical burdens and risks of IVF were unequally divided between them. A few women said that they sometimes became irritated or upset about this gender inequality, as, for example, when one said indignantly, 'It is me who has to undergo all this and not him!' Usually, however, such observations were followed by remarks such as, 'But there is nothing that we can do about that' or 'It does not help us when I complain that I have to undergo all this and not him'. Women thus sometimes expressed their dislike of having to bear the major part of the burden, yet they also felt they had 'no other choice', as they wanted a child of their own with their current partner. In fact, for several couples in this study with male-factor infertility there would have been the option to go for the use of donor sperm (AID), which would have been a much less intrusive and intensive treatment for the women. Yet almost all women and men in this study strongly expressed their wish to have a child of 'the two of us together'. They saw this as an expression or confirmation of their love for each other, and in the hope that they would recognize each other's and their own features in their child. This viewpoint reflects the importance of having a shared genetic link to their off-spring – the essentialization of genetics – instead of importing genetic links whose origins you do not know, and underlines the role they attribute to genes in a child's constitution. One man, for example, stressed that it has been proven that some behaviour, like criminality for example, is genetically defined, and that made him hesitant to use donor semen (and the use of adoption alike), because 'you never know what you will get in your house'. In addition, some of the men dreaded that if their wife conceived with donor semen they would feel that the child was more connected to their wife than to them, and that they would not consider it to be their own child (see also Ngemera 2001).

However, one man, Bert (see introductory case in this chapter), deviated from this general picture of essentializing a shared genetic bound. Bert was an older man, who was already a father and grandfather himself; he had been sterilized and had to undergo PESA, as the attempt to undo the sterilization had failed. He suggested that he would have preferred that his wife had attempted to conceive with/ from another man, instead of going through all the trouble of IVF. For him it was more important that his wife could have the experience of a pregnancy and that *her* kinship links with the prospective child were guaranteed than that he should have genetic links with the child. Though he uttered this suggestion a bit jokingly, there was definitely a serious undertone in his offer. His wife, however, would not think of this, as she definitely wanted to have a child with him. Having the child of her husband, whom she loved and whose characteristics she hoped to see in her future child, made this woman – and most other women in this study – willing to accept an unequal part of the risks and the burdens of IVF. In their case and probably in most other cases, 'accepting the risks of new reproductive technologies is less a patriarchal bargain than an act of connubial love and commitment' (Inhorn 2003:187). Sharing genes matters.

The Imperative of Conjugal Communication

The uneven gender distribution of the burdens of IVF had an important implication. As most men felt bad – and some even guilty, especially in the case of male-factor infertility – that their wife had to undergo the major part of the treatment in order to achieve their communal goal (cf. Nachtigall et al. 1992; Verdurmen 1997), most of them considered supporting their wife as the major contribution they could make in the IVF process, and many of the men in the study were fully dedicated to that role. We have seen that most were at home when their wives took the injections; they helped to prepare the injection needles and sometimes actually administered the injections themselves. Most men also tried to accompany their wives to the clinic as much as their work permitted and they were always present during the ova pick-up and the embryo transfer (their presence at these two interventions was a requirement from the clinic). Some men explicitly insisted on being present at all clinic visits, as they disliked the idea of their partner being unexpectedly confronted with bad news in their absence. Men closely watched their wives (and the screens) in the treatment rooms; they held their hands and showed compassion with what they had to go through. Men often complimented their wives for being brave and able to stand the pain. Moreover, and this was apparently crucial for many women, back home most of them shared with their wives their experiences, anxieties and hopes. When doing the pregnancy test, men made sure that they were at home to share their emotions and be there for each other. The meaning for the women of their partner's support throughout the treatment process should not be undervalued. On several occasions women showed that they were pleased when their partners acknowledged that they (the women) were bearing the majority of the physical burden of treatment and when they were concerned and caring for them. The recognition of the gender inequality alone seemed to alleviate their burden somewhat. In this context, several men and women also expressed the feeling that going through the fertility treatments, which in itself was a difficult process and sometimes brought conjugal problems, in the end had brought them closer together as a couple, a feeling that has also been observed by other authors in this area.[26]

Being able to communicate well as a couple – to exchange feelings, thoughts and hope – seemed to be paramount for successfully going through the treatment process. This ability reflects current day expectations of intimate partnerships in the Netherlands, where 'the survival of partnership increasingly hinges on the willingness to take the other partner's well-being into consideration' (Van den Troost 2005: 19). Great demands are placed on the emotional side of conjugal relationships (Dykstra et al. 2006). Both men and women are supposed to be able to communicate freely and extensively about emotions, and actively contribute to each other's well-being (cf. Greil 1991). If the partner does not live up to these expectations, this may lead to conjugal tensions or divorce.[27] Such tensions were clearly visible among some of the couples in this study.

The situation of Fleur and André illustrates this unmistakably. Fleur, while on the IVF waiting list, anticipated that her partner André could never give her the support she thought she would need when undergoing all steps in IVF and therefore decided to withdraw. Fleur frankly said that she dreaded both the physical pain and the emotional demands of IVF treatment, but emphasized that the main reason for withdrawing was that she felt that her partner was inconsiderate of her anxieties:

> I feel that after every hospital visit I have to do it on my own. I do not like to have my blood pricked, I do not like those tests and I do not like the idea that they watch me from the inside. But it is part of it, so I accept it. And I think it is very stressful, because imagine that it [fertilization] is not possible or you are half way and you find out that the embryos are not good. I will have to bear it on my own. He accompanies me to the hospital. Yes, he does. But after that day it is finished – we do not talk about it anymore.

André, whose sperm was frozen years ago, before he underwent cancer treatment, had previously undergone IUI treatments at the Radboud Clinic with his former partner. These treatments had failed and soon after this André and his former wife had divorced. Some years later André met Fleur (who was much younger than her partner) and after a while they decided to go for treatment together. André compared Fleur's reaction with the way his former partner had undergone the treatment: '[Name of former partner] did not bother at all about it'. He explained Fleur's refusal to further pursue

IVF by saying that she is 'far more sensitive' and that she had 'to quit smoking, lose weight, inject herself [what she dreaded] and visit the clinic frequently'; but he did not consider his own role in this, namely that she did not feel supported by him. Fleur repeatedly told me that if he would have shown more understanding and support, then she would have been willing and able to stand the burdens. As she anticipated, however, that this would not be the case, she did not want to do the IVF. The last time I spoke with them I interviewed them separately (on Fleur's request) because she was angry with him, saying, 'He really does not understand why I do not want to pursue the IVF treatment'. André thus did not live up to the standards of support and communication about intimate and personal issues, which not only Fleur expected from André, but – as was apparent in several of the other interviews – also reflected the desired communication style of most study participants, and certainly of the women (cf. Van den Troost 2005; Dykstra et al. 2006). Without her partner's empathy and support Fleur was not prepared to bear the heavy toll of treatment; she refused to bear the burden on her own (cf. Greil 1991).

Of the couples participating in this study, André and Fleur were the only one for whom the (anticipated) lack of support and empathy had such far reaching consequences. Some other couples did, however, also go through difficult phases together.[28] Chris, for example, stated in the third interview (after he and his wife had gone through three failed IVF cycles) that their inability to conceive had seriously threatened their relationship. Mireille much more than Chris wanted to talk through things and initially he had not been at all open to that. In the first interview he even said to me, 'Talking does not resolve any problems' (an expression I heard only two other men say during the interviews). He had only 'learned to talk' after a tough and serious conjugal crisis which – as Chris said – 'could have ended differently', pointing to a divorce. At the moment I spoke with them, both said that their relationship had changed for the better: they now talked a lot and Mireille stressed that she could now share her pain and emotions with him. Several other women and men expressed in a similar way that the infertility problems brought them closer together.

Greil (1991), who found a similar pattern of increased conjugal communication and bonding in his own study, questions why going through IVF may bring people together, and argues that this might result from two interrelated factors. First, he contends, couples in his study considered infertility a major life crisis they were forced to confront together, to 'weather the storm' (ibid.: 115). While any major life crisis may potentially strengthen the quality of intimate relationships, Greil further argues that infertility – as it is generally seen as a couple's problem – may enhance that feeling. In addition, as was also the case with Chris and Mireille, the need to frequently talk together – so, improved conjugal communication – may simply lead to better rapport. Greil (ibid.: 118) emphasizes that this does not mean that all relationships of couples struggling with infertility turned into 'idyllic marriages'. Rather he argues that those couples who considered it to be a common problem requiring communication, felt that it was strengthening their relationship; while couples in which one of the partners was unwilling to accept their infertility as a shared problem or to communicate about it, tended to grow apart. A similar analysis may well apply to my study findings as well.

Strikingly, none of the couples ever spoke in terms of guilt in my presence.[29] Still, I got the strong impression that for Chris – and for a few of the other men as well – the fact that he was the cause of the fertility problem complicated their situation: his wife had to undergo the major burdens of treatment for 'his failure' and even then he was (initially) not able to support her well. Why then would she not leave him and try to have a child with another man? This question was never spoken aloud in my presence, but still I can imagine that it conceivably passed through the study participants' minds or entered their conversations.

Conjugal problems resulting from the infertility and subsequent treatments were also discussed at the monthly social-work meetings of the Radboud Clinic. In these meetings it was observed that conjugal problems were often related to the divergent expectations and needs of women and men, or when they were not able to communicate about their experiences and feelings. The importance of the man's role in supporting his wife was recognized and encouraged by clinic staff. At the information evenings, for example, explicit attention was paid to the partner's role. The couples who shared their experiences with the public at the information evening (in two out of the three evenings I attended the man told the major part of the story) emphasized the significance of, as one of the men put it, 'Going together through the treatment process and sharing your feelings with each other, even when most of the actual treatment is done on the woman's body'. Sharing the experience and talking about your feelings with your partner was one of the messages couples took home from the information evening, a message that many of the study participants referred to in the interviews

and seemed to underline. Clinic practices thus reflected and reconfirmed notions of intimate relationships and the gendered (divergent) needs and expectation for support and communication in
contemporary Dutch society (cf. Thompson 2005).

'She Has to Decide'

Margriet: I dreaded to start the treatment again, to do all this to
myself again.
TG: Have you ever considered not starting another treatment because
of that anxiety?
Hein: She had to make the decision. She herself had to choose for it.
Because she has to undergo it and it brings much more stress for her
than for me . . . It all happens in her body, so . . .
Margriet: Yes and for the woman there is not a second that it does not
occupy you, because you feel every sign, every bit, yes, everything,
every time.

In the first interview I had with Margriet and Hein they recalled
how they had decided to start another IVF treatment cycle, in the
hope of having a second child (their first child was born after four
IVF cycles). Hein emphasized a number of times that Margriet had
to make the decision as she had to bear the majority of the burden.
In the literature it is sometimes suggested that women are put under
pressure from their husbands to undergo IVF instead of opting for
less invasive artificial insemination with donor semen (in case of
male fertility problems), as men are said to be more committed to
biological parenthood than women (e.g., Lorber 1989, cited in Greil
1991: 69). This is not, however, what I learned from my contacts
with the participants in this study. Rather, I found that most men
– aside from being concerned about the health of their partners –
insisted that their wife should decide on whether and when to start
(another) IVF treatment (cf. Verdurmen 1997: 187, in her study
among Dutch couples with fertility problems).

The men in the current study frequently stated explicitly that
their wives had to be ready for treatment (again). If this was not the
case, then they did not want to start treatment. In a few cases the
men preferred to stop further treatment, even though the women
still wanted to continue, as they thought the prognosis was too
bad to allow their wives to suffer once more; in these cases of conflicting views, the preference of the women was always followed.
However, while men may not have pressurized their wives, women
still might have felt some form of indirect pressure as they realized
that whether or not their husband could become a father would

depend on their decision. José, for example, four months after she had a miscarriage from her second full treatment, wrote me the following e-mail:

> Recently, we saw on TV a series of interviews with six women about their fertility problems – very recognizable. We ourselves, after the initial happiness that it [the treatment] was successful in May and the miscarriage in June, have slowed things down . . . In fact, I continue feeling bad when I think of IVF and everything around it. At one moment I think 'once more' and at another moment I do not want to do it again. For Tim things are different, but he does not have to undergo all this. He leaves me the choice. How will our life look if we stop . . .? Will not we regret this later?

José felt ambivalent about doing one more treatment, in particular because she hated going, again, through the hassle of treatment. Still, she felt it was hard to make the decision not to pursue a third treatment, because, among other reasons, she could not foresee what that would do to their life in the future. Would she and her husband later on not regret that they had not taken all available chances? José in her email did not bring up the question whether her husband would later on blame her for not continuing. Another woman, though, explicitly said that she found it a huge responsibility that she had to make the decision about future treatments and she questioned whether her husband would not later on reproach her if she did not do another treatment. In this way, for these women, while bearing the major burdens of treatment gave them the privilege to have the final say in decision-making, this privilege also added to their heavy toll as this made them also responsible for a (communal) future with or without a child.

Conclusion

The detailed stories about the physical and psychical effects of IVF presented in this chapter undoubtedly confirm the idea that women are more physically affected by these treatments than men (see, e.g., Greil 1997; Becker 2000; Thompson 2005; Verhaak et al. 2005). While new reproductive technologies, such as PESA and TESE, have the potential to increase the bodily involvement of men (Inhorn 2003), in the current study this was hardly the case. Thus the gender inequality with regard to the burdens of IVF – a major point of feminist critique – to a large extent continues to exist.

This gender inequality had some major implications. First, it turned (most) men into supportive and understanding partners. In turn, women were prepared to bear the burdens, even when the cause of the infertility problem lay with the man, as long as they felt supported by a concerned and committed partner with whom they could share their experiences and feelings. The Radboud Clinic stressed the importance of husbands being strongly involved, supportive and communicative. This emphasis on partner involvement and communication – from the point of view of the clinic and the couples – reflects and confirms contemporary Dutch (gendered) values about intimate relationships. Further, women were prepared to bear the burdens of treatment, as it kept alive the hope of a child from the two of them, their preferred goal, one that they could not achieve without IVF. Going for IVF instead of for the less intrusive option of AID (in case of male-factor infertility) underlines the importance ascribed to genetic relatedness of offspring and couples' preference to be part of a 'traditional family' (cf. Becker 2000). The fact that the Radboud Clinic did not offer donor treatment at the moment the study was conducted reconfirmed this genetic essentialization. Finally, the gender inequality left the woman to decide whether she was prepared to undergo (once more) the burdens of treatment. While the men in this study did not seem to pressure their wives to undergo treatment against their will, women might still have felt some form of (internal) pressure as they realized that their husband's future – with or without a child of their own – depended on their decision. The freedom to decide thus added another burden onto the woman's shoulders.

The stories in this chapter have also shown that IVF may affect different couples – and in particular the women – extremely differently. While these different experiences may be partly explained by the fact that the hormonal treatments and medical interventions actually do affect their bodies differently, I have argued that the way couples experience and respond to treatment is to a certain extent socially constructed. The way treatment affects women and men is, for example, related to: the meaning and intensity of their wish for a child, which was different when they, or one of them, were already parents; their experiences with hormonal medicines in former fertility treatments and their views about hormonal medicines in general; and the 'normalizing' information couples received about the treatment, possible side effects or pain, which shaped their views and expectations and may have put them at ease.

Finally, this chapter has given profound insight into the multiple effects of the patient-centred practices provided at the Radboud Clinic. Before starting IVF treatment, couples were well informed about all facets of treatment and well prepared for what was going to happen. Once in treatment, (most) couples had the experience that clinic staff put a lot of effort into diminishing the burdens of treatment and they were and felt well monitored. Without any doubt, such a supportive clinic environment helped couples to bear the burden of treatment. However, looking at these patient-centred practices from a disciplinary perspective, the clinic's intensive preparation and support also have a number of other (unintended) effects (cf. Cussins 1998; Pasveer and Heesterbeek 2001; Sawicki 1991). Throughout the IVF treatment, couples – and again women more than men – were disciplined to live their lives according to the requirements of the IVF treatment (such as injecting themselves, frequent clinic visits and producing sperm) and they learned to continuously, carefully watch their bodies. They thus became 'bureaucratic objects' (cf. Thompson 2005) and constantly sharpened their 'medical gaze'. Over the course of time they became better at all this, even when they disliked doing it (cf. Pasveer and Heesterbeek 2001). They thus became experts on their own bodies and on IVF procedures, which allowed them to undergo the treatments. They also came to internalize the idea that experiencing pain and stress was a normal part of IVF. While women did suffer from and complained about the pain and burdens, they were also inclined to relativize the burdens of their experiences, compared to others, compared to what they were prepared for and in view of the intended goal. The normalization of the heavy tolls of IVF, I have argued, makes couples more willing to accept the pain and emotional demands when they actually occur (cf. Benjamin and Ha'elyon 2002). In addition, the careful monitoring during the IVF cycle increased the feeling among couples that they were well monitored by considerate clinic staff. This diminished their concern and at the same time enhanced the trust couples had in the clinic staff, as I discussed in Chapter 5. Since considerate staff would not let them undergo treatments if this were irresponsible, the increased trust may in turn have made them more prepared to bear the burdens once more. In sum, I argue that while these patient-centred practices aim at *and* succeed in preparing and supporting couples, at the same time they have the unintended – ambiguous – effect of keeping most couples on the treatment track, even when they consider it to be a substantial burden. Only in extreme situations of an unsupportive partner, negative treatment experiences, distrust in staff and/or bad prospects, as discussed in this and previous chapters, might women (or couples) decide not to be prepared to bear the burdens any longer.

Notes

1. One study has shown that men with male factor infertility experience a more negative emotional response and a higher state of anxiety over time than those without (see Hardy and Makuch 2002).
2. For the first fourteen days, women at the Radboud Clinic injected Decapeptyl®, a hormonal medicine suppressing their normal hormonal cycle. Once they reacted satisfactorily, they started the next series of medicine, Puregon®, a follicle growth stimulating medicine. From that day onwards women had to take two different injections daily, one with Decapeptyl® and one with Puregon®. Eight days later they had to return to the clinic to check the follicles' growth by means of ultrasound; from that day on the growth of the follicles was monitored. When the follicles were big enough to be aspirated (which might take a further two to six days) women had to take a Pregnyl® injection, a hormonal medicine that stimulates the process of ripening and releasing of the eggs in the follicles. Thirty-six hours after this Pregnyl® injection, the ova pick-up took place. On the day of the ova pick-up women started taking Progestan®, a medicine that increases the chances of successful implantation of the embryo. Progestan® medicines came in the form of capsules, which had to be placed in the vagina on a daily basis for a period of fifteen days or up to the day that the woman started menstruating.
3. A medicine used to stimulate the growth of follicles in IUI treatments
4. In total I followed forty IVF cycles with nineteen couples: in about half of these cycles women mentioned adverse effects from Decapeptyl® and also in about half of the cycles women (not always the same ones) mentioned the adverse effects of Puregon®. In addition, a few women mentioned side effects of the Pregnyl® injection and the Progestan®. Only one woman said that she had not faced any adverse effects at all in the three IVF treatments she had undergone.
5. OHSS only occurs *after* ovulation when the follicles with ripe eggs have already been aspirated. It can occur when, behind the follicles with ripe eggs, a second cohort of small hidden follicles is present, which start growing as a result of the Pregnyl® injection (containing the hormone that stimulates the ripening of the eggs and the ovulation). As these follicles continue growing after the ova pick-up, the ovaries can become very big (up to ten centimetres in diameter) and liquid from the ovaries enters the belly and the peritoneum. In extreme cases this can lead to serious consequences such as thrombosis and shock (Sagasser 2001).

6. The Estradiol level gives an indication of the number of follicles present, even when they cannot yet be seen.

7. Though the head of the IVF clinic told me that bodily signs are not in fact important for detecting OHSS in that stage.

8. In 2006 3.2 per cent of all IVF cycles at the Radboud fertility clinic were cancelled; it is estimated that 1–2 per cent of all cycles are cancelled because of an over-reaction to the hormonal medication (personal information, Prof. Dr J. Kremer).

9. In addition, two women had experienced a threatening OHSS in previous IVF cycles: one woman when she did IVF treatment in another hospital, and one who did a series of four IVF treatments at the Radboud Clinic, which led to the birth of a child.

10. Women could choose any time between 2 P.M. and 12 A.M. to take the Decapeptyl® and Puregon® injections. However, once they had chosen a certain time they had to stick (approximately) to that time. It was recommended that they took the medicines out of the fridge at least half an hour before injecting, as this makes injecting the liquid less painful. They could keep the medicines out of the fridge for about one day, as long as they were not kept in direct sunlight.

11. The Radboud Clinic was in that period involved in the conduct of a study 'IVF, work and stress', Bouwmans, et al. (2008).

12. Some couples contrasted this with their experiences in the preceding period, when they underwent fertility examinations and low-tech treatments, during which waiting times were often longer. Some couples also complained about miscommunication between the fertility department and other clinic departments (such as the urology department where the PESA procedure took place or the department where habitual miscarriage examinations were carried out), which sometimes caused long waiting times and the loss of patient files.

13. In many other clinics a (partial) narcosis is a standard procedure during the ova puncture.

14. This resembles the discourse around deliveries in the Netherlands, where epidurals are not regularly provided and women are also complimented for being brave.

15. Only one man did not join his wife during the ova pick-up, as he dreaded that he would immediately faint.

16. Benjamin and Ha'elyon (2002: 677) further argued that only when the women felt that the treatment really 'endangered their physical or mental existence' did the meaning of the pain change and women started to consider quitting their IVF treatments.

17. As mentioned in the previous chapter men whose sperm had been previously shown to be of bad quality and who were therefore indicated for ICSI were, however, sometimes concerned and tense about its quality on the day of the ova pick-up and this certainly added to the stress couples experienced at this stage of the treatment.

18. TESE normally takes place under full narcosis, but was not yet carried out at the Radboud Clinic at the time of the fieldwork.
19. The discrepancy with Inhorn's study, in which she found that men were strongly bodily affected, can be explained by the fact that in Egyptian clinics, in general, men are more often operated on and get more medicines compared to men in the Radboud Clinic, and many more men in her study underwent PESA or TESE (Inhorn 2003: 188).
20. In the Netherlands cycling is one of the main modes of transportation.
21. Peanut butter and *hagelslag* are both typical Dutch sandwich filling.
22. In the current study this was the case for four of the nineteen couples undergoing IVF treatment. The majority of couples participating in the study – and this can be generalized for the wider group of people undergoing IVF treatment – were not immediately successful or were not successful at all even after repetitive treatments.
23. Personal information Prof. Dr J. Kremer.
24. It irritates Layne (2003) that the implication of this increased attachment on those who lose their pregnancies has not been taken into consideration in clinical practices, as only the benefits of increased attachment are considered in these practices. She argues that it might psychologically be better for parents 'not to determine their pregnancies so early, not to start investing in the social construction of fetal parenthood until a later date' when the chances of a successful pregnancy are larger (ibid.: 101).
25. Margriet had worked with children with mental retardation, including children with Down syndrome, and this experience strengthened her and her husband's view that a child with Down syndrome was more than welcome (cf. Rapp 2000: 224).
26. See, e.g., Greil 1991; Becker 2000; Inhorn 2003; Franklin and Roberts 2006.
27. Communicational problems scored highest in the list of reasons for divorce by Dutch women and men (Van den Troost 2005).
28. Five couples participating in my study reported tough and troublesome periods in their relationship, which were partly due to fertility problems and treatment. One of them separated during the course of the study.
29. This might be because I interviewed the couples together, though I really regret not having brought up the topic myself in the interviews.

References

Aalten, A., N. Van Amsterdam and M. Van der Linden. 2008. *Het verhaal van pijn. Wat het lichaam ons vertelt en waarom wij (niet) luisteren.* Rotterdam: Codarts/Rotterdamse Dansacademie.

Becker, G. 2000. *The Elusive Embryo. How women and men approach new reproductive technologies.* Berkeley: University of California Press.

Benjamin, O. and H. Ha'elyon. 2002. 'Rewriting fertilization: Trust, pain and exit points', *Women's Studies International Forum* 25(6): 667–78.

Bouwmans, C.A., Lintsen, B.A., Al, M., Verhaak, C.M., Eijkemans, R.J., Habbema, J.D.F., and Hakkaart-Van Roijen, L. 2008. 'Absence from work and emotional stress in women undergoing IVF or ICSI: an analysis of IVF-related absence from work in women and the contribution of general and emotional factors', *Acta Obstetricia et Gynecologica Scandinavica* 87(11): 1169–1175.

Cussins, C.M. 1998. 'Ontological choreography: Agency for women patients in an infertility clinic', in M. Berg, and A. Mol (eds), *Differences in Medicine: Unraveling practices, techniques, and bodies.* Durham, NC: Duke University Press, pp. 166–200.

Dykstra, P., M. Kalmijn, T. Knijn, A. Komter, A. Liefbroer and C. Mulder. 2006. *Family Solidarity in the Netherlands.* Amsterdam: Dutch University Press Logo.

Franklin, S. 1997. *Embodied Progress: A cultural account of assisted conception.* London: Routledge.

Franklin, S. and C. Roberts. 2006. *Born and Made: An ethnography of preimplantation genetic diagnosis.* Princeton: Princeton University Press.

Greil, A.L. 1991. *Not Yet Pregnant: Infertile couples in contemporary America.* New Brunswick: Rutgers University Press.

———— 1997. 'Infertility and psychological distress: A critical review of the literature', *Social Science and Medicine* 45(11): 1679–704.

Greil, A.L., K. Slauson-Blevins and J. McQuillan. 2010. 'The experience of infertility: A review of recent literature', *Sociology of Health and Illness* 32(1): 140–62.

Hardy, E. and M.J. Makuch. 2002. 'Gender, infertility and ART', in E. Vayena, P.J. Rowe and P.D. Griffin (eds), *Current Practices and Controversies in Assisted Reproduction.* Geneva: WHO, pp. 272–80.

Helman, C.G. 2000. *Culture, Health and Illness* (fourth edition). Oxford: Butterworth-Heinemann.

Inhorn, M. C. 2003. *Local Babies, Global Science: Gender, religion and in vitro fertilization in Egypt.* New York: Routledge.

———— 2012. *The New Arab Man: Emergent masculinities, technologies, and Islam in the Middle East.* Princeton: Princeton University Press.

Layne, L. 2003. *Motherhood Lost: A feminist account of pregnancy loss in America.* New York: Routledge.

Lupton D. 1997. 'Foucault and the medicalisation critique', in A. Petersen and R. Burton (eds), *Foucault, Health and Medicine.* London: Routledge, pp. 94–110.

Lorber, J. 1989. 'Choice, gift, or patriarchal bargain? Women's consent to in vitro fertilization in male infertility', *Hypatia,* 4(3): 23–36.

Nachtigall, R.D., G. Becker and M. Wozny. 1992. 'The effects of gender-specific diagnosis on men's and women's response to infertility', *International Journal of Gynecology and Obstetrics* 39(1): 77–78.

Nettleton, S. 1995. *The Sociology of Health and Illness*. Oxford: Blackwell Publishers.

Ngemera, D.B. 2001. 'Dutch men experiencing infertility, infertility treatment and involuntary childlessness.' Amsterdam: University of Amsterdam (MA thesis). Retrieved 23 March 2016 from dare.uva.nl.

Pasveer, B. and S. Heesterbeek. 2001. *De voortplanting verdeeld. De praktijk van de voortplantingsgeneeskunde doorgelicht vanuit het perspectief van patiënten*. The Hague: Rathenau Instituut.

Rapp, R. 1999. *Testing Women, Testing the Fetus: The social impact of Amniocentesis in America*. New York: Routledge.

Sagasser, J. 2001. *IVF*. Houten: Van Holkema and Warendorf.

Sawicki, J. 1991. *Disciplining Foucault: Feminism, power and the body*. New York: Routledge.

Thompson, C. 2005. *Making Parents: The ontological choreography of reproductive technologies*. Cambridge, MA: The MIT Press.

Van den Troost, A. 2005. *Marriage in Motion: A study on the social context and processes of marital satisfaction*. Leuven: Leuven University Press.

Van der Ploeg, I. 1998. *Prosthetic Bodies: Female embodiment in reproductive technologies*. Maastricht: Maastricht University Press.

Verhaak, C.M., Smeenk, J.M.J., Van Minnen, A., Kremer, J.A.M., and Kraaimaat, F.W. 2005. 'A longitudinal, prospective study on emotional adjustment before, during and after consecutive fertility treatment cycles', *Human Reproduction* 20(8): 2253–60.

Verdurmen, J. 1997. 'Keuzes bij onvruchtbaarheid. Besluitvorming bij onvruchtbare paren'. Ph.D. dissertation. Amsterdam: University of Amsterdam.

Chapter 8

BIOETHICS IN PRACTICE

Reproductive autonomy refers to the freedom to make essential choices affecting one's reproductive life, including choosing whether or not to have children, with whom, when and under what circumstances (Bateman 2001). When women and men with fertility problems visit a clinic with a request for medically assisted procreation, their reproductive autonomy may be jeopardized, as third persons – in particular doctors – become involved in the realization of their wish for a child. Specific (physical) conditions of the prospective parents may raise concerns about the appropriateness of having children. Moreover, ARTs enable procreation for women and men in circumstances other than a heterosexual relationship or within 'normal' reproductive age (including singles, lesbian and gay partners, divorced or widowed women and men and menopausal women), leading people to also question the appropriateness of procreation in these less conventional family situations (Bateman 2001; Bolt et al. 2004). While prospective parents may perceive their own (physical) condition and social situation as appropriate for conceiving and raising a child, medical professionals may feel unease or be reluctant to offer medical assistance when confronted with a request from the same prospective parents.

Since the early introduction of ARTs there has been much debate about the criteria by which decisions about the appropriateness of its use for special patient groups should be made and who should decide in the case of disagreements (Bateman 2001; Bolt et al. 2004; Hunfeld et al. 2004; Jones and Cohen 2004). Worldwide, governments, clinic staff, ethicists, feminists, religious leaders, the public in general and women and men with fertility problems themselves have highly diverging (moral) views about this (cf. Jones and Cohen 2004). These debates and views 'are deeply embedded within particular "local moral worlds" of religion and culture' (Inhorn and Birenbaum-Carmeli 2008: 184, Kleinman 1995, Thompson 2005; see also the Special Issue of *Culture, Medicine and Psychiatry* 30(4), 2006).[1] In addition, as Franklin and Roberts (2006: 209) observed, there is a tension between the 'near-unanimous recognition of a social, legal, political, economic, and moral need for clear and established limits to technical "assistance" to human reproduction and heredity' and 'the desires of individuals in extreme circumstances to break, defy, or transcend these same boundaries'.

In clinical settings, deciding who will decide in the case of disagreement involves weighing the doctor's responsibility for the safety and well-being of his/her patient (the prospective mother) and for the prospective child, versus the patients' freedom to make their own reproductive choices.[2] The fact that the future child is not able to express his/her views makes such situations more complicated. This chapter discusses how clinic staff at the Radboud Clinic handled the tension that may exist between individual reproductive autonomy and medical responsibility and authority.

In Chapter 2 I provided an overview of the governmental legislation and professional guidelines that have regulated access to ARTs in the Netherlands over the last three decades. These regulations, though, do not cover all possible requests for medical assisted procreation (cf. Stern et al. 2003); even more so as these requests are taking place in a constantly evolving field of medical and scientific innovation, in which new sorts of requests are constantly emerging. In these cases it is left to clinic staff to decide whether or not to provide ARTs. Yet the role and authority of doctors in deciding the appropriateness of the use of ARTs in certain situations has been questioned, as this is considered to be beyond their direct professional competence and responsibility: since the values at stake are more about 'moral convictions regarding what constitutes "good" life in terms of sexuality and procreation, family life, health and handicap' (Bateman 2001: 321) than about medical-technical issues. Thus, the legitimacy of medical authority in this domain has been strongly questioned. On the other hand, the dominance of the individual autonomy principle in contemporary 'liberal society' and medical practice has also been questioned (Heesterbeek and Ten Have 2001; Muller 1994). Firstly, as Heesterbeek and Ten Have

(2001) have argued, doctors, as autonomous individuals themselves, cannot be forced to fulfil each and every request for IVF or
any other treatment if they are not in favour of such a treatment in
a particular situation. Secondly, fulfilling the requests of individuals
based on the principle of personal autonomy may in the long term
have unforeseen consequences for other individuals, for (kinship)
relationships between people and for society at large. Such possible consequences are, however, not taken into consideration if
decisions are only based on the principle of personal autonomy.

   This chapter thus addresses how the tension between medical
authority and individual reproductive autonomy was dealt with in
the Radboud Clinic: it discusses how clinic staff actually deliberated
and handled requests for medically assisted reproduction that they
– or some of them – considered ethically sensitive. The dominat-
ing framework in bioethics guiding doctors' decision-making is the
four principle approach, including the principles of patient autonomy, beneficence, non-maleficence, and justice (Beauchamp and
Childress 1994). The strict application of this approach has been
criticized for being 'a-contextual, ethnocentric, reductionistic, and
sterile' (Muller 1994: 451). A contextualized approach, in contrast,
takes into consideration the many factors that shape particular circumstances and decisions. This chapter, by looking at 'bioethics in
practice' starts from the position that both the definition of an ethical
dilemma *and* the way it is handled is constructed in its context –
political, institutional, sociocultural and religious – and that this is
continually evolving (cf. Hoffmaster 1992; Muller 1994: 453–59).

   The current chapter is mainly based on information collected
during the multi-disciplinary ethics meetings at the Radboud Clinic
and on conversations with staff attending these meetings. Contrarily
to the previous chapters, in this chapter the views of the couples
discussed in the meetings are not presented as I did not personally
speak with them. A slightly different version of this chapter has
been published in *Social Science and Medicine* (Gerrits et al. 2013).

Multi-Disciplinary Ethics Meeting

At the Radboud Clinic the situations of couples requesting medical
assistance in procreation which raise concerns or doubts with
regard to further examination and treatment are discussed in multi-
disciplinary ethics meetings. At the time of the fieldwork these ethics
meetings were held bi-monthly; in a period of one and a half years

(from September 2003 until January 2005) the requests of twenty-nine couples were discussed. It should be noted that the clinic sees more than 1,700 new couples per year; thus in fact only a very small percentage of couples was discussed in these meetings.

The ethics meeting is interdisciplinary, meaning that doctors, nurses, a clinical psychologist, a medical ethicist and a social worker (and incidentally an embryologist or laboratory technician) participate. Theoretically, all participants could propose couples for discussion; however, in practice it turned out that it was almost always the medical doctors who proposed couples for discussion, as they were the ones who did the intake of new couples and were therefore the first to observe information in the background of their patients that might raise ethical concerns. Couples concerned were informed that their case would be discussed in the meeting.[3] Most of the couples proposed for discussion were indicated for IVF and related high-tech treatments, though some of them were still early on in the examination phase or had been indicated for low-tech treatments.

Situations that raised concerns among clinic staff and were presented in the ethics meetings in the study period included couples of which one or both partners were (potential) carriers of genetic diseases or suffered from serious psychological problems; where the man was terminally ill or of an advanced age; where the couple did not fulfil the clinic's criterion for a stable relationship; and some other situations (see Appendix 2: Table A2).[4] The case chosen for presentation below – a couple of which the woman was a carrier of a cancer gene – illustrates how clinic staff at the interdisciplinary ethics meetings (and thereafter) discussed and handled ethically sensitive cases in actual daily practice. In the sections thereafter I first discuss how the concerns expressed about this and other cases presented at the ethics meetings reflect the specific context in which the use of ARTs was requested; next I discuss the practices the clinic staff employed to address and resolve their concerns.

Case Study: Woman Carrier of a Cancer Gene

Monday morning, 11 o'clock. The bi-monthly interdisciplinary ethics meeting of the Radboud Fertility Clinic is starting. Ten staff members, including gynaecologists, IVF doctors and nurses, a clinical psychologist, a medical ethicist, and a social worker, are sitting round the table in the office of the head of the ObGyn Department. Today's agenda is exceptionally full, with ten cases to be discussed.

Reaching case number six on the agenda, one of the IVF doctors introduces the couple. She talks about her patients Mr and Mrs P, both in their
late twenties, who came to visit the clinic because they had not managed
to conceive on their own. After having gone through a series of diagnostic procedures, the doctor indicated them for IVF treatment. During
the diagnostic process it came to light that the woman is the carrier of a
cancer gene, which was also the reason the doctor proposed their case
to be on the agenda for the meeting.[5] The doctor briefly presents the
family's disease history: the woman's father is a carrier of the same gene
(he had actually suffered from the particular type of cancer), and – most
probably – her grandfather as well (he died from a disease with similar
symptoms, though at that time the origin of his disease was not identified). When the woman herself was in her teens, she was screened for
the cancer, and when the test had proved positive she underwent an
operation, removing the vulnerable body part as a preventive measure.
The doctor ends her introduction by saying that she referred the couple
to the clinic's genetic centre for advice from the geneticist.

As soon as the doctor finishes her presentation of the case a lively
discussion starts, with several concerns and thoughts expressed by the
attendees. One of the doctors refers to a similar past case: 'I remember, at that time we refused treatment here in the hospital. In that case,
the couple went to another hospital in the Netherlands, and they were
immediately treated on the condition that they undergo prenatal diagnosis (PND). I remember that afterwards, we felt we had been rather paternalistic'. Remarks about the seriousness of this type of cancer are made:
one doctor observes that this specific disease can manifest itself in various
degrees of seriousness, and another suggests that the fact that the woman
had been screened and immediately operated upon might indicate that
the woman is the carrier of a serious form of the disease. Someone else
questions whether this type of cancer presents an indication for PND in
their hospital, or rather for pre-implantation genetic diagnosis (PGD) in
the academic hospital in Maastricht (the only hospital in the Netherlands
where PGD is allowed to be performed). Nobody is certain about the
answer to these questions; it has to be looked at further.

Then one of the doctors raises the following question: 'Imagine that
PND is an option, and that it is found that there is a 50 per cent chance
that the future child will be affected. In that case, an induced abortion
would be an option. Can we then still speak of an emergency case, if we
know beforehand that there is a 50 per cent chance that the foetus will
be aborted?'[6] The discussion switches to the issue of responsible parenthood. 'What are parents doing to their children?' the same staff member
is questioning. 'If you are a carrier of this disease, you are 100 per cent

sure you will get cancer. Even when you have a preventative operation done, this does not guarantee that you won't get cancer elsewhere
in your body!' 'The clinical psychologist comments, 'But the woman is
suffering from it herself. She knows what it is, and she apparently feels
it is bearable'. 'That may be true, but isn't this a known form of denial
among carriers of certain genetic diseases?' 'Yes, but denying may be
an effective mechanism'. 'Okay, when it concerns yourself. But this is
about someone else . . . I cannot imagine that you want this for your
child!'

At a certain moment, the doctor who introduced the case and who
has been watching the discussion silently is asked directly what she
feels about the case. She answers: 'For me it is important to know if the
patient is fully informed. I think differently about PND and pregnancy
termination than some others here do'. The social worker then suggests
that they ask the couple what they themselves feel about PND and a
possible termination of the pregnancy. This may also provide an indication of how they would feel if they had an affected child. This suggestion is agreed upon. The discussion ends with the following remark by
the attending gynaecologist: 'You know, if people do conceive without
medical assistance, it is their responsibility. But now we are involved, it
is our responsibility as well'. It is decided that no decisions will be made
before the information from the geneticist is available, and the case will
be discussed in the next meeting.

Two months later Mr and Mrs P's name is again on the agenda of the
ethics meeting. The clinic's genetic centre has not yet sent any information about the couple to the doctor, and therefore the case cannot be
discussed. One of the staff members expresses her surprise about the fact
that this case is being discussed at their interdisciplinary ethics meeting,
because 'being a carrier of this particular cancer gene in our hospital
is not an indication for pregnant women to undergo PND. I wonder
whether this would be different in the case of a medically assisted pregnancy'. Thereafter, one of the doctors again refers to the similar past
situation, where the couple was immediately treated in another hospital
in the Netherlands, and where in retrospect they had felt paternalistic.
However, they all agree not to make a decision about the case until they
receive the information from the geneticist.

Some weeks before the next interdisciplinary ethics meeting takes
place, the information from the geneticist becomes available, and the
attending doctor sees Mr and Mrs P to discuss the results. Both the
couple and the doctor receive a copy of the geneticist's letter. The letter
states that the children of carriers of this specific cancer gene have a
50 per cent chance of being a carrier as well; however, it is impossible

to predict the seriousness of the disease, the age of onset, and other possible complications. Moreover, the letter states, removing the 'vulnerable' body part at a young age cannot always prevent cancers in other places in the body. In cases where the exact 'genetic error' is known, it is possible to do a PND in the twelfth or sixteenth week of the pregnancy to find out whether the embryo is affected or not. The exact genetic error in their family is not yet known. Research to detect this has been initiated with the woman's father, but this may take six to eight months. However, even if this information becomes available, Mr and Mrs P told the geneticist – and he in turn had written it in his letter – they would not be interested in doing a PND in the event of a pregnancy. They both feel they could live with the idea of having a child with this disease.

Based on the information of the geneticist and her conversation with the couple, the attending medical doctor writes in the medical dossier that there are no arguments for withholding IVF, as the couple is well informed about and aware of the possible risks. The doctor contacts the head of the department who agrees with this position; thus the couple is put on the IVF waiting list. The couple's case is not brought up in the next interdisciplinary ethics meeting.

Concerns in Context

The concerns clinic staff expressed when discussing the above case and other cases related to the physical health and/or psycho-social well-being of the prospective child and/or the impact of the treatment or pregnancy on the physical or mental health of the prospective parents.[7] In this section I discuss which situations raised what sort of concerns and how these concerns reflected the specific context in which the requests for assisted procreation were discussed, namely in a clinic (where clinic staff thus becomes involved in decision-making) residing under Dutch legislation and 'rooted' in a Catholic community and will. With regards to the Catholic roots of the Radboud Clinic it should be noted that the clinic – obviously – does not adhere to the formal position of the Catholic Church that completely condemns IVF.[8] However, some positions taken by the clinic staff affecting the use of ARTs, as we will see, might be related to the roots of the clinic, even when the clinic staff never explicitly referred to 'Catholicism' in their reasoning about ethical concerns (cf. Thompson 2006).[9]

The Physical Health of the Future Child

The physical health of the future child was found to be a major concern for the clinic staff when – as we saw in the case of Mr and Mrs P – one or both prospective parents were (potential) carriers of serious genetic diseases.[10] This concern is in line with the governmental regulation stipulating that in cases of assumed medical contraindications for ARTs, further examinations are required; and medical doctors have the right to withhold treatment when they think that the outcome of these examinations is worrisome (Gezondheidsraad, 1997). We are so used to doctors dealing with issues of physical health that this concern is hardly surprising. However, if one thinks of the way most children are conceived – in a private place – one realizes that this health concern can only acquire such a central position precisely because reproduction is taking place in a hospital setting and is assisted by medical doctors.

The impact of procreation taking place in a clinical setting becomes even more obvious when doctors expressed their concerns (though to a lesser degree) about the possible physical harm to the future child when the prospective father was an elderly man. In these cases it was questioned whether the semen of elderly men may negatively impact on the physical health and psycho-social well-being of the future child, a question that most probably would not have been raised if conception had taken place outside the clinic. The concern expressed in the cases of elderly men did not result directly from governmental guidelines, as in the Netherlands no maximum age is set for men taking part in medically assisted reproduction. However, in the past some staff members had felt uneasy when confronted with elderly men in the IVF treatment rooms and therefore clinic staff had agreed to discuss all couples involving men older than fifty-five at the multi-disciplinary ethics meetings. By discussing the cases involving elderly men in the multi-disciplinary ethics meetings, clinic staff aimed to better understand their own personal discomfort and better position themselves towards them. To gain insight into the possible effects on children (including also effects on their psycho-social well-being) when they are conceived by and grow up with elderly fathers, clinic staff carried out a literature review (Römkens et al 2005).

The Psycho-Social Well-Being of the Future Child

As mentioned before, according to governmental regulations factors related to the psycho-social well-being of the prospective child may be considered contraindications for medically assisted procreation, on the conditions that the assumed risk is serious and very well grounded (Gezondheidsraad, 1997: 89–90; Bolt et al. 2004: 7). Clinic staff expressed their concerns about the psycho-social well-being of the future child in a number of situations: when one or both prospective parents were or had been suffering from serious psychological problems; when the prospective father was an elderly man or terminally ill; and when they had doubts about the stability of the couple's relationship. These concerns were based on the view that for children's well-being it is important that they know the identity of both parents and – ideally – that they also grow up with both of them. This particular view about children's psycho-social well-being is suggested to have a psychological basis, rather than a moral one (cf. Hunfeld et al. 2004), and has also been reported elsewhere (see, e.g., Patel and Johnson 1998; De Geyter et al. 2010). While this view may also have been influenced by Catholic values of what constitutes a proper family, this was never referred to by the clinic staff.

This particular view about children's psycho-social well-being had a number of implications related to access to treatment. In the first place, for a couple to have access to any form of fertility treatment, the Radboud Clinic in principle required the prospective parents to be in a stable relationship, which was defined as the couple having been together and residing at the same address for at least one year (below we will see that in practice clinic staff were not always strict in applying this criteria). Secondly, this view explained and informed clinic staff member's concerns about offering treatment to elderly or terminally ill prospective fathers: they questioned whether there were any (major) psycho-social risks for children if their father died before they were born or while they were still very young. Thirdly, this view was also reflected in the hospital's policy regarding the post-mortem use of gametes and embryos. If one of the partners had or would have passed away before treatment could take place, but frozen semen or embryos were still available, the clinic would not allow the surviving woman or man to use these frozen materials. In this regard, hospital policy deviated from governmental regulations that allow post-mortem use of gametes and embryos under certain, carefully stipulated conditions (Modelreglement Embryowet, 2003: 39–44). Finally, the clinic's standpoint that the child should know the identity of both parents was also a reason why the clinic – at the time of this study – did not work at all with donor gametes, as the identity of anonymous donors could not be traced. Thus in this regard the clinic's policy was also more restrictive than governmental legislation prescribed. As of January 2008, this clinic's policy changed.

The Physical or Mental Health of Prospective Parents

Finally, clinic staff expressed concerns about the impact of fertility treatments on the physical and/or mental health of one or both prospective parents. For example, they questioned whether there was a chance that the burden of treatment or a treatment failure (in particular in a demanding IVF treatment) could lead to deterioration or a relapse if the prospective father or mother had been or still was suffering from serious psychological or psychiatric problems. This concern was for example raised in the case of a couple of which the woman had recently attempted to commit suicide. Health professionals also questioned – as we will see – whether it would be acceptable to expose a woman who already had four children, and whose deliveries had been complicated, to the risks and burden of an intensive IVF treatment and another (possibly) complicated delivery. Further, they questioned what the stress of fertility treatment would do to the health of prospective fathers who were terminally ill at the time of the request for medical assisted reproduction, and to their partners.

All these concerns may be seen as a reflection of the core tasks of doctors and hospitals: taking care of the health of people and avoiding doing harm. Yet if these couples had been able to conceive without medical assistance, they would not have needed the authorization of anybody else. Entering the clinic thus rendered couples dependent on another party in the decision-making process regarding their process of conception. Still, the fact that these couples' situations were presented and discussed at the ethics meeting by no means implied that they were all denied access to treatment. On the contrary, despite health professionals' initial ethical concerns, only four out of the twenty-nine couples presented in the meetings were not offered treatment in the Radboud Clinic on the basis of ethical concerns (see Appendix 2: Table A2). Three other couples were not offered treatment because additional medical examinations revealed that their prognosis was too bad to justify treatment, and in two cases no final decision was made as the couples did not return to the clinic. Thus for most couples, the initial ethical concern only formed a temporary obstacle to further treatments and not a final constraint.

Addressing Ethically Sensitive Requests

While contextual features clearly set the agenda for the multi-disciplinary ethics meetings, they did not fully determine what decisions were made. Governmental regulations and clinic policy left an area of ambiguity and uncertainty and it was in this area that the clinic's multi-disciplinary ethics meetings functioned. Over the past years clinic staff developed and employed a number of practices in order to address their concerns; these practices will be discussed in this section.

Consulting Professionals

Radboud Clinic staff, when discussing the situations of couples presented in the interdisciplinary ethics meetings, in many cases acknowledged that they did not have the competence in a specialized field, nor sufficient information about the specific woman and man, to be able to assess the seriousness of the presented ethical concern. In most cases, therefore, a first action was to request additional information from other (health) professionals such as geneticists, oncologists, general practitioners, psychiatrists, psychologists and social workers, who had been or still were involved in the treatment of one or both partners. Professionals were consulted for all couples with genetic diseases and serious psychological problems, and when the prospective father was suffering from a serious disease (in all three cases the men suffered from cancer and therefore their oncologist was consulted); in some cases gynaecologist colleagues experienced in giving preconception advice were asked to see a couple. Couples were always asked for their consent before another professional was consulted.

The responses provided by the consulted professionals often demonstrated a high degree of uncertainty. Information that the geneticists provided generally entailed several uncertainties and ambiguities, e.g., about the seriousness and age of onset of some of the genetic diseases (cf. Rapp 1999).[11] Predicting the course of mental problems was also found to be extremely difficult. When no hard predictions on serious future risks could be made, and/or when the genetic disease in 'normal' pregnancies was not considered an indication for prenatal diagnosis (PND) in the Radboud Clinic, the principle of patient autonomy gained weight in the decision-making process. However, in these cases two conditions had to be fulfilled: the attending doctor had to be convinced that the couple was well informed about the genetic disease and showed that they had 'sensibly thought about' the possible implications of their decision. This was, according to the attending doctor, the case with Mr and Mrs P, where we saw that the principle of 'patient autonomy' overruled the doctor's initial concerns about potential harm being done to the prospective child. Mrs P and her relatives (had) lived with this disease themselves and felt that living with this disease was acceptable/ bearable. They were thus able to resist the focus on statistics that is required by '[t]he powerful language of risk attached to age, ethnic background or family genetic history' (cf. Rapp 1999: 73); rather they were able to interpret and respond to the statistics based on their own experience, which the clinic staff permitted them to do.

Similar considerations, in combination with collegial consultation, were also decisive in the case of a couple of Turkish background, who already had four daughters and who wanted to have a fifth child.[12] The woman had had three complicated and risky deliveries and in addition some other health conditions might further complicate pregnancy and delivery. Some of the clinic staff clearly demonstrated that they did not understand this couple's request, particularly as they initially assumed that the couple desired a boy. They felt that the woman – 'due to her culture' – was obliged to undergo intensive IVF and endure the risks of another probably complicated delivery in order to bear a son. The consulted gynaecologist, who specialized in preconception advice, replied however that the potential complications during delivery could be well monitored (if known beforehand) and therefore that was not a reason to deny IVF treatment. Moreover, the doctor in charge of the couple stated that she had had some 'intensive talks' with them and reported that she had encountered a 'sensible couple' that was well aware of all the ins and outs of the treatment, the limited success rates and possible complications; further, they stated that they would be happy to have a daughter and were aware that the chance of having a son was equal to the chance of having a girl. Given that the number of children that a couple already has is not defined as an exclusion criterion for IVF (neither at clinic level nor stipulated by Dutch policy nor for health insurances), the fact that the couple already had four children could not be justified as a reason to deny them access to treatment. Thus the couple was allowed access to treatment. In this case the clinic staff – despite the fact that at least some of them still did not comprehend why this woman would take any risks at all and suffer the burden of treatment, given that the estimated success rate was small and the couple already had four children – accepted the gynaecologist's preconception advice and respected the autonomy of the 'well informed and sensible' couple.

For other couples, the advice of consulted professionals had other implications. This was particularly striking in the case of two couples where the women had serious psychological problems and were still in therapy when they requested fertility treatment. In both of these cases the woman was consulting more than one (health) professional – a psychiatrist and/or psychologist, a general practitioner, and/or a social worker – and the doctors attending the couples at the fertility clinic asked these providers to give their views on the couples' requests for medically assisted procreation. In both cases the consulted providers came up with mutually conflicting information and advice: one supporting and the other not supporting the request for fertility treatment. This conflicting advice meant that the clinic staff decided not to offer fertility treatment to these couples at that particular moment, as they did not dare take the risk and be held responsible for jeopardizing the health and well-being of the women involved and – if treatment was successful – of the future children. In one of these cases it was stated explicitly, however, that the decision was provisional; if the woman's condition continued to improve, the couple was invited to return to the clinic after a period of about six months for further examinations and possible treatment. Collegial advice thus played a crucial role in the assessment of the seriousness of a certain condition.

Offering Medical Tests: PND or PGD?

When prospective parents are – potential – carriers of a serious genetic disease, prenatal diagnosis (PND) or pre-implantation genetic diagnosis (PGD) can be performed to detect the genetic abnormality at an early phase and avoid the birth of an affected child. PND is a test performed in the sixteenth or twentieth week of pregnancy; in the case that the embryo is affected, the prospective parents may decide to terminate the pregnancy. PGD, a screening that has to be combined with IVF treatment, is performed *before* the pre-embryo is transferred; couples at risk of having children with a known genetic abnormality can have their pre-embryos screened, allowing only unaffected pre-embryos to be selected for transfer and affected pre-embryos to be 'discarded'. Thus, a choice has to be made to abort an affected foetus (after PND) or to discard a similarly affected but not-yet-transferred pre-embryo (after PGD).[13] Preference (or probably it is better to speak of 'less dislike') of both potential users and clinic staff for one or the other was related to people's moral views about the status of the pre-embryo and foetus (cf. De Wert, 2003). In addition, parents might emotionally prefer 'to terminate an eight-cell embryo' than a three-month old foetus (cf. Franklin and Roberts 2006: 157).[14] Moreover, as we saw in the case of Mr and Mrs P, couples may – based on their own experiences with a certain disease – have their own ideas about whether living with a certain condition is bearable or not (which may differ from the staff's view), and based on this view be unwilling to have any test performed.

While the Catholic roots of the Radboud Clinic does not prevent the clinic from performing IVF, the clinic's restricted policy on induced abortion (that is, not on social indications, but only in cases of existential or other emergencies) results in the clinic staff's inclination to prefer PGD over PND. In the words of one of the doctors: 'We cannot really speak of an emergency abortion if we know *beforehand* that there is a 25 per cent chance that our treatment will lead to an abortion'. Subsequently, some couples were advised to do PGD, for which they had to be referred to the academic hospital in Maastricht, as this was the only Dutch clinic allowed to conduct PGD (as part of a clinical trial) at that time.

While in some cases the testing options resolved the question of access to treatment, for two couples this was not the case. These couples, who were carriers of cystic fibrosis, a serious genetic disease indicated for PGD, could not be screened at the Maastricht hospital as they both would have had to make use of IVF with PESA (Percutaneous Epididymal Sperm Aspiration). PESA is a procedure used in extreme cases of male infertility that at the time of the study in the Netherlands could also only be offered as part of a clinical trial (among others, at the Radboud Clinic). As combining two treatments that were both part of clinical trials would disturb the outcomes of the trial, the Maastricht Hospital rejected these two couples for PGD. The Radboud Clinic staff maintained their position and did not offer the IVF-PESA treatment without PGD. Yet they informed the couples about the possibility of combining PESA and PGD in Belgium (as both procedures were allowed at that time in Belgium), and about the possibility of combining PESA and PND in two other fertility clinics in the Netherlands. Both couples themselves also preferred PGD to PND – for emotional reasons – and therefore opted for IVF-PESA and PGD in Belgium, even though this meant that they had to travel cross-border, and that they would have to pay for the entirety of the treatment themselves. Clearly, here, Dutch legislation and the clinic's ethical stances affected the clinic staff's decisions on access to treatment.

Summarizing the obstacles to testing discussed so far, we see that medical-technical solutions (PGD and PND) do exist to overcome concerns about the physical health of a future child. Yet PND confronted the interdisciplinary meetings with another dilemma related to the particular moral stance of the hospital (avoiding a non-emergency abortion), resulting in clinic staff advising couples to go for PGD, which in turn meant that they had to refer them to other hospitals where it could be done. Subsequently, we see that the implementation of this technical solution was impeded by two other constraining factors, namely government legislation regarding the experimental status of PGD and PESA treatments and a decision of the Maastricht hospital not to have their study results on PGD distorted.

In addition, financial obstacles also impeded a technical solution to ethical problems. For example, a financial obstacle emerged for a couple where the woman was a carrier of a serious genetic disease and who had in the past given birth to a child seriously affected with that particular disease. The couple was referred to the Maastricht hospital for IVF-PGD treatment. At that very moment, however, they were confronted with a (temporary) new government policy stating that people would have to pay for their first IVF treatment themselves; however, the couple were not able to bear these costs. They therefore returned to the Radboud Clinic with the request to do a low-tech, less expensive treatment (ovulation induction by means of hormonal treatment). When doing this low-tech treatment, however, PGD cannot be performed (as PGD has to be combined with IVF), meaning that the only option left for screening was PND. For this couple the clinic staff made an exception and allowed them access to treatment, although they knew that they intended to do a PND and that this may lead to an induced abortion. In this case, understanding and human compassion from the side of the medical professionals clearly played a role in resolving an ethically complex situation (when a technological solution was hampered by financial constraints) and even overruled the clinic's principle to avoid induced abortion other than in the case of an emergency.

Referral to Other Clinics

Informing couples about treatment options that were not offered in the Radboud Clinic, and referring them to other hospitals, was another practice that was sometimes employed to resolve ethical concerns. Above we have seen that some people were referred to do IVF with PGD-PESA or PND-PESA in another Dutch clinic or in Belgium. In addition, some couples – where the man or the woman was the carrier of a genetic disease – were advised to use donor gametes to avoid transferring the disease to the future child. However, as the Radboud Clinic did not work at all with donor gametes at the time the study took place, this would have required these couples to go to another fertility clinic.[15]

Searching Scientific Evidence

Searching scientific evidence in the literature is another practice the Radboud Clinic staff used to support decisions in ethically problematic cases, perfectly fitting with current-day evidence-based medicine ideals. In the period the study took place scientific evidence was sought for couples involving elderly men and for cases where one of the partners suffered from severe mental problems.

As previously mentioned, clinic staff members conducted and published a literature review to assess the possible risks of elderly men taking part in fertility treatment (Römkens et al. 2005). The main question addressed in this article is the same as posed during the multi-disciplinary ethics meetings: what are the potential physical and psycho-social risks for a child that is conceived by and grows up with an elderly father?[16] Though none of the reviewed studies focused explicitly on children conceived through ARTs, it was concluded that the risks for children conceived by and/or growing up with an elderly father were very limited, and could not be reason alone to withhold fertility treatment. The authors, however, emphasized that this did not automatically imply that all elderly men should immediately gain access to treatment; medical professionals might still judge otherwise in particular cases if they could foresee serious harm to the future child. In the period when I conducted my study, none of the elderly prospective fathers, ranging from sixty-four to sixty-nine, were denied access to fertility treatment for this reason. Regarding couples where one of the partners suffered from severe mental/psychiatric problems, the clinical psychologist searched for scientific information about the chances of and conditions under which a relapse of that particular condition may occur, and about the impact that parents with the particular condition might have on the well-being of their children. As the consulted literature did not provide any substantial or specific information, no conclusions could be drawn. Thus in all situations in which mental problems were involved, the advice obtained from collegial consultation was of primary importance.

Moreover, in the period the study took place Dutch researchers (not based at the Radboud Clinic) published literature reviews to gain insight into the psycho-social development of children living in single-parent or lesbian families (Bolt et al. 2004; Hunfeld et al. 2004). The first (Bolt et al. 2004) showed that in lesbian families the psycho-social development of children and the quality of parenting were not different from those in heterosexual two-parent families. The authors of the study argued that withholding fertility treatment from lesbian families on the assumption that this would not be in the best interests of the future child was not justified (ibid.: 75); in the second review, for single-parent families, no conclusions could be drawn due to lack of relevant studies. It was therefore concluded, 'that singles should not be excluded from IVF treatment but individually screened by a psychosocial expert' (Hunfeld et al. 2004: 287). The results of these studies formed an impetus for the Radboud Clinic to change their access policy towards lesbian couples.

Getting Additional Medical Information

Often, the couples were still undergoing examinations at the moment when their situation was first presented in the inter-disciplinary ethics meetings and therefore not all relevant medical information was yet available. When the results of these examinations became known, a few couples could not continue further treatment because the results showed conditions that were too unfavourable for conception. In these cases, medical findings overruled the ethical questions before they were 'resolved' (even though for some of the couples the decision on ethical grounds might have been a negative one). It was apparent that the medical professionals sometimes felt relieved that they did not have to make a decision on ethical grounds, making remarks such as: 'Nature [or God] was with us!' This type of relief was particularly expressed when there was more than one concern at stake, yet each one in itself was not serious enough to deny access to treatment; in these situations, clinic staff felt uneasy and uncertain. The previously mentioned couple (where the man was sixty-eight) is an example of this: aside from the prospective father being elderly, he also suffered from a genetic disease (though not a life-threatening one); both the man and the woman had life histories full of severe psychiatric problems (though the woman's psychiatrist did not advise against fertility treatment); and they did not live together at one address for financial reasons (they were in a long-term relationship, but they did not fit the formal Radboud criterion of a stable relationship).

Mirroring Concerns

During the multi-disciplinary ethics meetings, the question, 'What does the couple think or feel about it?' was regularly posed. In addition, the attending medical doctor was at times explicitly requested to mirror the staff's concerns to the couple, to gain insight into the couple's views. This mirroring seemed to serve two purposes.

Firstly, mirroring such concerns enabled doctors to check if the couples were well informed about and aware of the possible risks or implications for the future child. When couples demonstrated that they were indeed well informed, and in particular when they seemed to be 'sensible, well intentioned' people it became easier for clinic staff to respect their autonomy and to leave the decision-making to the prospective parents.[17] The importance of couples being 'sensible, well intentioned' people was repeatedly referred to; however, in the period when I conducted fieldwork the staff never explicitly defined or discussed the meaning of this expression and it was left to the attending doctor to decide whether this 'criterion' was met. Overall, it seems to refer to the capability of parents not only to – obsessively – think of their own wish for a child, but also to consider the future child's well-being. In particular with regard to some genetic diseases, the prospective parents' views were deemed important, especially when one of the partners knew what it meant to live with the disease (as we saw in the case of Mr and Mrs P). A few times doctors in the ethics meetings mentioned that later on children may feel that it would have been better not to have been conceived, and may claim 'wrongful life'. To date in the Netherlands no jurisprudence regarding wrongful life claims from children conceived by medically assisted procreation exist and fear of wrongful life claims did not (yet) guide the Radboud Clinic staff's decisions. Still, it was occasionally referred to as one more reason to fully inform prospective parents about possible implications.

A situation in which mirroring concerns to check the sensibility of the prospective parents was crucial was the case of a young woman who suffered from cancer at the moment she requested medically assisted conception. The woman had to undergo chemotherapy and wanted to do part of an IVF treatment before starting the cancer treatment, in order not to lose the opportunity to get pregnant later in her life (at that time freezing ova was not yet possible). Instead of immediately transferring the fresh embryos into her uterus, she wanted all embryos to be frozen for later use (cryopreservation) when she would be fully recovered from her illness. The woman had requested that her boyfriend – whom she had only known for half a year – provide the sperm, and he agreed. While this couple thus did not fulfil the clinic's criteria for a stable relationship, after some serious talks – that is mirroring concerns – with both the woman and her boyfriend separately, the doctor concluded that they were both 'sensible people' and that the young man was well informed. For these reasons they were granted access to IVF. The clinic staff felt it would not be fair for her to risk losing the opportunity to conceive for the rest of her life because they had strictly applied the clinic requirement of being in a relationship for a minimum of one year.

A second purpose of mirroring concerns was that health professionals sometimes hoped that by expressing their concerns, the couple would become more conscious of potential problems and subsequently might decide to refrain from treatment. This intention in particular seemed to play a role in more complex situations, for example when one or more concerns were at stake at the same time (each in itself not big enough to withhold treatment) or in combination with a non-favourable medical situation.

In a number of situations the medical doctor reported having satisfactorily mirrored the staff concerns to couples, achieving one or both of the above-mentioned purposes. In some other situations, however, medical staff reported being dissatisfied about their efforts to mirror their concerns (in a few cases they felt that language barriers complicated a thorough communication of ideas about complex medical and ethical issues). Two couples did not return after a first or second visit to the clinic, which included a couple of which both partners were mentally disabled and it might be that they felt discouraged by the questions raised by clinic staff.

Subjective Values

Bolt et al. (2004) found that many a time, when making judgements about access to fertility treatments, doctors in Dutch fertility clinics would base such decisions on intuition and past clinical experience; in other words, they were guided by what they personally thought was right. While the Radboud Clinic had developed a set of practices – namely in the form of the inter-disciplinary meetings – to handle and decide on ethically sensitive situations, in order to avoid individual doctors making overly subjective and arbitrary decisions, clinic staff's personal values and viewpoints still played a role. Personal viewpoints expressed in the meeting varied from outspoken sympathy and understanding for a couple's request for medically assisted conception to – a few times – candid irritation and disagreement. Thus while the inter-disciplinary ethics meetings served in a way to control the impact of these personal values on decision-making, such values still definitely – and probably unavoidably – interacted with the way ethical problems were defined and resolved.

We saw this, for example, in the situation described above of the couple referred to the Maastricht hospital for IVF-PGD, but who returned to the Radboud Clinic to do low-tech treatment (and PND) because they were not able to pay for the first round of treatment themselves. The couple's distressing situation definitely played a role in this. At a young age the woman had delivered a child affected with a serious genetic disease and she was sterilized immediately after the delivery of her second child (this had probably occurred under pressure from her family). Attempts to undo the sterilization had not been successful and in the end she and her husband had been caught out by the new health insurance policy, as they could not afford the first IVF.[18] Based on this personal history, clinic staff argued that if this woman was to become pregnant through low-tech treatment and if by means of PND she found out that she was pregnant with an affected child, her possible subsequent decision to induce an abortion would be understandable and acceptable. The inter-disciplinary ethics meeting therefore agreed to allow her and her partner access to treatment, in the hope that the woman would give birth to a healthy child. At the same time, the doctor in charge of the couple put in a request to their health insurance to make an exception in their case and pay for their first IVF-PGD, as PGD remained a priority above PND. Here we clearly see that understanding and sympathy for the couple's situation overruled a major ethical concern of the clinic, namely to do the utmost to avoid an induced abortion. Likewise, in the case discussed above, of the young woman who suffered from cancer at the moment she requested medically assisted conception, we saw that another hospital criterion was bypassed.

While in this latter situation compassion for the woman's request made clinic staff flexible in the application of the clinic criterion for a stable relationship, in another case they were not at all inclined to be flexible on this point. This concerned the situation of a man who had undergone an IVF-ICSI treatment with his former wife using his sperm (that had been frozen several years ago before the man had undergone cancer treatment). His wife had become pregnant and delivered a child, but one month after the delivery of the baby he had left his wife and they divorced. Now he had returned to the clinic with his new partner – whom he had known for half a year – with the request to use his remaining frozen sperm. Some of the clinic staff became irritated when confronted with this request (they apparently had a different view on what responsible parenthood entailed) and one of them commented that it was 'as if it is simply about fetching another roll from the bakery'. In this case they decided to be strict about the one year relationship criterion and some of them seemed almost relieved when further medical examinations revealed that the woman's condition (an extremely high FSH level) did not justify IVF treatment.

These examples clearly show that the individual subjective values of clinic staff did affect which cases were presented in the inter-disciplinary meeting, the way they were spoken about and dealt with, but not really the decisions made. Feelings of sympathy for a couple's situation – which were more easily induced when doctors and couples shared ideas about the wish for a child and responsible parenthood or relationships – to an extent opened up the clinic's ethical boundaries, and the space that clinic rules allowed for ambiguity was then used in favour of the couples. In cases where clinic staff were less understanding towards a couple's request, clinic criteria seem to be applied somewhat strictly. Yet (as we saw previously in this chapter), even when clinic staff did not really understand or agree with a couple's request, the professional principle of patient autonomy was still applied as long there were no hard grounds upon which to deny access to treatment. At times, however, clinic staff expressed some form of relief if people in these ambiguous situations could not be treated on medical grounds or when people withdrew from treatment after the clinic staff had mirrored their concerns.

Conclusion

In this chapter I have shown that concerns expressed by clinic staff about couples requesting medically assisted procreation who were living with certain (physical) conditions or in particular social situations, resulted from the specific context in which these requests took place and that in some cases the Radboud Clinic had a more restricted policy and practice than governmental legislation prescribes. By looking at 'bioethics in practice' at a series of multi-disciplinary ethics meetings, this chapter has provided insight into the complex and dynamic interplay between particular couples' situations, contextual features, bioethical principles, the employ-ment of various clinical practices and doctors' subjective feelings and views.

We have seen that the multi-disciplinary ethics meetings provided a space for clinic staff to express and reflect on their personal views and feelings of unease regarding certain requests for fertility treat-ments, while at the same time diminishing the risk that decision-making was (too heavily) shaped by these feelings and views. While Bolt et al. (2004) report that doctors in Dutch fertility clinics often based their decisions about access to fertility treatments on intuition and past experience, this study suggests that while personal feelings and subjective views to a certain extent inform the agenda of the multi-disciplinary ethics meetings, in the end these personal views did not determine the final decision taken in these cases.

The ethics meetings seem to function as a space where staff members can (freely) express and reflect on their personal feelings, thoughts and doubts. By discussing the cases they were concerned about, clinic staff were constantly exploring the boundaries of what they considered ethically acceptable. They became more conscious of their personal views and related values, which helped them to better position themselves towards couples' requests. In addition, I contend, staff members were constantly reassessing their own values and norms – which are socioculturally constructed – regarding what is acceptable and not acceptable in the field of reproductive medi-cine. By doing so, they were involved in the creation of new medical culture: a decision taken about a certain ethically sensitive case (and the way they reflected on this decision afterwards) thus became part of the staff's shared experiences and practices and influenced the way they would address a similar case in the future. The exact role the multi-disciplinary ethics meeting plays in the creation of medical culture is a theme that certainly needs further exploration.

Examining real-life cases of which many details are known, as I did in this chapter, shows that it was exactly the particularities of couples' situations and experiences (that are unknown in studies that presented only hypothetical cases to clinic staff)[19] *and* the way they reflected on their own situation that seemed to convince clinic staff to place couple's autonomy above their own discomfort. The obser-vations of the meetings revealed that neither staff's subjective views, nor bioethics principles, fully determined the decisions made. An important new insight emerging from my observations of the prac-tices at these meetings is that clinic staff members, when confronted with particularly complicated cases, employ a number of routine medical practices with the intention of carefully resolving the concerns they are confronted with. These practices are typical doctors' ways of resolving clinical problems, including: collegial consultation; searching for scientific evidence in the literature; obtaining more medical information; offering medical tests and screening; referring couples to other clinics; and ensuring informed consent. In the midst of bioethical uncertainty, these medical practices provide the staff with a sense of control over the issues at stake. Rather than examining hypothetical cases, which evoke principles, observations of practice in sites of interaction between clinic staff over time in a series of multi-disciplinary ethics committees has allowed the identification of the influence of routine medical practice on ethical decisions.

To what extent was couples' reproductive autonomy at the Radboud Clinic jeopardized? Who, then, finally decided on the solution to ethically sensitive issues? We have seen that in several cases risks (physical or psycho-social for the future child or for the prospective parents) could not be predicted with a degree of certainty that justified withholding access to fertility treatment (cf. Bateman 2001). When the consulted colleagues or scientific literature were not overly negative about possible future risks, or when they could not make a 'hard enough' prediction to justify withholding access to treatment, the principle of patient autonomy received more weight in the decision-making process. In these cases, it was left to the couples themselves to decide whether they wanted to take a certain risk or not, as long as they showed that they were 'sensible people' and the criteria for informed consent were fulfilled. Thus, in these cases the principle of patient autonomy preceded health professionals' authority or responsibility. Only in a few cases (four out of twenty-nine) did health professionals' authority take precedence over couples' reproductive autonomy, and the doctors decided to withhold treatment in their clinic on ethical grounds. Thus, despite initial concerns from the side of the medical professionals (some of which might be regarded as paternalistic), the reproductive autonomy of most couples seeking ART was not jeopardized and they could decide for themselves whether or not to start treatment.

Notes

This chapter was reprinted from *Social Science and Medicine* 98, T. Gerrits, R. Reis, D. M. Braat, J. A. M. Kremer and A. P. Hardon, 2013, 'Bioethics in practice: Addressing ethically sensitive requests in a Dutch fertility clinic', pages 330–39, Copyright 2013, with permission from Elsevier.

1. This Special Issue of *Culture, Medicine and Psychiatry* (30(4), 2006) is devoted to 'Sacred Conceptions: Religion and the Global Practice of IVF'. The articles in this Special Issue examine how religious people around the world – Muslim, Hindu, Orthodox Jew, Greek Orthodox and Catholic – negotiate 'technologies and modalities of conceptions' (Bharadwaj 2006: 423). Thompson (2006: 557) summarizes the various functions religion takes in the papers in this issue as follows: 'as a means for patients and practitioners to navigate technical procedures, helping doctors and patients to accept that the procedures sometimes don't work, appreciate the grounds on which such procedures might be permitted, and understand how technically assisted reproduction can sometimes be capable of reconstituting kin and nation'. In addition, as Layne suggests, the papers illuminate 'differences between orthodox dictates and lived experience' (2006: 537).

2. Several studies have dealt with this question (see, e.g., Apoola et al. 2001; Stern et al. 2002, 2003; Bolt et al. 2004; Hunfeld et al. 2004; Maheshwari et al. 2008; De Geyter et al. 2010). These studies show the variety of criteria that are taken into account when doctors judge the eligibility of prospective parents' use of ARTs, including the upper age limit (for women and sometimes for men as well), marital status, sexual preference, substance abuse, psychiatric history or a history of violence, being a carrier of serious genetic diseases and/or being HIV-positive. However, none of these studies gave insight into how these criteria are actually applied in daily practice, which is the focus of the current chapter.

3. Notes are jotted down in the medical dossier of the patient concerned. No minutes are taken and therefore no file of ethical cases discussed is available. The current review is the first systematic overview of cases discussed at the clinic's inter-disciplinary ethics meetings.

4. During the period in which the study was conducted, the Radboud Clinic did not make use of donor gametes or embryos, thus ethical dilemmas resulting from donation and surrogacy were not discussed.

5. To protect the privacy of the couple I do not mention the exact name of the disease and some other data have been slightly changed.

6. The clinic's policy is to only perform terminations on an 'emergency' basis, and it is questionable here whether this would be considered to be one.

7. It should be noted that in some cases prospective parents shared (part of) the concerns with clinic staff.

8. The Catholic Church condemns IVF for two reasons, namely because it involves the destruction of embryos and because by means of ARTs 'humans are technologically interfering with a process that should remain under God's dominion' (Ratzinger 1987 in Roberts 2006: 507).

9. Reflecting on her own study in the USA, Thompson (2006: 560) also states that staff and patients hardly made any explicit appeals to religion (even while most of her respondents claimed religious affiliation). Still, she refers to some instances in which patients made (more or less implicit) appeals to religion reflecting that 'religion is alive and well here, too'. One of the couples in this study (members of an orthodox Protestant Church) whose case was discussed in the ethics meeting at the Radboud Clinic (included in the category 'Other') was firmly against discarding embryos and therefore only wanted to fertilize a very limited number of ova. The doctor attending this couple had presented the couple at the ethics meeting as she questioned whether it was justifiable (medically speaking) to let a woman undergo an intensive IVF treatment, while diminishing her chances of success to such an extent. In addition, among the study participants I followed over a longer period, I came – a very few times – across appeals to (moral) values that could be related to religious beliefs as well.

10. Potential carriers here means that the gene is present in the family of the man and/or the woman requesting medical assistance, though they have not (yet) been and/or do not want to be tested themselves.

11. In a similar vein Rapp (1999), in her seminal book about amniocentesis, discusses the way that the testing leads to 'a cascade of statistically expressed possibilities which the pregnant woman and her supporters must assess' (ibid.: 73), which they find extremely difficult. She also argues that all diagnosis appear to be ambiguous, both for the pregnant women and 'inside of biomedicine' (ibid.: 188).

12. This is one of the couples belonging to the category 'Other'.

13. Rapp (1999: 130–34) discusses why women are often ambivalent about doing a selective abortion. First, she contends that many of the women she spoke with did not have problems with abortion in itself (and some even had had an abortion previously), but with the fact that they had to give up a *desired* pregnancy and that they realized that they had to go through some form of labour. Further, deciding about selective abortion forced the women to rethink their view about disability – 'to act as a moral philosopher' – and assess their own role as mother of a disabled child. Finally, most women knew a child that was affected with retardation, mostly a child with Down syndrome. They often felt that the child had a reasonable live; yet the price was paid by the relatives. These experiences and insights also affected their thoughts.

14. However, choosing PGD does not necessarily exclude PND. Franklin and Roberts (2006: 158) describe how in the clinic where they conducted their study couples were offered PND after a pregnancy was established (by means of IVF and PGD) to ensure that the genetic diagnosis was accurately done. For the couples concerned, the thought of endangering their pregnancy was absolutely 'unattractive', the

authors write, as they opted for PGD exactly to avoid such a 'tentative pregnancy' (Rothman 1986).

15. To my knowledge none of the couples followed up this latter suggestion.

16. Becker (2000: 146) remarks that in her study context – the USA – the question whether a man who becomes a father at on older age will live long enough to educate the child through childhood is rarely asked. She suggests that this may reflect the persistent cultural assumption that women are primarily responsible for child rearing. The fact that this question is asked in the Radboud Clinic may reflect a changing view of the role of fathers in child rearing in Dutch society (Jacobs 1998).

17. As this chapter is only based on observations of the ethics meetings and conversations with staff members and not on observations between staff and couples I cannot indicate on what grounds the attending doctor determined that men and women were 'well informed', 'sensible' or well intended'.

18. The Radboud Clinic lobbied against this newly introduced treatment policy.

19. Studies that presented hypothetical 'ethical sensitive' cases to clinic staff are, for example, Bolt et al. (2004) and Stern et al. (2003).

References

Apoola, A., J. Tenhof and P.S. Allan. 2001. 'Access to infertility investigations and treatment in couples infected with HIV: questionnaire survey', *British Medical Journal* 323: 1285.

Bharadwaj, A. 2006. 'Sacred conceptions: clinical theodicies, uncertain science, and technologies of procreation in India', *Culture, Medicine and Psychiatry*, 30(4), 451–465.

Bateman, S. 2001. 'When reproductive freedom encounters medical responsibility: Changing conceptions of reproductive choice', in E. Vayenna, P.J. Rowe and P.D. Griffin (eds), *Current Practices and Controversies in Assisted Reproduction: Report of a WHO Meeting*. Geneva, Switzerland: WHO, pp. 320–32.

Becker, G. 2000. *The Elusive Embryo: How women and men approach new reproductive technologies*. Berkeley: University of California Press

Beauchamp, T. and J. Childress. 1994. 'The four principles', in R. Gillon (ed.) *Principles of Health Care Ethics*. New York: John Wiley, pp. 3–12.

Bharadwaj, A. 2002. 'Conception Politics: Medical egos, media spotlights and the contest over test-tube firsts in India', in M.C. Inhorn, and F. Van Balen (eds), *Infertility around the Globe: New thinking on childlessness, gender and reproductive technology*. Berkeley: University of California Press, pp. 315–33.

Bolt, L.L.E., M.A.J.M. Buijsen and J.A.M. Hunfeld. 2004. *Morele contra-indicaties voor ouderschap? Een psychologisch, ethisch en juridisch onderzoek naar de selectie van hulpvragers voor een IVF-behandeling.* Ethiek and Beleid NWO. Budel: Uitgeverij Damon.

De Geyter, C., B. Boehler and S. Reiter-Theiler. 2010. 'Differences and similarities in the attitudes of paediatricians, gynaecologists and experienced parents to criteria delineating potential risks for the welfare of the children to be conceived with assisted reproduction', *Swiss Medical Weekly* 140 (w13064): E1–E8.

De Wert, G.M.W.R. 2003. 'Handelingen met geslachscellen en embryos', *Signalering: Ethiek en Gezondheid.* The Hague: Gezondheidsraad.

Franklin, S. and C. Roberts. 2006. *Born and Made: An ethnography of preimplantation genetic diagnosis.* Princeton: Princeton University Press.

Gerrits, T., R. Reis, D. M. Braat, J. A. M. Kremer and A. P. Hardon. 2013. 'Bioethics in practice: Addressing ethically sensitive requests in a Dutch fertility clinic.' *Social Science and Medicine* 98: 330–39.

Gezondheidsraad. 1997. *Het Planningsbesluit.* Publicatienummer 1997/03. The Hague: Gezondheidsraad.

Heesterbeek, S. and H. Ten Have. 2001. 'Het normatieve spanningsveld tussen autonomie en paternalisme', in S. de Joode (ed.), *Zwanger van de kinderwens: Visies, feiten en vragen over voortplantingstechnologie.* The Hague: Rathenau Instituut, pp. 138–54.

Hoffmaster, B. 1992. 'Can ethnography save the life of medical ethics?', *Social Science and Medicine* 35(12): 1421–31.

Hunfeld, J.A.M., J. Passchier, L.L.E. Bolt and M.A.J.M. Buijsen. 2004. 'Protect the child from being born: Arguments against IVF from heads of the 13 licensed Dutch fertility centres, ethical and legal perspectives', *Journal of Reproductive and Infant Psychology* 22(4): 279–89.

Inhorn, M.C. and D. Birenbaum-Carmeli. 2008. 'Assisted reproductive technologies and culture change', *Annual Review of Anthropology* 37: 177–96.

Jacobs, M.J.G. 1998. *Vaders in spe: over de kinderwens van mannen en hun voorstelling van het vaderschap.* Amsterdam: Swets and Zeitlinger.

Jones, H.W. and J. Cohen. 2004. 'IFFS Surveillance 04', *Fertility and Sterility* 81(5), Suppl. 4: S1–S54.

Kleinman, A. 1995. *Writing at the Margin: Discourse between anthropology and medicine.* Berkeley: University of California Press.

Modelreglement Embryowet. 2003. *Modelreglement Embryowet.* Utrecht: Kwaliteitsinstituut voor de Gezondheidszorg CBO.

Maheshwari, A., M. Hamilton and S. Bhattacharya. 2008. 'A survey of clinicians' view on age and access to IVF and the use of tests of ovarian reserve prior to IVF in the United Kingdom', *Human Fertility* 11(1): 23–27.

Muller, J.H. 1994. 'Anthropology, bioethics and medicine: A provocative trilogy', *Medical Anthropological Quarterly* 8(4): 448–67.

Patel, J.C. and M.H. Johnson. 1998. 'A survey of the effectiveness of the assessment of the welfare of the child in UK in-vitro fertilization units', *Human Reproduction* 13(3): 766–70.

Rapp, R. 1999. *Testing Women, Testing the Fetus. The social impact of Amniocentesis in America.* New York: Routledge.

Ratzinger, C.J.C. 1987. "Instruction on Respect for Human Life in its Origin and on the Dignity of Procreation", Congregation for the Doctrine of the Faith, the Feast of the Chair of St. Peter, the Apostle, February, 22.

Roberts, E.F. 2006. 'God's laboratory: Religious rationalities and modernity in Ecuadorian in vitro fertilization', *Culture, Medicine and Psychiatry* 30(4): 507–36.

Römkens, M., B. Gordijn, C.M. Verhaak, E.J.H. Meuleman en D.D.M. Braat. 2005. Geen onderbouwing voor maximale leeftijdsgrens voor mannen bij in-vitrofertilisatie of intracytoplasmatische sperma-injectie. *Nederlands Tijdschrift voor Geneeskunde* 149(18): 992–95.

Rothman, B. 1986. 'Reflections on hard work', *Qualitative Sociology* 9: 48–53.

Stern, J.E., Cramer, C.P., Garrod, A., and Green, R.M. 2002. 'Attitudes on access to services at assisted reproductive technology clinics: Comparisons with clinic policy', *Fertility and Sterility* 77(3): 537–41.

Stern, J.E., Cramer, C.P., Green, R.M., Garrod, A., and DeVries, K.O. 2003. 'Determining access to assisted reproductive technology: Reactions of clinic directors at ethically complex cases', *Human Reproduction* 18(6): 1343–52.

Thompson, C. 2005. *Making Parents: The ontological choreography of reproductive technologies.* Cambridge, MA: The MIT Press.

_____ 2006. 'God is in the details: Comparative perspectives on the intertwining of religion and assisted reproductive technologies', *Culture, Medicine and Psychiatry* 30(4): 557–61.

CONCLUSION

This book began with the words of a Dutch couple in the midst of their fertility treatment, reflecting on the inclination of infertile people to shift their boundaries – in terms of what they would be prepared to do and how far they would go – once they enter the biomedical domain. I set out to understand what makes many infertile couples so willing and even eager to continue treatment, despite the many drawbacks of ARTs; a question that has interested several social scientists before me. In particular, I intended to examine how – in a context where ARTs are highly regulated and in a clinic that is strongly geared towards offering high quality and empowering patient-centred care – ARTs are offered in actual daily clinic practices, and how this form of medicine co-shapes the experiences, views and decisions of the women and men using these technologies. Throughout the book, I have portrayed several aspects of the quest of infertile couples in the Netherlands to have 'a child of their own', zooming in from the macro level of the situation of Dutch IVF, through the mid level of the daily clinical practices at the Radboud Clinic, to the micro level of the women and men visiting the clinic: their experiences, hopes, views and pains. After delving into these aspects in depth in the preceding pages, in this final chapter I intend to wrap up the key findings and arguments of the book, and present some after-thoughts and reflections about the future of IVF services in the Netherlands and internationally.

Dutch IVF

The most notable feature of Dutch IVF is perhaps its emphasis on 'equality': in principle, all Dutch people with fertility problems from all socioeconomic classes have equal access to IVF and do not have to endure any financial hurdles (up to three IVF treatments per child). Dutch ART policies do not 'stratify reproduction' on economic grounds, as has been noted in several other countries worldwide.[1] However, the 2013 change in health insurance coverage – whereby IVF for women over the age of forty-three is no longer paid for – might be considered discriminatory against older women.

The equality principle goes beyond socioeconomic class: in the Netherlands, ARTs are theoretically equally accessible and financed for women and men in all sorts of family situations and relationships, including unmarried and lesbian couples and single women. This reflects the dominant – though not unanimous – acceptance of non-traditional relationships and families in present day 'progressive' Dutch society. In practice, however, only a limited number of Dutch clinics do actually offer fertility treatments using donor material (which lesbian couples and single women need). Treatment for lesbian and single women has become even more complicated since identifiable gamete donation was made mandatory in 2004, which had the effect of further limiting the availability of donor material, and additionally some clinics privilege heterosexual couples in need of donor material above lesbian and single women. The Dutch government allows such privileging practices as long as there are other clinics in the country where lesbians and singles can access treatment, a situation that – understandably – is highly contested by the groups concerned.[2] Such practices show partiality towards traditional (heterosexual) family models and can be seen as a form of 'stratified reproduction'.

Another core feature of Dutch IVF is its non-profit character: the number of clinics licensed to offer ARTs is highly restricted and all of them (with the exception of one) are situated in public hospitals. In the Netherlands, IVF is thus not a privatized and competitive 'industry' geared towards making maximum profit (in strong contrast to many places worldwide, including the USA). The non-profit basis of Dutch fertility clinics, in combination with mandatory transparency about clinic success rates, thwarts the practice of attracting – and exploiting – infertile women and men by means of vague or manipulated success rates. Commercialization of third-party involvement in conception is also strictly prohibited, and this certainly prevents the exploitation of donors and surrogates. However, it further increases the shortage of donor material and leads to cross-border reproductive tourism to countries with less restrictive policies, shorter waiting lists and/or more donor material and surrogates available (Pennings et al. 2009; Gürtin and Inhorn 2011).[3] This may lead to unethical and undesired practices, in particular the exploitation of third parties in resource-poor countries, where ARTs are often less regulated and strongly commercialized. Maintaining 'high ethics' in the Netherlands may thus lead to the involvement of Dutch citizens in non-ethical practices abroad. In an ever more globalizing world, this leads to new ethical dilemmas and a situation of transnational 'stratified reproduction' that cannot be resolved at the national level.

Dutch ART policies, while enabling the use of ARTs to a large extent, also set a number of strict boundaries based on medical-technical, cost-efficiency, ethical and/or juridical considerations. The Netherlands is internationally known for its restrictive ART policies: not all technologically possible treatments are allowed and made readily available. In addition, the professional organization NVOG has stipulated 'restrictive' medical measures, which aim to increase cost-efficiency and decrease the risks and burden of treatment for the women involved. Such restrictive measures may, in a way, be considered as 'de-medicalizing', since they intend to postpone the actual medicalization of fertility problems in some cases or diminish the intensity of medicalization. Clinic staff at the Radboud Clinic seemed to adhere fairly strictly to these measures; the 'expectative policy', for example, was fairly strictly applied, and when one IVF cycle gave poor results, couples were not allowed to start another. The willingness to accept such limitations, from the side of both staff and users, in part reflects a tendency in Dutch society not to over-medicalize bodily problems (doctor visits and medication use are low compared to neighbouring countries) and to base medical regimes on efficacy and efficiency (De Vries 2003). The typical Dutch birth system, through which one-third of deliveries take place in people's homes (which is unique in the Western world), is another example illustrating the tendency to not necessarily pursue all available medical technologies. On the other hand, and despite the restrictive policies and measures, it is a fact that the total number of IVF cycles in the Netherlands is increasing on a yearly basis. This increase might be related to a growing number of people confronted with fertility problems (due to the postponement of childbearing to a later age) and to the continuously expanding treatment options. The technical imperative is hard to resist.

Finally, while in principle ARTs are accessible to all, on an individual basis some people may be excluded, for instance in case of serious concerns about the well-being of the potential future child. There is a general professional protocol instructing infertility clinic staff on how to handle requests for assisted procreation that are considered 'sensitive', emphasizing that clinics and doctors should be extremely cautious when making such judgments and avoid basing them on (often) highly subjective opinions (NVOG 2010). The protocol indicates that decisions should be taken in multi-disciplinary meetings, and gives instructions about the process of decision-making. However, the protocol does not prescribe moral views and leaves space for (individual) considerations, which are likely to vary between clinics as well as staff members. The avoidance of imposing a top-down moralistic standpoint has been referred to as a typical feature of Dutch health care (De Vries 2003). While not everyone may agree with the outcome of ethical deliberations in particular situations, Dutch ART policy and the system of multi-disciplinary deliberation does avoid the systematic exclusion from treatment of certain categories of people. Health professionals' responsibility for the well-being of the future child are recognized (as they are involved in the creation of the child); yet the principle of autonomy of the women and men in treatment forms the starting point of the ethical deliberations.

Bioethics in Practice

Clinical practices at the Radboud Clinic are definitely not without boundaries (Braat 2000). With regard to medical-ethical issues, I have shown that the Radboud Clinic (with its roots in a Catholic community) was, at the time of my research, in some aspects more restrictive than national policy. The clinic did not make use of donor semen, based on the principle that for the well-being of a child it is important to know the identity of both parents, and that ideally the child should grow up with both parents. This principle – which was said to be founded on psychological insights rather than moral considerations (Hunfeld et al. 2004) – implied that lesbian couples and single women did not have access to treatment at the Radboud Clinic (this policy partly changed in 2008, based on more recent scientific insights). The clinic also deviated from national policy as a result of its moral attitude towards induced abortion, which was allowed only in 'emergency' cases. This had implications for the way in which the requests of couples with genetic diseases were addressed.

In most of the cases discussed at the clinic's inter-disciplinary ethics meetings, the principle of 'patient autonomy' overruled staff's concerns or health professionals' authority or responsibility. This was particularly so when the consulted health professionals or scientific evidence were not overly negative about possible future risks, or when it was impossible to make a 'hard enough' prediction to justify withholding treatment. In these cases, it was left to the couples themselves to decide whether they wanted to take a certain risk or not, as long as they could demonstrate that they were responsible people and the criteria for informed consent had been fulfilled.

Patient-Centred Practices

Highly Appreciated – A Good Example

Throughout the book, I have portrayed various aspects of the patient-centred practices of the Radboud Clinic. Overall, women and men visiting the clinic appreciated the way in which the fertility services were offered. They felt properly informed, prepared and supported to bear the burden of IVF treatment, and were pleased that clinic staff invested a lot of time in them and that they were not merely seen as a number. The couples partaking in the Digitale Poli experienced it as a valuable additional service, as it gave them unlimited access to their personal medical files and allowed them to communicate with staff and other women and men in treatment. Without a doubt, the support and empowerment achieved through such patient-centred practices increased – as intended – the ability of women and men to carefully consider the pros and cons of (further) treatment and make informed choices. This confirms the importance of the introduction of patient-centred practices in fertility clinics more generally, as has been observed by various scholars in the field. The patient-centred practices described in this book thus firmly illustrate that the Radboud Clinic has overcome the problems outlined by critics of the early days of IVF, whereby doctors were accused of purposively duping, misleading and/or pushing women (and men) in treatment to use ever more medical technologies.

The Radboud Clinic's patient-centred practices may even serve as an example of 'good practice' for other fertility clinics, both in and beyond the Netherlands. For me, as a Dutch citizen myself, I was not overly surprised by the clinic staff's transparency and straight-forwardness about potential risks and limited success rates (though I was struck by the doctors' explicit openness about the limitations of reproductive technologies and the many uncertainties they shared with couples). However, when presenting my research findings to international audiences, I became aware that such transparency is far from obvious for people coming from other countries, in particu-lar when IVF and related technologies in these countries are mainly or solely offered in private and commercial clinics (Hampshire and Simpson, 2015). Such transparency is, I believe, of prime impor-tance in order to enable informed consent, even when – as I have suggested – the concept of informed consent is in itself problem-atic when dealing with such complicated medical subjects and technologies.

Missed Opportunities

I have also pointed to 'missed opportunities' in the practice of patient-centred medicine, related to doctors' and couples' inclination to start and continue treatment. This inclination results from a combination of factors or processes, including the unspoken assumption that people come to the clinic to 'have their problem fixed', the insight that 'doctors are doers' and the 'imperative' of three IVF treatments. As a result, women and men are not always explicitly asked if they indeed want to start treatment and/or switch to another treatment type or cycle. Doctors, when I spoke with them about these 'missed opportunities', often recognized them and felt challenged to avoid them in the future; they felt, for instance, that it would be better to explicitly ask couples if they want to start treatment and/or go from one treatment to another.

I have, nevertheless, also questioned whether routinizing treat-ment might not be preferable – from the point of view of couples – to repeatedly asking them whether they want to go on, as they would not have to re-think their position each and every time. Routinized treatment might give couples more peace of mind, in particular as they (largely) place their trust in the doctors' judgement. Giving people in treatment more choice and a voice should therefore not be considered better per se, or better for all, as this may also add to the burden and responsibility that they experience, as has been argued elsewhere (see Mol 2006; Trappenburg 2008).

The Paradox of Patient-Centredness

Finally, in my analysis of the daily practices of the Radboud Clinic, I have revealed a paradox at the heart of the approach of patient-centredness. The amount of information and support provided; the intensive monitoring; the ongoing visualization of the process of conception mediated by medical technology and the Digitale Poli; the empathic treatment and support; the bonds created between doctors and couples; and the trust couples have in clinic staff, all strengthen lay people's 'medical gaze' and normalize the burdens of IVF. Couples come to trust in the fact that clinic staff will not allow them to do (further) treatments and bear the burden and risks of treatments if it were not responsible. The normalization of pain, the relativizing notion that it could always be worse, and the faith in and bonds with clinic staff may render couples more inclined to continue with treatment, even in the face of uncertain prognoses and/or significant corresponding physical and emotional toll. While patient-centred practices can definitely be seen as a significant improvement over previous clinical encounters infused with paternalism, they may also bias patient decision-making towards (further) medical treatment, a phenomenon that I have labelled 'the paradox of patient-centredness'. This paradox may seduce couples to pursue (further) treatments – and thus draw them onto the medical treadmill or make them more persistent in their use of medical treatment – despite clinic policy and doctors' firm disposition not to do so.

Patient-centred practices do not therefore provide an easy escape route, solving the problem of medicalization. On the contrary, and as Foucauldian scholars have argued (cf. Lupton 1997), providing lay people with more information and knowledge may actually increase their clinical gaze and intensify the medicalization of their condition, rather than the opposite. The analysis I have provided in this book illustrates well the point that these Foucauldian scholars have made. In particular, two of the dynamics of patient-centred practices as observed in the Radboud Clinic – the ever increasing number and quality of visualizing technologies and the trust-building between couples and staff – are especially important for understanding this potential paradoxical effect.

Regarding the former, the way in which IVF and related technologies split the process of conception into various stages, the way that outcomes are visualized and interpreted at each treatment step, and the meaning that these outcomes assume for couples in treatment may lead couples to be more inclined to do further treatments (cf. Sandelowski 1991, 1993). Couples' initiation into the medical understanding of bodily processes and medically assisted conception enables them to better follow and understand the outcomes of IVF treatments at the various treatment steps, which may make them more eager to do further treatments. Furthermore, various patient-centred practices, with their strong emphasis on the provision of information and interpretation of in-between steps, further increase this dynamic. For instance, the visualization of the process of conception, in particular of the embryo and embryo transfer, mediated by medical technology and the interpretations of staff – in the case of the Radboud Clinic, this includes making a picture of the transferred embryo available through the Digitale Poli – means that couples feel a sense of being 'close' to pregnancy. This increases their hopes and expectations, and having been 'so close', if and when the treatment fails it is hard for them to say no to the option of making one more attempt.

Uncertainty and Trust

Couples' decisions to pursue fertility treatment are at least partly based on feelings of trust in the judgement of the health professionals providing the treatment, even when abundant information is provided. Their trust in doctors is strengthened by doctors' transparency about the possible risks, limited success rates, and uncertainties involved in reproductive technologies. Franklin and Roberts (2006) found a similar pattern in their ethnographic study of PGD: openness about the many uncertainties of PGD technology among medical staff strengthened the feeling among potential users that they were in good hands. As mentioned before, these findings can be understood in light of the views of the philosopher O'Neill (quoted in Franklin and Roberts 2006: 203–4), who underlines the importance of providing layered and repeated information as an important step in trust-building, since it enables people to critically scrutinize the information provided. In a similar way, in the Radboud Clinic the feeling of trust experienced by several of the research participants may be induced by the intensive provision of information and committed interaction between staff and couples, where uncertainties and risks are not hidden but rather explicitly mentioned and explained.

This is not to say that being open about uncertainties is always valued in contemporary medicine. The positive assessment of the Radboud Clinic's openness by couples using ARTs may have much to do with the long-term relationships that are built up between couples and the clinic doctors, which may make it easier to discuss uncertainty (as suggested by Gordon et al. 2000). In addition, being open about uncertainty may be more positively evaluated in contexts where users are generally satisfied with other aspects of patient–staff interaction, as was strongly the case in the Radboud Clinic. Finally, for people who do not need to pay for their own treatments, it might be more acceptable to live with some uncertainty compared to people who have to invest their own (scarce) resources to attempt at least one IVF.[4]

The finding that couples' decisions to pursue fertility treatment are, at least in part, based on feelings of trust in the health professionals providing the treatment also points to a dilemma in the application or rather the meaning of the notion of 'informed consent' within contemporary biomedicine. The more complex biomedicine and biomedical technologies become, the more dependent lay people become on professionals who can interpret and translate the insights and findings (cf. De Joode and Fauser 2001). I see this as a major challenge for the future practice of patient-centred medicine. For now, I suggest that 'informed consent' should not be seen as the result of a purely rational and autonomous process of decision-making, based on a profound understanding and assessment of the information that professionals provide to women and men attending their clinic. In fact, it may be more realistic to speak about consent based on information and trust in the medical professional. Considering informed consent in this way underlines its relational and interactional aspects, and at the same time points to its potential perils, namely the possibility of abuse of this trust.

Gender Inequality and the Imperative of Genetics

Couples' accounts of the experienced burden of fertility treatment in the current study confirm accounts presented in ethnographic studies about this topic in other Western countries (see, e.g., Greil 1991; Sandelowski 1993; Franklin 1997; Becker 2000). Gender inequality with regard to the burdens of IVF definitely continues to exist. Marcia Inhorn (2003) has pointed to the increasing suffering of men with fertility problems, because their bodies have become more and more doctored (mainly as a result of new technologies such as PESA and TESE). In the current study, however, physically speaking it was still women who suffered more than men (and

both women and men agreed about this). Most men were nevertheless found to be intensively involved in the treatment process
and also mentally and emotionally affected by it, as well as by the
infertility problem itself. This certainly also applied to those men
confronted with a late miscarriage or the death of a prematurely
born child. I have suggested that in the case of male infertility, men
may feel more emotionally affected (see also Lechner et al. 2007).
In addition, I suggest that for Dutch men the psychological and
emotional impact of fertility treatments may also increase due to
changing gender role expectations; for many Dutch men, fatherhood is increasingly becoming an important part of their male
identity in which they want to invest time, energy and emotions,
at the expense of paid labour. However, to date, limited insights
into the meaning of male infertility in the Netherlands exist and
how this relates to current and changing notions of masculinity
and fatherhood. The topics and issues mentioned here definitely
deserve more scholarly attention. Marcia Inhorn's recent book on
'emerging masculinities' among Arab men confronted with infertility and ARTs may form a source of inspiration for such studies,
starting from the notion that 'manly selfhood is not a thing or a
constant; rather, it is an act that is ever in progress' (Inhorn 2012:
31).

Gender inequality with regard to the burdens of IVF have some
major implications. First, in my study it meant that (most) men
became overtly empathetic and supportive partners, with women
more ready to bear the burdens as long as their partner is supportive, involved and committed (cf. Greil 1991). The Radboud Clinic
strongly encourages men's involvement. The weight given to partner
involvement and communication both reflects and confirms Dutch
values about intimate relationships: men and women are expected
to communicate. Second, I found that women are prepared to bear
the heavy toll of treatment as it keeps alive the hope of having a child
that is genetically and biologically from them and their partner. This is
something that is both men's and women's preferred goal, and cannot
be achieved without IVF. For women and men, it is very important to
recognize traits of their partner in their child as a confirmation of the
conjugal bond. In case of male-factor infertility, they would rather opt
for a burdensome IVF-ICSI than for the less intrusive option of AID.
Despite the fact that in contemporary Dutch society many non-traditional family forms and relationships exist and are widely accepted,
and many children grow up in a blended or patchwork family, the
couples' (in this study) preference to have a child 'of the two of them'

points to the imperative of genetics and couples' preference to be part of a 'traditional family' (cf. Becker 2000).

Final Thoughts:
Implications for the Field and Future Research

The major contribution of this book is that it enhances our understanding of the persistence of couples with fertility problems in seeking medical help and in the process of medicalizing their fertility problems. I have further shown that a fertility clinic's patient-centred practices, aside from empowering and supporting couples, (may) also seduce them to pursue (further) treatment. What can such insights mean for the field of reproductive medicine?

First of all, it is important to mention that the persistence in help-seeking of couples with fertility problems – the fact that many find it hard to say no to further treatment – is a widely recognized phenomenon among health professionals and couples in treatment (and among the public in general). The insights put forward by this book may help to further sensitize health professionals and couples about this persistence and aid them to better understand how such persistence evolves. In particular, the 'paradox of patient-centeredness' may be a good concept 'to think with' (Green and Thorogood 2004: 197) and 'to talk with'; that is, to raise it as an issue in interactions among women and men visiting the clinic with fertility problems and doctors and staff when discussing further steps in treatment, in particular when couples express ambivalence about whether or not to continue. By no means do I intend to claim that medical practices should be less patient-centred in order to avoid the paradoxical effect of increasing lay people's medical gaze. Rather, I see the latter as an unavoidable side effect of patient-centred practices, which should be made explicit and talked about. In particular, I argue that patient-centred practices should not be viewed as solving the problem of ongoing medicalization.

Another interesting point worth highlighting is that despite the numerous studies that have been conducted looking at various aspects of infertility treatments, still very little is known about how fertility clinics actually provide their services. The research upon which this book is based is therefore unique in that it provides an in-depth account of the actual daily practices in a particular contemporary fertility clinic. While many studies have been conducted to measure women's and men's satisfaction with fertility

services offered, none of these studies give insight into actual practices, which makes it impossible to relate people's satisfaction levels
to the way in which practices are actually offered (Dancet et al.
2010). While I do not expect numerous hospital ethnographies to be
undertaken in other fertility clinics in the future (as this would be
too time-intensive), I would suggest that researchers who carry out
patient satisfaction studies could endeavour to provide more insight
into the particular clinical practices with which women and men are
(dis)satisfied. They could look at what sort of information is actually given, and at what moment. How much time do doctors and
couples spend together? How are privacy issues dealt with? While
Blonk et al. (2006) have taken patient satisfaction studies one step
further, by not only measuring people's satisfaction but also the perceived importance of the aspects of care they measure, a description
of actual practices would further enhance the value of such studies.

Previous (mainly quantitative) studies have looked at the reasons
why people with fertility problems do not pursue further treatment
or – as it is often put – what makes them 'drop out' of treatment.
These studies have the tendency to reduce the reasons for drop out
to one single factor. In this book, I have drawn attention to the complexity of reasons, considerations and circumstances of the couples
who did not pursue (further) treatment. I suggest that future studies
intending to understand drop-out should allow space for multiple
answers and/or for qualitative descriptions of individual situations,
as this may enhance insight into actual reasons and – if so desired
– provide more concrete leads regarding further interventions.
Moreover, following up on what has been suggested by Smeenk et
al. (2004: 267), voluntary drop-out from treatment should not per
se be considered a negative outcome, but can also be seen as a 'self-
protective measure', and may be the result of a lengthy and conscious process of considering pros and cons.

Finally, I want to raise an issue stemming from the restrictions
set by Dutch ART policy and the Radboud clinic. In this study, I
have not pictured how couples confronted with ethical restrictions experienced this situation, and what they subsequently did
when they were discouraged or actually prohibited from accessing
further treatment at the Radboud Clinic. Did they visit another
clinic in the Netherlands or abroad? If yes, were their requests for
medical assistance honoured in these other clinics/countries? In
other words, what are the (international) implications of Dutch
policies and practices regarding restrictions and boundaries? IVF
and reproductive tourism, I believe, is an issue that deserves

more (qualitative) research and scholarly attention (cf. Inhorn and Gürtin 2011). As new reproductive technologies will continue to develop and thus new (ethical) questions and dilemmas about their use will continue to evolve – both in national and international contexts – the area of ARTs constitutes 'fertile ground' for social science research.

Notes

1. See, e.g., Sandelowski (1993); Becker (2000); Bharadwaj (2002); Inhorn (2003); Gerrits and Hörbst (2016). De Vries (2003: 47) has pointed to the importance of the value of 'solidarity' in Dutch society and in the health care system, as well as in other Western European countries, compared to the more individualistic market-driven USA. While this may still be true (in comparison with the USA), many concerns are currently being expressed about the decrease in solidarity in Dutch society.
2. See: ww.meerdangewenst.nl.
3. See *Reproductive BioMedicine Online* 23(5), November 2011, for a Special Issue on Cross-Border Reproductive Care.
4. This remark was made by an Indian participant in an international conference, who claimed that such transparency about limited results and potential side effects would not be appreciated by most Indian couples visiting private clinics.

References

Becker, G. 2000. *The Elusive Embryo: How women and men approach new reproductive technologies.* Berkeley: University of California Press.

Bharadwaj, A. 2002. 'Conception Politics: Medical egos, media spotlights and the contest over test-tube firsts in India', in M.C. Inhorn, and F. Van Balen (eds), *Infertility around the Globe: New thinking on childlessness, gender and reproductive technology.* Berkeley: University of California Press, pp. 315–33.

Blonk, L., J.A.M. Kremer and T. ten Haaf. 2006. 'Het ontwikkelen van een patiënttevredenheid vragenlijst.', *Tijdschrift voor Verpleegkundigen* (7–8): 54–57.

Braat, D.D.M. 2000. 'Donor-eicellen: Wanneer en bij wie?', in W.C.M. Weijmar-Schultz (ed.), *Fertiliteit en ethiek, een kind tot (w)elke prijs?* Symposium WPOG, 10 November 2000. Groningen: Instituut Wenckebach.

Dancet, E.A.F., W.L.D.M. Nelen, W. Sermeus, L. De Leeuw, J.A.M Kremer, and T.M. D'Hooghe, 2010. 'The patients' perspective on fertility care: A systematic review', *Human Reproduction Update* 16: 467–87.

De Joode, S. and B. Fauser. 2001. 'Keuzes, verantwoordelijkheden en dilemma's van een gynaecoloog', in S. De Joode (ed.), *Zwanger van de kinderwens: Visies, feiten en vragen over voortplantingstechnologie*. The Hague: Rathenau Instituut, pp. 84–102.

De Vries, R. 2003. 'Can the Dutch way of birth teach us to do health care reform better?' *Society* 40(3): 43–48.

Franklin, S. 1997. *Embodied Progress: A cultural account of assisted conception*. London: Routledge.

Franklin, S. and C. Roberts. 2006. *Born and Made: An ethnography of preimplantation genetic diagnosis*. Princeton: Princeton University Press.

Gerrits, T. and V. Hörbst. 2016. 'Entrepreneuring Barren Grounds', in: L. Manderson, A. Hardon and E. Cartwright (eds),*The Routledge Handbook of Medical Anthropology*. London: Routledge, pp. 345–50.

Gordon, G.H., S.K. Joos and J. Byrne. 2000. 'Physician expressions of uncertainty during patient encounters', *Patient Education and Counseling* 40(1): 59–65.

Green, J. and N. Thorogood. 2004. *Qualitative Methods for Health Research*. London: Sage Publications.

Greil, A.L. 1991. *Not Yet Pregnant: Infertile couples in contemporary America*. New Brunswick: Rutgers University Press.

Gürtin, Z.B. and M.C. Inhorn. 2011. 'Introduction: Travelling for conception and the global assisted reproduction market', *Reproductive Biomedicine Online*: 23(5): 535–37.

Hampshire, K. and B. Simpson (eds). 2015. *Assisted Reproductive Technologies in the Third Phase: Global encounters and emerging moral worlds*. Oxford: Berghahn Books.

Hunfeld, J.A.M., J. Passchier, L.L.E. Bolt and M.A.J.M. Buijsen. 2004. 'Protect the child from being born: Arguments against IVF from heads of the 13 licensed Dutch fertility centres, ethical and legal perspectives', *Journal of Reproductive and Infant Psychology* 22(4): 279–89.

Inhorn, M.C. 2003. *Local Babies, Global Science: Gender, religion and in vitro fertilization in Egypt*. New York: Routledge.

———— 2012. *The New Arab Man: Emergent masculinities, technologies, and Islam in the Middle East*. Princeton: Princeton University Press.

Inhorn, M.C. and Z.B. Gürtin. 2011. 'Cross-border reproductive care: A future research agenda', *Reproductive Biomedicine Online* 23(5): 665–76.

Lechner, L., C. Bolman and A. Van Dalen. 2007. 'Definitive involuntary childlessness: Associations between coping, social support and psychological distress', *Human Reproduction* 22(1): 288–94.

Lupton, D. 1997 'Foucault and the medicalisation critique', in A. Petersen and R. Burton (eds), *Foucault, Health and Medicine*. London: Routledge, pp. 94–110.

Mol, A. 2006. *De logica van het zorgen. Actieve patiënten en de grenzen van het kiezen*. Van Gennep: Amsterdam.

NVOG. 2010. *Richtlijnen voortplantingsgeneeskunde. Onverklaarde subfertiliteit.* Retrieved 1 March 2015 from www.nvog.nl.

Pennings, G., C. Autin, W. Decleer, A. Delbaere, L. Delbeke, A. Delvigne, D. De Neubourg, P. Devroey, M. Dhont, T. D'Hooghe, S. Gordts, B. Lejeune, M. Nijs, P. Pauwels, B. Perrad, C. Pirard and F. Vandekerckhove. 2009. 'Cross-border reproductive care in Belgium', *Human Reproduction* 24(12): 3108–18.

Sandelowski, M. 1991. 'Compelled to try: The never enough quality of conceptive technology', *Medical Anthropological Quarterly* 5: 29–47.

_____ 1993. *With Child in Mind: Studies of the personal encounter with infertility.* Philadelphia: University of Pennsylvania Press.

Sandelowski, M. and S. De Lacey. 2002. 'The use of a "disease": Infertility as a rhetorical vehicle', in M.C. Inhorn and F. van Balen (eds), *Infertility around the Globe: New thinking on childlessness, gender and reproductive technology.* Berkeley: University of California Press, pp. 33–51.

Smeenk, J.M.J., C.M. Verhaak, A.M. Stolwijk, J.A. Kremer, and D.D. Braat. 2004. 'Reasons for dropout in an in vitro fertilization/intracytoplasmic sperm injection program', *Fertility and Sterility* 81(2): 262–68.

Trappenburg, M. 2008. *Genoeg is genoeg. Over gezondheidszorg en democratie.* Amsterdam: Amsterdam University Press.

Appendix 1: Methods

Is this study only being done in one clinic? And why in Nijmegen? (Study participant)
Is the number of couples that you intend to follow not too small? (Doctor)
I prefer to talk with you instead of completing questionnaires. (Study participant)
What are you looking at: the patients or us? (Nurse)
What happens with the results? Are you going to write a book? (Study participant)
What are you actually writing down in your notebook? (Nurse)
For me, this study approach is far too vague. (Doctor)
Interesting topics, but how are you going to analyse all this? (Doctor)
(Questions and comments raised during the course of the fieldwork)

This book is based on an intensive ethnographic study that I conducted in the Radboud Clinic, an academic hospital in Nijmegen, the Netherlands from September 2003 until August 2006. Data were collected by means of ethnographic observations in the Radboud Clinic and prospectively following twenty-three couples with fertility problems who visited this clinic.

It has been observed that in many publications presenting qualitative research results scarce attention is given to an adequate description of the research design and research procedures (see, e.g., Green and Thorogood 2004; Inhorn 2004: 2096; Wester 2005: 9–10). I fully share these authors' opinions that such description is crucial for the reader to assess the validity and credibility of the presented study findings and interpretations, even more so as this book may reach a multi-disciplinary audience, who might not be familiar with the anthropological approach as applied in the study on which this book is based (as the questions and remarks on the top of this page demonstrate). Secondly, I share Inhorn's view that 'discussion of [methodological and ethical] challenges may be instructive for future ethnographers, who will study IVF in other hospitals around the world' (Inhorn 2004: 2106). These are the reasons that I provide below detailed insights into methodological issues (in addition to what I presented in Chapter 1).

Ethnographic Observations

With the head of the department I had agreed that I would initially have a period of three months to familiarize myself with the people working at the clinic, its organization, functioning, and culture. Based on this first introduction, I would then be able to further develop my study approach, including the sampling of couples. During this period I was present at the whole range of possible events going on in the clinic: I observed a large number of consultations, examinations, and treatments, and listened to the IVF nurses when they responded to patients' requests on the phone; I attended several staff meetings, such as the daily IVF staff meetings, the interdisciplinary ethics meetings, and the social-work meetings. In this period I also attended information evenings for IVF/ICSI patients, and I spent some time in the laboratory to gain insight into lab procedures, and in the operating theatre watching gynaecological operations.

In this first period I had plenty of informal talks with all types of staff in the coffee room, at the reception desk, in offices, and also before, during, and after consultations and meetings, and I collected and read all kinds of documents (ranging from brochures for patients to detailed instructions for staff members). All of these activities and encounters provided me with a basic insight into what was going on in the clinic, the medical terminology and technologies, and in the diagnostic and treatment procedures. Observing the consultations also gave me a good first impression of the concerns and questions of women and men with fertility problems, and the way in which professionals and patients communicated and interacted in these clinical encounters.

In the initial stage, building good working relationships with clinic personnel was paramount. At the start of this period the head of the fertility clinic introduced me to several staff members, individually and at meetings, as 'a medical anthropologist from the University of Amsterdam', saying something like 'she is going to study how we are dealing with the patients and how patients go about treatment'. In this period several staff members – who were being observed by me and saw me taking notes – questioned me about the study. Their queries were about the research objective, the study methodology, what I was taking notes about, how I was going to analyse my notes, and so on. Though they were not at all used to this method of doing research, they were all very willing to collaborate to help me find my way, allowing me to attend their consultations, and on my request they explained various medical issues and procedures. Only once did a trainee gynaecologist (whom I had not met before) say she did not want me to observe her consultations because she felt extremely tired and expected it to become a difficult and tiresome afternoon. However, once I had explained to her a bit more about the study, and that I was just watching, not intervening or judging, she agreed, and afterwards commented that she had not felt my presence as a burden. At the end of December 2003 I e-mailed a newsletter to the clinic staff members explaining the study objective and approach, to be sure that all of them were – or at least could be – fully informed about the study and the reason for my presence. At a later moment in the study – when I had started following couples – I presented the study aims and methods in a meeting with clinic staff. In the initial period contacts with women and men visiting the clinic – as agreed with the head of the department – were superficial. I did not approach patients for extensive talks or interviews.

During the period when I followed the couples (see below), I continued doing overall ethnographic observations, though less intensively than in this initial phase. The focus of data collection then shifted to the couples, and I only attended consultation and treatment sessions in which one of 'my couples' was involved. Based on analysis of the observations during the first period, and in close deliberation with the study supervisors, I slightly revised the initial study proposal, developed topic lists for interviews and observation and developed and defined the sampling strategies. Using this revised study proposal I requested and was granted permission from the regional medical-ethical commission (CMO Regio Arnhem-Nijmegen) to conduct the study. From this moment onwards I was able to approach study participants.

Selecting and Recruiting Couples

The second fieldwork stage in which I approached couples for participation in the study and followed them throughout their treatment trajectory started in February 2004. Two distinctive groups of couples were approached: the first group consisted of couples who were visiting the clinic for the very first time with their fertility problem (beginners); the second group was made up of couples who were starting their first IVF in a new episode (beginners IVF) (see Chapter 1 for more information about the criteria and motivation for the sampling strategy). The study aimed at following eight couples belonging to the category 'beginners' and sixteen 'beginners IVF'.

Couples were approached through the sending of a patient information letter, in which the study objective and methodology were explained, and their participation was requested; a contact number was given in case they wanted additional information about the study or their participation. The 'beginners' received the information letter about the study together with some other information about the clinic, after they had made their very first appointment at the clinic, but before that appointment took place. 'Beginners IVF' received this letter the moment they were invited for their pre-IVF consultation (which takes place about one month before starting actual IVF). Couples that intended to participate in the study were requested to fill in, sign, and return an agreement form. Couples that did not want to participate in the study were requested to complete and return a 'form for non-participants', which included questions about background variables and a question regarding their reasons for not participating in the study. All letters contained return envelopes.

The information letters were sent for as long as was estimated necessary in order to reach the planned number of study participants. In total, ninety-eight letters were sent over a period of two to three months; twenty-five couples (eight 'beginners' and seventeen 'IVF beginners') reacted positively to the request to participate in the study. One of the couples was excluded from participation in the study as the woman spoke too little Dutch, and another couple did not turn up at the hospital for their appointment. Thus, in total twenty-three couples participated in the study.

My first contact with the couples took place in the clinic (with twelve couples) or at their homes (with eleven couples). When I spoke with them for the first time – at the clinic or on the phone – and we arranged the first appointment, I once more asked them to confirm that they both were willing to participate in the study, and I provided some additional information about the study objective and approach. All of them confirmed that they were still definitely willing to participate.

In-depth Interviews

Over the course of the study two to three interviews were held with almost all of the couples, at intervals of five to six months. The interviews were held at their homes. The couples lived within a circumference of approximately 75 km around the city of Nijmegen (a city in the mid-eastern part of the Netherlands), a region stretching from the north of the province of Limburg to the east of the province Noord-Brabant and up to the Achterhoek, a region in the province of Gelderland. Many of them lived in villages or small towns, with only a few living in the city of Nijmegen. Generally, I travelled to their homes by means of public transport, and many times the couples picked me up from the bus or train station, sometimes at quite some distance from their house. On the way to their home, we chatted about all kind of topics, related and not related to the reason for my visit, which certainly contributed to an informal ambience.

Before starting the first interview I pointed to a number of issues: once more I briefly explained the study objective, that the study was a collaboration project between the University of Amsterdam (UvA) and the Radboud Clinic (with the UvA being the financer), and my intention to write my dissertation based on the study. I emphasized the importance of hearing both the woman and the man's stories and views, encouraging them both to make their contribution. I asked their permission to record the interviews (they all agreed with this), guaranteed their anonymity (all names used in this book to indicate the study participants are fictitious), and promised confidentiality with regard to the issues we would speak about. I stressed that – as I was not part of the clinic staff – I was not in a position to answer questions regarding their specific medical situation. Finally, I mentioned the themes of the first interview, told them that the interview would take at least one hour and a half, and that they were free to not talk about any issue if they did not want to.

In practice, many of the interviews – including the second and third interviews – lasted more than one hour and a half (sometimes up to four hours). Overall, people seemed to be very willing to talk in depth and openly about their experiences, thoughts, and concerns. All interviews were recorded, and my impression is that this did not – or at the most only in the very beginning – hinder the study participants in telling their story. Many a time, the women and men told me that they were pleased to share their stories with me, and that they enjoyed the way the interviews were conducted.

The interviews were semi-structured, and use was made of topic lists, though ample space was given for couples to tell the stories in the way they chose to share them. Many of them voluntarily shared connected stories which provided me with valuable contextual insight into their personal circumstances and lifestyles. The three successive interviews covered partly the same themes, as the intention was to follow experiences and the development of thoughts over time.

The first interview covered five main topics: their reproductive life histories; couples' experiences in the hospital thus far, with an emphasis on how they felt they were treated by the clinic staff; their thoughts about examinations and treatments in the near future, including their ideas about their own limits – if any – with regard to the use of reproductive technologies; their sources of information about fertility problems, examinations, and treatments used thus far; and their sources of 'stress and support' related to their fertility problem, examinations, and treatments.

Besides asking questions and following up on the answers given, I used two projective techniques – the construction of a time line and the sorting of cards – to facilitate and stimulate people in talking about their experiences and perceptions. The timeline helped in elaborating reproductive life histories, giving an overview of the events and the process from the beginning of their relationship – or starting at any time before that when anything related to their wish for a child occurred – up to their first visit to the Radboud clinic (Box A1). When the couples constructed their timelines and told me their stories, they constantly deliberated together about the various events, trying to recall how, when, and/or why things happened or steps had been taken, which provided valuable insight into the way they saw their own process, and details on why and how decisions were made.

A card-sorting technique was used to gain insight into the sources of information women and men used, or had used, related to their

> ## Box A1: Timeline:
> ## A Focused (Reproductive) Life History
>
> When discussing the period before they visited a hospital I asked the couples to compose a timeline on a long piece of paper. I gave them a number of yellow post-it notes on which I had written moments or events that might be related to the process of their wish for a child, such as 'start relationship', 'wish for child', 'stop using contraceptives', 'visit general practitioner with wish for child', 'visit alternative healer', 'miscarriage', etc. I asked them to compose their timeline of important events from the beginning of their relationship (or starting at any time before that when anything related to their wish for a child occurred) up to their first visit to the Radboud hospital. I also provided blank post-it notes and encouraged the couples to add moments/events that were specifically relevant in their own history. On my request they added the dates. Pointing to the timeline, I asked additional questions in order to fully understand their story up to the visit to the clinic. These stories form the basis for the presentation of the couples in Chapter 3.

fertility problem, and to determine what type of information they had sought and from which source, enabling me to make a major distinction between factual medical information and experience-based information (Box A2).

Card sorting was also used to discuss issues related to 'stress and support' (Box A3). This gave me insight into people's concerns – what made them feel stressed – regarding their fertility problem, the threat of childlessness, and the coming or ongoing treatments, and the way they felt they could be best supported – or how they actually were supported – in this process.

About half a year after the first interview the second interview took place with all the couples except one. Just before the second interview was planned to take place, one couple withdrew from the study because the man perceived the interview as an extra burden on top of the already burdensome IVF treatment (and due to some other personal circumstances). With regard to two other couples, I spoke individually with the man and the woman, because one of these couples had separated since the first interview, and the other couple disagreed about further treatment.

I had spoken with most of the couples at the clinic in between the first and second interview, and with some I had had – sometimes lengthy – talks on the phone. I initiated the second interview by

> **Box A2: Sorting Cards:**
> **Women's and Men's Sources of Information**
>
> I provided a set of cards (sixteen) to both the man and the woman. Each card contained the name of one source of information, including written, audio-visual, and personal sources of information, both from within and outside of the clinic. I asked the man and the woman to individually pile the cards containing sources of information which they (had) used, and to order the cards in sequence of the most to least important source of information. I also gave them some blank cards on which they could write any additional sources of information they themselves had used. Once the man and the woman had both finished sorting the cards, we first went through the man's list, and subsequently through the woman's list. I asked both of them to explain how they had used the different sources of information – in terms of patterns and frequency of use, but also in terms of the type of information they had got from a specific source – allowing me to make a major distinction between factual medical information and experience-based information. This method provided insight into the patterns of information-seeking of women and men separately, as the literature suggests that women and men have different ways of seeking information on infertility related problems.

asking the couples to brief me about what had happened in terms of examinations and treatment since I had last spoken with them. Then I asked them to tell me about their experiences in the clinic, in terms of how they both experienced the way they were dealt with by clinic staff, and how they experienced the examinations and treatments and their effects – physically and emotionally/psychically. In addition, the content of the second interview was inspired by interim analysis of the data collected thus far, in particular through observations in the clinic. The observations made me question the following issues:

- How the couples experienced the amount and type of information they received from the clinic – as I had noticed that a lot of information was given, among others about possible side-effects and risks.
- To what extent they felt they could, if they so wanted, have any impact on the course of their treatment and deviate from the more or less standardized treatment regime trajectory – as I had got the impression that people's suggestions for adaptations,

Box A3: Sorting Cards:
Stress and Support

Another set of cards (forty) contained words that a) might be negatively associated with the experience of fertility problems, examinations, or treatments ('stress words'), such as maternity visit, physical examination, side effects of medicines; or b) might refer to a means of overcoming these problems ('support words') like 'talking with others', 'talking together', 'social worker', 'distraction', 'pets', 'adoption', 'patient organization', 'praying', and 'yoga'. The words were taken from infertility literature, though did not pretend to cover all possible stress and support factors. The men and women were asked to select cards with stress and support words relevant to them. Again, they got blank cards to add their own words, if they wanted. I explained to the couples that by using this tool they could set the agenda for the rest of the conversation, clarifying to me what made them concerned or sad, and how they tried to comfort themselves or make themselves feel better. We spoke about the cards they selected with negative and positive associations.

By broaching this topic in this way I intended to achieve two goals. First, while the meaning and experience of the fertility problem, and the threat of childlessness in itself, were not issues for the current research, I understood that it might be a major concern for the couples participating in the study. Therefore I felt I should allow people space to share their concerns and feelings, if they so wanted. It provided me with an idea of what they felt concerned about, and it was also part of building a long-term relationship with the study participants. Most of this information, however, has not directly been used in this book, as my focus is not on the experience of infertility per se. Secondly, this exercise provided insight into what people dreaded with regard to the (coming) fertility examinations and treatments – e.g., about hyperstimulation, frequent hospital visits, and physical examinations – and how they thought this affected them, or how they could be best supported in this.

often based on information from the Internet or hearsay, were rarely honoured.
- How they felt about the doctors sharing uncertainty or showing the limitations of technology and state of the art of medicine – as I had noticed they regularly did, for example about the cause of the fertility problems, the amount of hormonal medication to be given, the unpredictability of treatment outcomes, and possible side effects.

Another line of questioning I pursued was about decision-making and taking steps for the future, which depended on the actual situation of the couples at that particular moment. With the couples who were pregnant, I spoke about how they experienced this pregnancy; whether they thought they would have gone for further treatment in case they had not become pregnant from the last one, and what they thought about treatment in the future, in case they would want to have another child. With those who were not yet pregnant but were not continuing examinations or treatments, I spoke about the reasons for this discontinuation: was it their own or the doctor's decision, how they felt about it, and how they had experienced the way clinic staff had dealt with this decision. When a man or woman expressed doubts about further treatment I elaborated on it, asking them how they themselves had dealt with these doubts, whether they had shown their doubts to the clinic staff, and how it was reacted upon. With the couples who had decided to continue examinations or treatments, I spoke about their considerations with regard to this decision, about their views on the next treatment, and about whether they thought they would do further treatment if the next one was unsuccessful.

The topic lists for the interviews also contained various topics I intended to put forward, if they had not already been covered. Most of these followed up on issues that had been extensively spoken about in the first interview, such as the woman and man's (changing) need for information and support and how they realized this, their experiences with the Digitale Poli, the impact of the treatment trajectory on the couples' relationship, and issues related to payment of the treatments and health insurance. In practice, many of these issues had often already been touched upon spontaneously in the course of the interview.

With the couples who had become pregnant (five) or who had definitely stopped treatments for other reasons (five) at the time the second interview was held, this interview was also the final one. With the other study participants (twelve) a third interview was held, in which some of the same topics were covered as in the second interview; the emphasis in this last interview, however, was on decisions made, their thoughts regarding future steps in the treatment trajectory, and about alternative ways of dealing with their fertility problem. Over the course of the study, fifty-seven in-depth interviews were held with twenty-three couples, in addition to many informal conversations.

Observations, Phone Calls, and E-mails

Besides the interviews, which provided information at more or less regular intervals of five to six months about a number of themes, couples' ongoing experiences and perceptions were grasped by means of observations at the clinic, phone calls and e-mails. Regarding the observations, I had planned to attend one-third of the couples' visits to the clinic. In the course of the first few months of the study, however, I realized that this was too ambitious and impossible to do, in particular in the periods when the couples underwent IVF treatments and visited the hospital frequently, at short notice, and spread over seven days a week. Therefore I reduced the number of observations per couple, and – though still attempting to observe different types of clinical settings – I gave priority to consultations during which plans were made and results evaluated (and thus considerations regarding stopping, pausing, or continuing treatment were made explicit). In addition, I followed couples' ongoing experiences by means of regular phone calls and emails, as long as the women and men agreed with this. To inform all participants about this slightly altered approach, and to keep them updated about the development/course of the study, I sent them a newsletter. While the interviews at the couples' homes were always held in the presence of both the woman and the man, this was not always the case for the other contact moments.

When observing consultations or treatment sessions I took handwritten notes, which I elaborated on as soon as possible – in most cases the same day – after the observation had taken place. I briefly described 'what happened' (events and actions) in terms of medical examination or treatment, and took extensive notes on the nature of the communication and interaction between the attending health professional(s) and the women and/or men visiting the clinic. I had prepared a checklist for observations; this checklist served as a kind of sensitizing instrument, and so was not meticulously employed at each and every observation. As the observed consultations and treatment sessions varied substantially with regard to content and duration, it was impossible to use a standardized observation form. Only one couple was not followed at all at the clinic, and this was because the woman told me during the first interview that she would like to participate in the study, but did not want me to attend her visits to the clinic: she already felt anxious about undergoing physical examinations in the presence of health staff, and disliked the idea of any extra person being present.

In phone calls and e-mail exchanges I asked the women and men to explain and write about recent events and experiences, such as how they had undergone a certain step in treatment, what the outcomes of the examinations or treatments had been, how they felt about it, what choices they had made or still had to make, and what were their doubts and considerations. Handwritten notes taken during the phone conversations were expanded on immediately after the phone call, and the complete e-mail messages were saved as text files.

Diaries

Couples participating in the study were also requested to keep a diary, in the hope of getting detailed insight into their (possibly changing) perceptions, feelings, and experiences with regard to their fertility problem and the examination and treatment trajectory. In the patient information letter the diary was mentioned as a potential, but certainly not mandatory, part of participation in the study, as I was aware that couples might consider keeping a diary as burdensome and for that reason might be inclined to renounce participation in the study altogether. During the first interview, I checked whether the man and/or the woman would be interested in keeping such a diary, but once more emphasized that they should feel free not to, and that they could do it in a way they felt good about. Therefore I did not give any detailed instructions on how to keep such a diary. In total, six women started to keep a diary on behalf of the study; incidentally one man – on the insistence of his wife – wrote a few passages in her diary. The level of detail and the time period covered in the diaries varied enormously: four gave detailed insight into the woman's changes of 'mood and mind' during the treatment process, and have been used in this study to illustrate and analyse these changes; the other two hardly provided any such information and are therefore not referred to in this study.

Overall, the frequency of contacts – interviews at home, at the clinic, by phone and/or by e-mail – I had with the different couples varied substantially. With six couples I had contact with them more than ten times; with seven couples I interacted seven to nine times; and with ten couples I interacted four to six times. All the couples in the last category belong to the group that I followed for a shorter period and only interviewed twice. The variation was not only with the frequency of contacts with the study participants, but also with the intensity of the contacts and the rapport built with them over the course of the study.

Data Analysis

The process of data analysis started with a close reading of all notes and interview transcripts. Data analysis was further aided by Atlas.ti, a computer programme for the analysis of qualitative data. Computer software programmes for the analysis of qualitative data are – much more than their counterparts for the analysis of quantitative data – used to aid systematic analysis, but cannot take over any of the intellectual or creative processes involved. The process of analysis is described below. All data collected during the study – the transcribed interviews, the expanded field-notes resulting from observations and phone calls, the emails, and the diary notes – were stored as separate files in Atlas.ti and coded. Many of the applied codes are index-codes, i.e., used simply to organize the material into themes and categories, such as rate, risk, side effects, adoption, health insurance, patient–doctor communication, and so on. Other codes are more conceptual, fixing meaning on the data, such as, for example, visualization and fragmentation (both concepts coming from social science theory and telling something about the impact medical technology may have on people's perceptions and experiences). Subsequently, I started analysing the data in detail and writing the chapters. Every time when starting a new chapter I defined what material – indexed and coded – I needed, and searched, retrieved, and printed the excerpts of the texts with selected codes. I re-read the texts pertaining to one code, divided themes into sub-themes and categories, and started to think about typologies/profiles and search for possible patterns and relationships among the data, with attention to how they related to theoretical ideas and concepts. Many a time when reading through the excerpts I went back to the original texts to fully understand the data in context and to select the cases that could best introduce and illustrate the arguments I intended to make. While analytic activities such as categorizing, summarizing, and making typologies of qualitative data are still rather structured and straightforward (Green and Thorogood 2004: 180), the steps of finding patterns and relationships among data and appropriate ways of presenting the data, and how to interpret them in the light of the research objective and to link them with theoretical notions are far less structured and straightforward. These steps are – even more than other steps in analysis – iterative and involve the application of social science imagination: the imagination to see links which are almost impossible to mark out (ibid.: 174). At the end, all these analytical and iterative steps – some of them taken very consciously and others somehow less intentionally – have informed and shaped the contents and outline of the current book.

References

Green, J. and N. Thorogood. 2004. *Qualitative methods for health research.* London: Sage Publications.

Inhorn, M.C. 2004. 'Privacy, privatization, and the politics of patronage: ethnographic challenges to penetrating the secret world of Middle Eastern, hospital-based in vitro fertilization', *Social Science and Medicine*, 59(10), 2095–2108.

Wester, F. 2005. 'De methodeparagraaf in rapportages over kwalitatief onderzoek', *Kwalon*, 10 (3): 8–14.

APPENDIX 2: TABLES

TABLE A1 Social and Demographic Background Data of Study Participants

		Men (N=23)	Women (N=23)	Total (N=46)
Year of birth (age)				
1947 (56)		1	–	1
1960–1964 (39–43)		5	3	8
1965–1969 (34–38)		11	10	21
1970–1974 (29–33)		5	7	12
1975–1980 (24–28)		1	3	4
Child(ren) before starting current treatment episode				
No children		17	19	36
Child from previous relationship		4	2	6
Child from current relationship		2	2	4
Level of education (highest completed level)[1]				
Low	Primary School	1	–	1
	LBO	4	3	7
	MAVO	1	2	3
Middle	MBO	8	8	16
	HAVO	2	1	3
High	HBO	2	3	5
	University	5	6	11
Employment				
Part-time job		7	12	19
Full-time job		15	4	19
Own firm		1	2	3
Unemployed		0	5	5
Income level per month (net income)				
No income		–	2	2
< 1000 euros		–	8	8
1000–1500 euros		9	8	17
1500–2000 euros		7	3	10
2000–2500 euros		4	1	5
2500–3000 euros		1	–	1
> 3000 euros		1	–	1
No information		1	1	2
Health insurance				
Public (Ziekenfonds)[2]		12	19	31
Private insurance		10	3	13
No information		1	1	2
Religion				
Roman Catholic[3]		14	13	27
Protestant		3	3	6
Other		0	4	4
None		6	3	9

Notes
1. LBO, MBO and HBO refer to lower, middle and higher vocational education respectively. MAVO and HAVO refer to middle and higher general education.
2. The division in public and private health insurance refers to the Dutch health insurance system until 2006 (see page 65–67).
3. All men and women who indicated to be baptized in the Roman Catholic Church, also reported to practice irregularly or not at all.

TABLE A2 Patients' or Couples' Characteristics or Situations Leading to Concerns among Clinic Staff and their Reasons for Withholding Treatment

Patients' or couples' characteristic(s) raising ethical concerns	No. of cases	No. of cases where treatment was offered	No. of cases where no decision was made[3]	No. of cases where treatment was withheld	
				Ethical reasons	Medical reasons
a) Carrier of genetic disease[1]	8	6	–	2	–
b) Serious psychological problems	5	3	–	2	–
c) Serious disease of the man	3	2	1	–	–
d) Elderly man	3	3	–	–	–
e) Instability of relationship	2	–	–	–	2
f) Multiple/other[2]	8	5	2	–	1
Total	29	19	3	4	3

Notes

1. The genetic diseases included: two cases of cystic fybrosis, *polyposis coli*, breast cancer, intestinal cancer, haemophilia-B, cadagil, *osteogenesis imperfecta*, and Lesch Nijham.

2. The category 'Multiple/other' includes couples with more than one of the previous mentioned characteristics (a–e) and various other cases: a couple of whom both partners had mental retardation; a couple of whom both partners were HIV+ and not co-habiting; a couple where the woman had recently had an induced abortion of twins; a couple that intensively used soft drugs and the man refused to visit the clinic to provide sperm; a couple who, for religious reasons, did not want to fertilize more than two ova to avoid discarding embryos; and a couple where the partners were suspected of having a close consanguineous relationship.

3. Not decided means that for these three couples the decision about access to further treatment was never made because the couple did not return to the clinic.

GLOSSARY

Assisted reproductive technologies (ARTs): All treatments that include the handling of eggs and/ or embryos, such as in vitro fertilization (IVF).

Chlamydia: A sexually transmitted disease; it is a common cause of pelvic infection and subsequent tubal damage and infertility.

Clomiphene (Clomid®): A hormonal medicine used to stimulate ovulation.

Corpus Luteum: A mass of yellow tissue formed in the ovary by a ruptured follicle that has discharged its ovum: if the ovum is fertilized, this tissue secretes the hormone progesterone, needed to maintain pregnancy.

Cryopreservation: The freezing of embryos created from one cycle, which may be stored and thawed for use in another cycle.

Decapeptyl®: A hormonal medicine that suppresses the woman's normal hormonal cycle.

Ectopic pregnancy: Pregnancy in which the fertilized egg implants outside the uterine cavity in the fallopian tube or the abdominal cavity. In some situations this requires immediate surgery to avoid risk of rupture.

Egg donation: A process in which a woman donates eggs through IVF to another woman.

Egg (ova) retrieval: A procedure used to obtain eggs from ovarian follicles. The procedure is performed by using a needle and ultrasound to locate the follicle in the ovary.

Embryo: A fertilized egg that has begun cell division.

Embryo transfer: Placing one or more embryos into a woman's uterus.

Endometriosis: The presence of endometrial tissue in abnormal locations, such as the fallopian tubes, ovaries and abdominal cavity. The condition frequently causes pain and discomfort during menstruation, or even chronic pelvic pain, and may also cause infertility.

Epididymis: Coiled tubing outside the testicles which store the sperm.

Estrogens (Oestrogens): Female sex hormones, a group of hormones that are produced mainly by the ovaries. They are essential for normal sexual development (the breasts, vagina, womb, broad hips and rounded figure, etc.) and for the reproductive system (make the cervical mucus amenable to the entry of sperm, prepare the endometrium and regulate the production of FSH and LH).

Follicle: A fluid-filled cyst in the ovary in which the egg develops.

Follicle aspiration: See egg retrieval.

FSH: Follicle stimulating hormone, which is secreted by the pituitary gland. It stimulates the growth of follicles in the female, and sperm production in the male.

Gamete: The male sperm or the female egg.

GnRH (Gonadotropin-releasing hormone): A hormone secreted by the hypothalamus. It stimulates the pituitary gland to release FSH and LH. GnRh preparations are produced synthetically.

GnRH analogues: A synthetic hormone similar to the natural Gonadotropin-releasing hormone. Two types are available: agonists and antagonists.

Habitual abortion: Repeat miscarriages.

hCG (human Chorionic Gonadotropin): A hormone that is produced in early pregnancy to stimulate the corpus luteum to produce the hormone progesterone and oestrogen, and is excreted in the urine (the substance detected in pregnancy tests). Also, hCG may be given by injection to induce ovulation and to support the luteal phase in females. It stimulates the production of the male hormone testosterone in males.

Hysteroscopy: Diagnostic procedure in which a lighted scope (hysteroscope) is inserted through the cervix into the uterus to enable the physician to view the inside of the uterus.

In Vitro Fertilization (IVF): A process in which an egg and sperm are combined in a laboratory dish (*in vitro*) to facilitate fertilization. If fertilized, the resulting embryo is transferred to the woman's uterus.

Intra Cytoplasmic Sperm Injection (ICSI): A micromanipulation procedure in which a single sperm is injected directly into an egg to attempt fertilization, used in cases of male infertility or couples with prior unsuccessful IVF fertilization.

Intra Uterine Insemination (IUI): Placement of washed sperm into the uterus.

Laparoscopy: Direct visualization of the ovaries and exterior of the fallopian tubes and uterus through a surgical instrument inserted through a small incision below the navel.

LH (Luteinizing hormone): A pituitary hormone that triggers ovulation and stimulates the corpus luteum to secrete progesterone.

Motility: The percentages of all moving sperm in a semen sample.

Oocyte (Egg, ovum): The female reproductive cell.

OHSS (Ovarian Hyperstimulation Syndrome): A possible side effect with some fertility drugs. It is characterized by swollen, painful ovaries and, in some cases, the accumulation of fluid in the abdomen and chest.

Ovulation induction: The administration of hormone medications (ovulation drugs) that stimulate the ovaries to produce multiple eggs.

Ovarian cysts: A fluid-filled sac inside the ovary. An ovarian cyst may be found in conjunction with ovulation disorders, tumours of the ovary, and endometriosis.

Polycystic Ovarian Syndrome (PCOS): Development of multiple cysts in the ovaries due to arrested follicular growth due to lack of ovulation.

Post Coital Test (PCT): An examination of a woman's cervical mucus after she has had intercourse to determine the number and motility (ability to move) of sperm in the mucus.

Preimplantation Genetic Diagnosis (PGD): A procedure performed in conjunction with IVF in which one or two cells are removed from an embryo prior to the initiation of pregnancy and screened for genetic abnormalities.

Pregnyl®: A fertility drug given by injection and consists of human Chorionic Gonadotropin.

Preimplantation Genetic Screening (PGS): A technique used to examine the embryo for aneuploidy (wrong number of chromosomes), and only transfer normal embryos.

Progestan®: A medicine that increases the chances of successful nestling of the embryo.

Progesterone: A hormone secreted by the corpus luteum in the second half of the menstrual cycle to stimulate the endometrium and prepare it for implantation and maintain it should pregnancy occur; progesterone is produced in large quantities by the placenta.

Puregon®: A recombinant follicle stimulating hormone; a 'fertility drug'.

Semen: The sperm and seminal secretions ejaculated during orgasm.

Semen donation: A process in which a man donates semen to an individual or couple.

Single embryo transfer: Placement of a single embryo into the uterus.

Sperm: The male gamete or sex cell that contains the genetic information to be transmitted by the male, also known as spermatozoon (plural spermatozoa).

Surrogacy: The situation in which a woman bears a child for another woman, either through artificial insemination by the other woman's husband or partner or by carrying until birth the other woman's surgically implanted fertilized egg.

Vaginal ultrasound: Ultrasound imaging of the female reproductive system through an ultrasound device inserted into the vagina.

INDEX